The Psychology of the Hum

Christopher Blazina · Güler Boyraz ·
David Shen-Miller

Editors

The Psychology
of the Human–Animal Bond

A Resource for Clinicians and Researchers

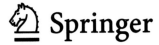 Springer

Editors

Christopher Blazina
Department of Psychology
Tennessee State University
Nashville, TN, USA
christex01@msn.com

Güler Boyraz
Department of Psychology
Tennessee State University
Nashville, TN, USA
gboyraz@gmail.com

David Shen-Miller
Department of Psychology
Tennessee State University
Nashville, TN, USA
dmiller20@tnstate.edu

ISBN 978-1-4419-9760-9 (hardcover)   ISBN 978-1-4419-9761-6 (eBook)
ISBN 978-1-4614-6196-8 (softcover)
DOI 10.1007/978-1-4419-9761-6
Springer New York Heidelberg Dordrecht London

Library of Congress Control Number: 2010928904

Printed on acid-free paper

Springer is part of Springer Science+Business Media (www.springer.com)

Now, as they talked on, a dog that lay there
lifted up his muzzle, pricked his ears...
It was Argos, long-enduring Odysseus' dog
he trained as a puppy once, but little joy he got
since all too soon he shipped to sacred Troy.
In the old days young hunters loved to set him
coursing after the wild goats and deer and hares.
But now with his master gone he lay there, castaway,
on piles of dung from mules and cattle...
But the moment he sensed Odysseus standing by
he thumped his tail, nuzzling low, and his ears dropped,
though he had no strength to drag himself an inch
toward his master. Odysseus glanced to the side
and flicked away a tear...

Homer, The Odyssey

Preface

There have been dramatic increases in the emotional, psychological, and financial investment of animal companions over the past four decades in the United States and abroad. It is estimated that more than 63% of homes in the United States own a pet, usually a cat or dog. Worldwide, the pet-related industry is predicted to top $65 billion in the coming year. North America, Western Europe, Asia Pacific, and Latin America lead the way in pet-related expenditures. The growing importance of animal companions in people's lives has resulted in an emergent number of investigations within academic literature; a rising number of books and scholarly articles published in recent years attempt to explain the bond from various vantage points, within mental health fields and beyond. One way to integrate the diverse number of perspectives within academia involves the use of *context*.

From a psychological perspective, *context* has become an ever-increasing salient consideration among both practitioners and researchers. Context provides clarification of the meaning of a variable or theme by providing a nuanced understanding of how other factors converge and interact with the factor one wishes to explore. Contextual factors include but are not limited to socioeconomic status, race, ethnicity, individual differences related to developmental issues across the life span, and unique dynamics within and across cultures.

In an attempt to provide a contextual foundation for readers interested in the human–animal bond, this book introduces students and professionals in mental health and related fields to the manner in which the bond is studied among multiple disciplines such as anthropology, sociology, philosophy, literature, religion, and veterinary medicine. Although this anthology uses psychology as the focal point, assimilating perspectives from other fields will enhance readers' conceptual appreciation of the bond in new and important ways. In addition to the contextual elements noted above, the way we perceive nonhuman animals, the meaning we attribute to our relationships with them, and the ways we respond to their loss are potentially influenced by factors such as our own history of relationships, support resources, cultural and religious beliefs, values, and worldview. When we can successfully integrate these various perspectives in a thoughtful way, we achieve a unique view of the bond, and how it acts as a mirror, reflecting back our own struggles and triumphs concerning work and love on the individual, familial, and cultural levels.

Contemplating the significance of the human–animal bond is a complex endeavor. We argue that there are distinct benefits for doing so. Ultimately, *The Psychology of the Human–Animal Bond* strives for three goals: (1) raise awareness regarding the myriad influences that shape the experience of the human–animal bond, and how they may be studied, (2) enhance the explanatory power of clinicians, researchers, and clients regarding the meaning of the bond, and (3) increase agency among clinicians, researchers, and clients when acting upon the meaning of the bond. *The Psychology of the Human–Animal Bond* encourages the reader to appreciate the various ways the bond is formed, adds meaning, and ultimately can add to the unique mosaic of our understanding. We hope you find it useful in your work.

Editors' note: The black and white photographs that appear with each section preface are provided by photographer Sharon Lee Hart. Sharon made portraits of the various residents of farm animal sanctuaries across the United States. Farm animal sanctuaries provide life-long shelter for those who have been rescued from situations in which they have been abused, neglected, or otherwise mistreated. We include these photographs as a stimulus for reader; one of the many complex manifestations of the human-animal bond.

Contents

Contributors

Hiroko Arikawa Missouri State University, Springfield, MO, hirokoar@gmail.com

Christopher Blazina Department of Psychology, Tennessee State University, Nashville, TN 37209, USA, christex01@msn.com

Güler Boyraz Department of Psychology, Tennessee State University, Nashville, TN, USA, gboyraz@gmail.com

Todd J. Braje Department of Anthropology, San Diego State University, 5500 Campanile Drive, San Diego, CA 92182-6040, USA, tjb50@humboldt.edu

Michael E. Bricker Lakeshore Psychotherapy Alliance, Chicago, IL, USA, michael.e.bricker@gmail.com

Sue-Ellen Brown Paoletta Counseling Services Inc., Mercer, PA 16137, USA, sebi2i@aol.com

Helen L. Davis Murdoch University, Perth, Australia, hdavis@murdoch.edu.au

Sarah DeGue Centers for Disease Control and Prevention, Atlanta, GA, USA, sdegue@cdc.gov

Aubrey H. Fine College of Education and Integrative Studies, CA State Polytechnic University, 3801 W. Temple Ave. Pomona, CA 91768, USA, ahfine@csupomona.edu

Carol L. Glasser Department of Sociology, University of California, Irvine, CA, USA, cglasser@gmail.com

Lauren N. Hoffer Assistant Professor of Victorian Literature, Department of English & Theatre, University of South Carolina Beaufort, Bluffton, SC, USA, lauren.hoffer@gmail.com

Maria Andromachi Iliopoulou Animal Studies Program, Department of Sociology, Michigan State University, Ann Arbor, MI, USA, iliopoul@cvm.msu.edu

Linda Kalof Animal Studies Program, Department of Sociology, Michigan State University, East Lansing, MI, USA, lkalof@msu.edu

Laurel Lagoni World by the Tail, Inc., Fort Collins, CO 80525, USA; Argus Institute for Families and Veterinary Medicine, James L. Voss Veterinary Teaching Hospital, Colorado State University, Fort Collins, CO 80523, USA, llagoni@comcast.net; www.veterinarywisdom.com

Bronwyn M. Massavelli School of Psychology, University of Queensland, Brisbane, Australia, bronwyn.massavelli@uqconnect.edu.au

Samara McPhedran smcphedran@iprimus.com.au

Nancy A. Pachana School of Psychology, University of Queensland, Brisbane, Australia, npachana@psy.uq.edu.au

Camilla Pagani Institute of Cognitive Sciences and Technologies, National Research Council, Rome, Italy, camilla.pagani@istc.cnr.it

Rod Preece Faculty of Arts, Wilfrid Laurier University, Waterloo, ON, Canada, rodpreece@rogers.com

Sofia Robleda-Gomez School of Psychology, University of Queensland, Brisbane, Australia, sofia.robledagomez@uqconnect.edu.au

Lisa A. Ruff Blue Bell Elementary School, Blue Bell, PA, USA, lruff@wsdweb.org

Bruce S. Sharkin Department of Counseling and Psychological Services, Kutztown University, Kutztown, PA, USA, sharkin@kutztown.edu

David Shen-Miller Tennessee State University, Nashville, TN, USA, dmiller20@tnstate.edu

Judith M. Siegel Department of Community Health Sciences, School of Public Health, University of California, Los Angeles, CA, USA, jmsiegel@ucla.edu

Judy Skeen School of Religion, Belmont University, Nashville, TN, USA, judy.skeen@belmont.edu

Donald I. Templer Alliant International University, Fresno, CA, USA, donaldtempler@sbcglobal.net

David A.H. Wilson School of Historical Studies, University of Leicester, Leicester, UK, dw149@le.ac.uk

About the Editors

Christopher Blazina, Ph.D., is a licensed psychologist, researcher, and professor of psychology. He received his doctorate in Counseling Psychology from the University of North Texas. He has been a faculty member at the University of Houston and Tennessee State University, training graduate students to become counselors and psychologists. Dr. Blazina is the author of more than forty articles and four books, and serves in various capacities such as on the Editorial Board of the journal *Psychology of Men and Masculinity* and the Editorial Advisor Board for "The Routledge Series on Counseling and Psychotherapy with Boys and Men." In addition, Dr. Blazina has been a guest on numerous radio programs across the United States and internationally. He also produces and hosts a weekly radio program *The Secret Lives of Men* exploring gender and culture. Dr. Blazina has presented research on the psychology of pet ownership at the American Psychological Association. He is currently working on a self-help book for pet owners dealing with themes of attachment and loss.

Güler Boyraz, Ph.D., is Assistant Professor of Psychology at Tennessee State University. Since completing her doctoral training at the University of Memphis in 2008, she has conducted research on the topics of grief, loss, trauma, and cancer health disparities. Güler has had clinical experiences in both Turkey and the United States and worked with diverse populations. Her recent research projects focus on the process of meaning-making following the loss of a loved one, and her goal is to contribute to the well-being and adjustment of bereaved individuals and trauma survivors through her research and other professional activities.

David Shen-Miller received his doctorate in counseling psychology from the University of Oregon in 2008. From 2003 to 2006, he served as the Director of the University of Oregon Men's Center, engaging in clinical and administrative work and research on men's health. He has received grant funding for several research projects. In 2009, he received the Barbara A. Kirk award for outstanding dissertation research from the American Psychological Association's Society for Counseling Psychology. He is an assistant professor at Tennessee State University in the counseling psychology program and also engages in individual, couples, and group counseling and psychological testing. Dave conceptualizes and conducts clinical practice and research within an ecological framework. His research interests include the psychology of men and masculinity, diversity and multicultural issues, problems of professional competence in training, and qualitative research. He has authored peer-reviewed articles, book chapters, and more than 30 regional, national, and international presentations. Dave has also served as a consultant for work related to men's centers and trainee competence problems. He is a coeditor with Dr. Chris Blazina on the book *An International Psychology of Men: Theoretical Advances, Case Studies, and Clinical Innovations*, published by Routledge Press in 2010.

About the Authors

Hiroko Arikawa, Ph.D., received her B.S. in psychology from the University of Oregon in 1991, her M.S. in clinical psychology from Eastern Washington University in 1993, and her Ph.D. in clinical psychology from California School of Professional Psychology – Fresno in 1997. She has published her research in human–animal relationships, sleep paralysis, and international psychology. She was included in Marquis Who's Who Among America's Teachers in 2002 and 2005 and Who's Who in America in 2011. She is an adjunct faculty at Missouri State University and an advisory board member of Missouri Spinal Cord Injury Research Program. She lives with her mobility assistance dog. She is affiliated to Missouri State University, Springfield, MO.

Todd J. Braje is Assistant Professor of Anthropology at Humboldt State University. His research centers on the archaeology of maritime societies along the North American Pacific Coast, historical ecological approaches to understanding coastal hunter-gatherer-fishers, and maritime migrations. His first book, *Modern Oceans, Ancient Sites*, and many of his recent publications investigate human–environmental interactions and the deep history of human impacts on local ecosystems and animal communities.

Michael E. Bricker, Ph.D., is Co-Director of Lakeshore Psychotherapy Alliance, a group private practice in Chicago, Illinois. As a licensed clinical psychologist, Dr. Bricker maintains an active clinical practice where he serves both individuals and couples. Dr. Bricker is also an active presenter and trainer in the area of emotion-focused therapy. In addition, Dr. Bricker supervises and mentors mental health professionals in training as part of his duties as a consultant for a local agency.

Dr. Sue-Ellen Brown is a clinical psychologist and currently works at Paoletta Counseling Services in Mercer, PA. She sees clients of all ages and uses hypnosis when appropriate. She is certified in hypnosis through the American Society of Clinical Hypnosis. Three of her dogs are certified therapy dogs with Therapy Dogs International and they accompany her to see her clients. Dr. Brown worked as an assistant professor at the Tuskegee University School of Veterinary Medicine's Center for the study of human–animal interdependent relationships. From 1999 to 2010 she did research on the human–animal bond including the application of self-psychology to companion animals, ethnic variations in pet attachment, and dissociation and pet attachment. She practiced clinical psychology in Michigan and Pennsylvania from 1980 to 1999. In her private practice, she worked extensively with victims of childhood abuse. She was an assistant professor of psychology at the University of the Sciences in Philadelphia from 1986 to 1999. While serving as an assistant professor, she researched the ways in which animals enhance human health. Her focus was on the relationship between companion animals and stress, dissociation, and absorption in people. She earned her B.A. degree in psychology in 1977 and her M.A. degree in clinical psychology from Oakland University. She received the Psychology Doctorate (Psy.D.) degree in clinical psychology in 1986 from Central Michigan University. For several years Dr. Brown did extensive volunteer work with animal rescue and served on the board of directors for the Macon County Humane Society in Tuskegee, Alabama. She shares her home with five dogs she rescued off the roads in Alabama.

Helen L. Davis is Senior Lecturer in Psychology at Murdoch University in Western Australia. She received her Ph.D. from the University of Western Australia. Her background is in cognitive developmental psychology and individual differences. Since her appointment at Murdoch University, she has been involved in collaborative work with colleagues from clinical psychology and veterinary medicine in investigating the experience of bereaved animal owners from various religious backgrounds, how they understand and cope with the death of their companion animal. She and her colleagues have also investigated the impact of exposure to animal death and to bereaved clients on the job stress and job satisfaction of practising veterinarians.

Sarah DeGue received her bachelor's degree in psychology and sociology from the University of Michigan in 1999 and Ph.D. in clinical psychology from the University of Nebraska-Lincoln in 2006, specializing in violence research and forensic evaluation. Since 2008, Dr. DeGue has worked as a behavioral scientist in the Division of Violence Prevention at the Centers for Disease Control and Prevention in Atlanta, Georgia, conducting research related to the primary prevention of violence, with an emphasis on sexual, family, and youth violence. Prior to joining CDC, Dr. DeGue was an assistant professor of psychology at the John Jay College of Criminal Justice, CUNY. In addition to teaching and research activities at John Jay, she was actively involved in a large-scale program that trains NYPD officers to safely manage individuals with severe mental illness. Dr. DeGue has a strong interest in the relationship between animal cruelty and interpersonal violence. In 2009, she published a paper on this topic entitled "Is Animal Cruelty a 'Red Flag' for Family Violence? Examining Co-occurring Violence towards Children, Partners, and Pets" in the *Journal of Interpersonal Violence*. Dr. DeGue lives in Decatur, Georgia, with her husband, Andrew, and dog, Bear.

Dr. Fine has also been on the faculty at California State Polytechnic University since 1981. He is presently a professor in the Department of Education. In 2001, he was awarded the prestigious Wang Award, given to a distinguished professor within the California State University system, in this instance for exceptional commitment, dedication, and exemplary contributions within the areas of education and applied sciences.

Aubrey is the editor of *The Handbook on Animal Assisted Therapy,* which is now in its third edition (Elsevier/Academic Press, 2010).

Carol L. Glasser received her MA and Ph.D. from the Department of Sociology at the University of California, Irvine. Her current research focuses on the intersections of feminism and animal rights and the role of radicalism in the animal rights movement. Carol is currently the research director at the Humane Research Council, a nonprofit organization that conducts research to understand social attitudes toward animal-related issues, to evaluate the effectiveness of animal protection programs and campaigns, and to otherwise support animal protection organizations with research services. She serves on the editorial team of the *Journal for Critical Animal Studies* and the board of Band of Mercy and participates in various grassroots campaigns for animal liberation. Carol resides in sunny Southern California with her two amazing companions, Bug and Oliver.

Lauren N. Hoffer is Assistant Professor of Victorian Literature at the University of South Carolina Beaufort. She received her Ph.D. from Vanderbilt University. Her research specializations include Victorian literature and culture, the British novel, and gender studies. She is currently at work on a book-length study of manipulative forms of sympathy and the paid female companion in the Victorian period.

Dr. Maria Andromachi Iliopoulou received a B.S. degree in French and literature from the Aristotle University of Thessaloniki and has studied at the College of Veterinary Medicine of the Aristotle University of Thessaloniki and the Veterinary school of Alfort in France ("Ecole Nationale Veterinaire d'Alfort") on a Socrates scholarship. She graduated from the College of Veterinary Medicine at MSU in 2007. In 2009, she completed an MS in the Comparative Medicine and Integrative Biology at MSU on the quality of life in dogs treated with chemotherapy. She is currently pursuing a Ph.D. in the Department of Community, Agriculture, Recreation and Resource Studies at MSU (Animal Studies Specialization).

Linda Kalof is Professor of Sociology, a Fellow of the Oxford Centre for Animal Ethics, and founder of the Michigan State University's interdisciplinary graduate specialization in Animal Studies. She has published more than 35 articles and book chapters and nine books including *Looking at Animals in Human History* (2007), *The Animals Reader* (2007), and *A Cultural History of Animals* (winner of the 2008 *Choice* award for Outstanding Academic Title).

Laurel Lagoni is currently the President/CEO of World by the Tail, Inc., makers of ClayPaws®, the original paw print kit™. She also directs the development of pet loss-related information and resources found in the Veterinary Wisdom Support Center at www.VeterinaryWisdomforPetParents.com. Formerly, Lagoni was the cofounder and director of the nationally renowned Argus Institute for Families and Veterinary Medicine at Colorado State University's James L. Voss Veterinary

Teaching Hospital. Lagoni holds a master's degree in Human Development and Family Studies, with specialties in family therapy and grief education, from Colorado State University. She is the coauthor of four books, including the ground-breaking text *The Human-Animal Bond and Grief*. Lagoni has written over 50 book chapters and journal articles and has been an invited speaker at numerous national meetings, including the Smithsonian Institute. Lagoni is published in *Chicken Soup for the Pet Lover's Soul* and has been showcased twice on ABC television's *20/20* program.

Dr. Bronwyn M. Massavelli is a recently graduated Ph.D. student and active member of staff in the School of Psychology at the University of Queensland. She has also recently completed her postgraduate clinical training in psychology at the University of Queensland. Bronwyn has a keen interest in aging, mental health, and the impact of pets from a psychological perspective – this includes pet and animal-assisted therapy, and the impact that animals can have for social support, mental health, health, and general well-being. She also has research and clinical interests in mental health and psychopathology across the age span. Bronwyn has presented at a number of prestigious national and international aging conferences, and she hopes that one day she will make a difference for aged care in Australia through clinical work and research regarding the importance of pets and animal-assisted therapy in later life.

Dr. Samara McPhedran holds a Ph.D. in psychology, awarded by the University of Sydney (Australia). Dr. McPhedran has a long-standing interest in a range of criminological and social justice issues, including evidence-based policy, violence prevention, and family violence, and relationships between animal cruelty and inter-personal violence. Most recently, she has been critically evaluating methods used to "measure" attitudes toward animals and animal cruelty, from a psychometric and theoretical perspective.

Nancy A. Pachana is a professor in the School of Psychology at the University of Queensland, Australia, and co-director of its Ageing Mind Initiative network. She received her Ph.D. in 1992 from Case Western Reserve University in Cleveland, Ohio. She completed postdoctoral training in geropsychology at the UCLA Neuropsychiatric Institute in Los Angeles and the Palo Alto VAMC in California. She has taught and conducted research in geropsychology for over 15 years, with over 120 peer-reviewed publications and chapters in the field. Her research expertise includes clinical assessment of cognitive decline and driving skills in older adults, measurement and treatment of anxiety and mood disorders in later life, and novel intervention strategies in residential aged care, including animal-assisted therapy and therapeutic gardening.

Camilla Pagani is a researcher at the Institute of Cognitive Sciences and Technologies (ISTC) of the Italian National Research Council (CNR). She has a degree in Modern Languages and Literature, a Ph.D. in Anglo-American Literature, and a degree in Psychology. As the head of the project "The sense of diversity and its psychological implications," she has mostly been involved in the following research areas: child–animal relationship with special reference to empathy and violence; the relation between animal cruelty and bullying; the relation between animal cruelty and interpersonal violence in general; youth's attitudes toward multiculturalism; the perception of threat in cross-cultural relations; the role of knowledge, hate and resentment in racist attitudes; empathy in cross-cultural relations. She is the head of the research group "HARE" (Human–Animal Relations) in collaboration with Prof. F. Robustelli (ISTC) and Prof. F. R. Ascione (University of Denver). She is also the head of the research group "MIDI" (Multiculturalism, Immigration, Diversity, and Integration). She has published papers in national and international peer-reviewed journals and chapters in national and international books and coauthored a book. She is "Expert Evaluator" of European projects for the European Commission and Fellow of the University of Denver. She is a member of ISAZ (International Society of Anthrozoology) and of IAIE (International Association for Intercultural Education).

Rod Preece is author, coauthor, or editor of 21 books and numerous chapters in other books, as well as many articles in learned journals. His best-known books are *Animals and Nature: Cultural Myths, Cultural Realities* (University of British Columbia Press, 1999) and *Brute Souls, Happy Beasts and Evolution: The Historical Status of Animals* (University of British Columbia Press, 2005). He is retired and lives in London, Ontario.

Sofia Robleda-Gomez graduated with an honours degree in psychology in 2009 and is currently completing her doctorate of clinical and clinical geropsychology at the University of Queensland. She has been working as a research assistant for Nancy Pachana since 2010, and this has increased her knowledge and interest in therapeutic issues related to later life, including animal-assisted therapy.

Lisa A. Ruff received her J.D. from Mercer University School of Law and her master's n Library and Information Science from Drexel University. She is currently pursuing her master's in Education. Dr. Ruff served as Vice President and Adoption Coordinator for Delaware Valley Doberman Pinscher Assistance for over five years and fostered over fifty homeless Dobermans. She is the coauthor of an annual legal publication for practicing attorneys in Pennsylvania. She is the proud owner of two rescued Dobermans.

Bruce S. Sharkin received his Ph.D. in counseling psychology from the University of Maryland. Dr. Sharkin is a staff psychologist and associate professor in the Department of Counseling and Psychological Services at Kutztown University in Kutztown, Pennsylvania. Dr. Sharkin is the author or coauthor of over 25 journal articles, including two articles on pet loss. He has served as an editorial reviewer for the *Journal of College Counseling, Journal of Counseling Psychology,* and *Journal of Counseling and Development*. Dr. Sharkin is currently an editorial advisory board member for the American Counseling Association Publications office. He has done several presentations on pet loss for veterinary hospitals and has been involved in pet rescue work.

Judith M. Siegel earned a Ph.D. in social psychology in 1977 and a postdoctoral master's degree in epidemiology in 1981. Currently, she is professor of public health in the Department of Community Health Sciences, UCLA School of Public Health. She has a long-standing interest in behavioral predictors of disease, with an emphasis on cardiovascular disease. More broadly, she studies the impact of stress on health, both physical and psychological, as well as the factors that may mediate this relationship. Animal companionship is one such mediating factor. Siegel teaches graduate courses in social epidemiology and health-related behavior change.

Judy Skeen, Professor of Religion at Belmont University, was born in the northeastern United States, raised in south Florida, attended college in Alabama, completed two masters and a doctorate in Kentucky and Tennessee and found home in the Bitterroot Valley of Western Montana. Her graduate studies were bifocal in biblical foundations and applied psychology, with her dissertation bringing together her interest in early Christian writings and pilgrimage. She is a teacher, a spiritual director, and a developing horsewoman. These days she can be found daydreaming about Native American wisdom and environmental studies and communicating with horses.

Dr. Donald I. Templer is Retired Professor of Psychology at Alliant International University. He received his Ph.D. in clinical psychology at the University of Kentucky and his post-doctoral fellowship in physiological psychology at Washington University. He has well over 200 publications and well over 2000 citations. His Death Anxiety Scale has been translated into 18 languages and his original article was declared a citation classic by Current Contents. He is a diplomate of the American Board of Professional Psychology (ABPP) and a fellow of the American Psychological Association.

David A.H. Wilson is an honorary research fellow in the School of Historical Studies at the University of Leicester. Until recently he was course leader for History at the University of Cumbria. His specialist research area and publications concern both historical anthrozoology and the history of comparative psychology and other studies of animal behaviour (pure and applied) especially in Britain, including interdisciplinary, institutional, professional, ethical, recreational, literary, and military aspects.

Sharon Lee Hart was born in Washington, DC, and currently lives and teaches photography in Nashville, TN. She has been visiting farm animal sanctuaries all over the United States and making portraits of the residents. She began this project because of her love of farm animals. The animals at the sanctuaries have escaped from slaughterhouses and live meat markets and lived through animal testing and cockfighting. Hart chose to title the photographs with each animal's first name and the name of the sanctuary in which they reside. She hopes the portraits encourage people to see with compassionate eyes and view farm animals in a new light. More of her work and information about farm animal sanctuaries can be found on her web site, www.farmanimalsanctuaryproject.com.

Part I
Contextual and Cultural Issues

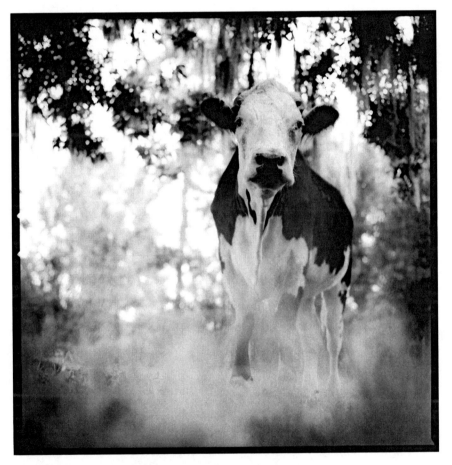

Aincho, Resident of Kindred Spirits Farm Animal Sanctuary
Aincho found his way to the sanctuary during a hurricane.

Chapter 1
Introduction: Using Context to Inform Clinical Practice and Research

Christopher Blazina, Güler Boyraz, and David Shen-Miller

Twenty years ago, "pet related issues" may have seemed an inconsequential matter or outside the scope of professional practice for many mental health practitioners and researchers. Yet, the 2006 *U.S. Pet Ownership & Demographics Sourcebook* found that 37.2% of US households have a dog and 32.4% have a cat. Today, there are more than 72 million pet dogs in the United States and nearly 82 million pet cats. In several research studies, between 87 and 99% of pet owners defined their pets as being "like a friend or family member" (Cain, 1983; Voith, 1985). If financial commitment can be considered as one level of emotional investment, it may be safe to assume that Americans have significantly invested in their pets. In 2005, US consumers spent more than $36 billion on their pets, more than double the amount spent ten years earlier (American Pet Products Association, 2005). The total US pet industry expenditures for 2009 was $45.5 billion. It is estimated that the trend will continue, with spending to top over $47.5 billion in the United States alone. Many may wonder how pet companions have obtained such important standing in contemporary times. Endenburg (2005) has suggested that this increasing investment and reliance on pets for companionship and social support is due to recent demographic and social changes, such as smaller family size, increased longevity, and higher incidences of relationship breakdown. For many, these increasing emotional and financial investments illustrate the depth and importance of the human–animal bond.

Psychological Relevance of the Human–Animal Bond

The changing role of companion animals in humans' lives has resulted in a growing emphasis on the human–animal bond research in the literature. Researchers have found that pet ownership has many measurable benefits, including enhancing psychological well-being, reducing feelings of loneliness in those who are living alone, and even aiding in recovery from illness and operations (e.g., Goldmeier, 1986;

C. Blazina (✉)
Department of Psychology, Tennessee State University, Nashville, TN 37209, USA
e-mail: christex01@msn.com

C. Blazina et al. (eds.), *The Psychology of the Human–Animal Bond*,
DOI 10.1007/978-1-4419-9761-6_1, © Springer Science+Business Media, LLC 2011

Marks, Koepke, & Bradley, 1995; Sharkin & Knox, 2003; Siegel, 1993; Wrobel & Dye, 2003). In addition, pet ownership has been found to be associated with lower levels of depression in bereaved elderly individuals who have minimal to no social support (Garrity, Stallones, Marx, & Johnson, 1989). Central to these positive effects is the resulting sense of attachment to another; that is, the human–animal bond allows for a sense of social relatedness and belonging. One may turn to pets to fill a range of roles from companion to child substitute that are experienced as psychologically comforting if not essential (Brown, 2004).

Some scholars have argued that the power and value of the human–animal relationship is based on a perceived nonjudgmental emotional support (Allen, Blascovich, & Mendes, 2002; Corson & Corson, 1981) or even "unqualified love and acceptance" (Nieburg & Fischer, 1982). Both Sigmund Freud and his daughter Anna wrote of their personal experiences with dogs and how this affiliation taught them about "pure love" relationships (Genosko, 1994). Although most people may benefit from a pure love relationship, based on their unique life contexts, some individuals may experience such relationships as particularly meaningful. For example, individuals with a personal history of emotional deprivation and abuse in their formative years, or trauma or loss in adulthood, may find that pets become more consistent and reliable others to which they can turn (see Brown, 2004 for a review). The relatedness encompassed within human–animal companionship may in turn foster an individual's ability to connect with others in more appropriate ways by increasing self-cohesion and -esteem (Brown, 2004). Pet companionship may also serve as a source of emotional sustenance for those who have no or limited connection (both physical and emotional) with other people (e.g., Brown, 2004; Sharkin & Bahrick, 1990). But even when the world does not seem like a dire place, we are all still in need of reliable ties that can be counted upon, ones that shape the very essence of who we are.

Just as connections with pets can foster well-being, the loss of a pet can lead to significant distress for their owners. When losing a pet, the intensity and duration of some pet owners' mourning mirrors or even surpasses the grief experienced when losing a human companion (Gosse & Barnes, 1994; Planchon & Templer, 1996; Wrobel & Dye, 2003). Unfortunately, societal mechanisms are not always in place to recognize or acknowledge this form of grief, leading to an experience of what Doka (1989) coined "disenfranchised grief," a loss that goes unrecognized by society as legitimate (Meyers, 2002; Sharkin & Bahrick, 1990; Stewart, Thrush, & Paulus, 1989). In such cases, the individual may not be afforded the proper grief support, which can have negative psychological consequences especially when bereavement is complex or prolonged. It is also important to note that pet owners lose their pets as a result of euthanasia, accidental separation, natural and unnatural causes, and even abandonment. Each of these circumstances can complicate the process of grieving, and pet owners may experience long-term significant distress. For mental health practitioners and researchers, attempting to understand of the importance of the human–animal bond through themes such as attachment, loss, and disenfranchised grief are essential clinical matters.

Moving beyond the immediacy of pet bonds and relationships, numerous other psychological themes also emerge in relation to human–animal interactions, some of which concern the influence of such interactions on human development. For instance, in the formative years, we may witness a pet companion's struggles toward achieving certain developmental milestones that may parallel our own maturation. One may even have the first incidence of loss and grief in the context of the bond. As Marie Bonaparte (1994/1940) once noted about dogs, one of our summers equals seven of theirs. There are certainly other considerations, not all of them normative, which also emerge within the familial domain. For example, there can be an interface of pet ownership with familial violence, neglect, and abuse. Clinicians and researchers likely will find understanding the relations between personal and societal attitudes as well as beliefs and experiences regarding animal cruelty and abandonment centrally important to their work with individuals for whom such issues are pertinent.

Thinking Broadly About the Human–Animal Bond: Cross-Cultural and Interdisciplinary Approaches

Considerations of the human–animal bond also need to consider the role of culture. There are various meanings attributed to pet ownership and the place of nonhuman animals in society, as well as significantly different perceptions of the human–animal bond for clients from diverse cultural backgrounds. Understanding cultural influences on the human–animal bond are an essential aspect of clinical work. Attention to the role of culture is important in terms of how the specific *elements* of a culture (e.g., its religions, histories, philosophies) contribute to the meaning of that bond in individual's or families' lives. Then also, cross-cultural comparisons—both within and across borders—are necessary to understand more of the diverse meanings of the bond. Such comparisons are made even more pertinent when examining cultural similarities and differences in their broader contexts. To comprehend how these and many other potentially different factors interface in shaping the psychological perception of the human–animal bond, a multidisciplinary perspective informed by context is in order.

   Although this anthology uses psychology as the focal point to integrate understanding of the human–animal bond, one of the important aspects of the text is the inclusion of interdisciplinary works from anthropology, philosophy, literature, religion, veterinary medicine, and social work. Adding these perspectives as part of our focus on the psychology of the human–animal bond allows for multiple vantage points that are rarely seen in clinically oriented texts, but that allow—and actually demand—the development of broad clinical conceptualizations and research models. The inclusion of multidisciplinary works helps form the big picture of the human–animal bond. For instance, understanding "The History of Animal Ethics in Western Culture" (Chapter 3) makes clear to the reader how a hierarchical frame of reference has often existed between humans and animals in Western civilization, with mankind usually being at the top. One potential scenario that can develop from this relationship is that humans assume the role of the "good steward" for animals placed in their charge. However, when a level of disconnection develops in terms of the interrelatedness of human–animal bond within this same hierarchical equation, it can justify for some the provision of less than proper care and treatment of animals, (i.e., "Animals are just property"). Similarly, when one considers the ways in which our relationships with animals are embedded in religious views (Chapter 5) or mirrored in literature (Chapter 6), one forms a broader and more complex portrait of the importance of the human–animal bond. Both perspectives help to contextualize and understand the developments that exist in social phenomena as the animal rights movement, and may help clinicians appreciate how a client's activism for animal rights is congruent (or incongruent) with their cultural norms. In other words, one can situate a client's presenting concern in the context of her/his cultural background. Themes begin to develop, and cultural (or cross-cultural) networks of meaning begin to emerge. These are just a few examples of the many elements that can underlie attitudes of clients, clinicians, and researchers.

Interfacing with multiple disciplines sheds additional light on the development of one's psychological experience of the human–animal bond that reaches beyond the pale of our traditional training as mental health professionals and researchers. The exchange asks us to think deeply about fundamental assumptions, attitudes, and beliefs that underlie our efforts as clinicians and researchers, and can ensure dialogue on topics that stimulate meaningful understanding, additional questions, and conversations. Figure 1.1 captures a sampling of the different disciplines which can inform the psychological perspectives of the human–animal bond.

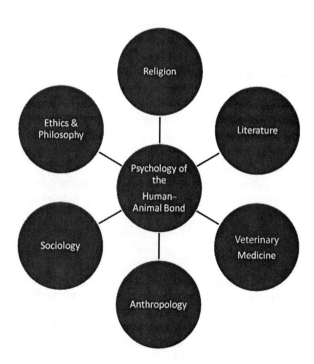

Fig. 1.1 Contextual Significance of the human–animal bond

Contextual Significance of the Human–Animal Bond

The inclusion of multidisciplinary works helps construct a broader view of the human–animal bond. However, the clinician and researcher also need a meaningful way to integrate seemingly divergent perspectives. If we establish psychology as one means to connect and interface with interdisciplinary works, then a contextual view of the work adds even more complex dimensions of thought. From a psychological perspective, *context* has become an ever-increasing salient consideration among both practitioners and researchers (e.g., Lewin, 1935). Context provides further clarification of the meaning of a variable or theme by providing a nuanced understanding of how other factors converge and interface with the one we wish to explore. Such factors include, but are not limited to, socioeconomic status, race, ethnicity, individual differences related to developmental issues across the life span, and power differentials within and across cultures and that affect individuals, families, groups, and organizations. Researchers and clinicians have developed numerous context-based conceptual models and approaches, such as multicultural frameworks (e.g., Fischer, Jome, & Atkinson, 1998; Sue, Arredondo, & McDavis, 1992; Sue, Bingham, Borche-Burke, & Vasquez, 1999), ones that call attention to issues such as gender (Enns, 2008; Falmagne, 2000; Heppner & Heppner, 2008; Stewart & McDermott, 2004; Wester, 2008), race/ethnicity (Helms, 1990), social class (Liu et al., 2004), sexual orientation (e.g., Cass, 1984), the psychology of men and masculinity, both in the United States and internationally (Blazina, 2003; Blazina & Shen-Miller, 2011; Connell & Messerschmidt, 2005), and many others, including intersections among multiple aspects of identity in their work.

Previous conceptual models and critiques within psychology and sociology that utilize context have also done so by conducting investigation at multiple levels of interest within a given society (e.g., Bronfenbrenner, 1979), as well as on an international level (e.g., Arnett, 2008; Blazina, 2003; Blazina & Shen-Miller, 2011; Connell, 1995; Leong & Savickas, 2007; Stevens & Wedding, 2004). We can see the emphasis upon multiple contextual foci within current theoretical approaches. For instance, psychodynamic/psychoanalytic traditions (e.g., Bowlby, 1982/1969; Winnicott, 1971) especially emphasize the individual and interpersonal context. Self is shaped, if not developed, in the relational context of another. The social constructionist approach (e.g., Connell & Messerschmidt, 2005) highlights the dialectic nature of self and culture when co-constructing the meanings of variables of interest within a society. Ecological models (e.g., Bronfenbrenner, 1979) argue for the interrelated and reciprocal influence of various systems. For instance, the individual may be influenced by family or social systems, but the culture is also affected by the individual and by interactions within other systems (Bronfenbrenner, 1979), leading to potential multiple systemic changes. Finally, a prominent aspect of multicultural models includes highlighting the interface of various sets of cultural values, beliefs, and actions.

In keeping with this growing contextual emphasis, we propose a multilayered focus in regard to the psychological study of the human–animal bond. This type of contextual approach is necessary if we are to understand the various meanings of the human–animal bond in an increasingly complex and sophisticated manner. Readers are encouraged to consider and challenge themselves by asking questions about each of the various proposed levels as they review the chapters that follow. In keeping with existing theoretical approaches that guide research and clinical work, we suggest that there is much to be gained by investigating single or multiple contextual foci that accentuate the bond's significance. Becoming more familiar with the distinctive contextual backdrop aids in our understanding of the unique experiences that helps shape the perception and meaning of the bond. We invite the contextual examination of the bond on the individual, interpersonal, cultural, cross-cultural, and professional levels. Each of these contextual perspectives is discussed further in this chapter.

Aims of the Model

The aim of this model is threefold: (1) raise awareness regarding the myriad influences that shape the experience of the human–animal bond, and how they may be studied, (2) enhance the explanatory power of clinicians, researchers, and clients regarding the meaning of the bond, and (3) increase agency among clinicians, researchers, and clients when acting upon the meaning of the bond. Each of these goals can be realized within the proposed levels of contextual study (i.e., individual, interpersonal, cultural, and cross-cultural) as well as across those levels, as noted below.

Raising Awareness

Awareness raising refers to deliberate efforts to bring attention to certain significant issues regarding the bond. We see its application on the cultural (and cross-cultural) level(s), where messages about the treatment and role of animals are brought to the attention of society. For instance, perceptions of the bond have evolved significantly over the past one hundred years in the United States and England in step with other social movements, advocating for better treatment of human and nonhuman others (see Chapter 2). But one must also be aware of more contemporary local and regional mores regarding the bond. In some instances, there are competing perceptions that are in significant conflict, such as issues concerning the reintroduction of wildlife into ranch or farmlands, or the status of dedicated sanctuaries when there are competing financial interests.

Raising awareness about the human–animal bond also involves issues pertinent to the family. This may be applicable in discovering the importance of normative developmental occurrences such as the impact of new pet ownership on the growth at the individual, interpersonal, and family levels. Some individuals discover their first reliable connection within the context of the bond. One may also expect the meaning of the bond to evolve over the course of time (e.g., a pet may become companion, become protector, provide an opportunity to reciprocate care for another). Concerning the interpersonal level, some couples may unwittingly approach the bond as a trial run for eventual parenting; or, in the case of an already-established family, a pet provides an opportunity for children to become socialized, including the prospect of learning how to care for another or about the importance and sanctity of all forms of life. Raising awareness of the multiple roles a pet may assume allows for deeper appreciation of the bond while the pet is living, and also aids the individual, couple, and family in understanding its significance when the pet has departed. Awareness raising in its many forms sets the stage for potential increases in explanatory power and a sense of agency on the part of the client, clinician, and researcher.

Enhancing Explanatory Power

Integrating the distinct vantage points that emerge from multidisciplinary work allows a unique and more comprehensive psychological understanding of the human–animal bond. For instance, on the cultural and cross-cultural levels, we are better able to assemble the various influences and patterns in a meaningful way, charting the rise of the current societal perception of the bond. One may also utilize the explanatory power in order to understand more about the bond's significance at the interpersonal and individual levels. For instance, certain pivotal happenings with the family set the stage for the bond to be experienced in a unique way. This may include messages conveyed in explicit and implicit fashion regarding the hierarchy or nature of the relationship between human and nonhuman others (e.g., "dogs are kept outside; inside of the house is for people only"). The bond may also be shaped by normative instances that occur across the life span, such as the loss of a pet as a child. The stage is set for one's understanding about life and loss through the experience of the bond. Likewise, unsettling occurrences, such as incidences of family violence, neglect, and abuse, are also significant. Harnessing explanatory power in these instances and others helps clients understand the descriptive and prescriptive messages that occur about the bond ("pet are only property," "abusing a pet is also a means of harming the family as a whole"). Within mental health fields, we can utilize our explanatory power to aid researchers and clinicians in constructing meaningful research models and therapeutic techniques. Clients benefit from more effective treatment and care that is provided, and also in developing their own ability to explore and articulate personal meanings regarding the bond. These advances aid the client in deconstructing and reconstructing one's personal narrative. Such investigations may assist clients to achieve deeper appreciation for the various contextual influences that shaped their experiences, helping them to articulate, "The bond was important to me because. . .".

Increasing Agency

Agency involves the ability to make independent choices for oneself and, when need be, advocate on behalf of another (human or nonhuman animal). On the individual level, agency concerns the ability to have say over one's own thoughts, feelings, and actions. For instance, one develops the wherewithal and ability to construct and reconstruct the personal narrative concerning issues of pet attachment and loss. Agency for instance, allows one to work toward forming a continuing bond after the death of a companion pet. At the same time, agency allows less tacit acceptance of other's perceptions that may be conveyed on the interpersonal, cultural, or cross-cultural levels. Instead, there is a progression toward developing a unique view of the bond. However, often the sequence of defining one's own personal meaning attributed to the bond occurs within the context of a helpful interpersonal relationship whose agenda is not to sway but rather aid in helping discover one's own unique experience. While this interaction may occur in many different forms, it can also happen in the therapeutic context; the client feels understood, supported, and impacted by the clinician. The clinician also develops therapeutic agency by being better able to effectively address the needs of the client. Likewise, the researcher experiences investigative agency by having more explanatory power. Certainly, one can also speak of agency in terms of intervening within a given social system or across cultures. One may advocate for the better treatment of animals, or work toward raising awareness about the importance of the bond, or the need for support when one has lost a beloved animal companion.

Contextual Layers

The depiction in Fig. 1.2 is meant to convey the kinds of potential interactions and interrelationships that occur across the proposed layers of context. For example, cultural norms certainly have an influence on the context of an individual, and on interpersonal norms and relationship expectations as well. As Bronfenbrenner

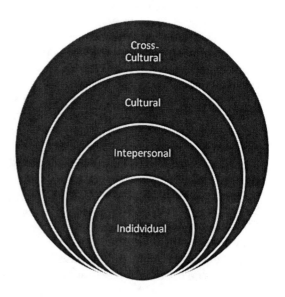

Fig. 1.2 A conceptual model of the human–animal bond

(1979) pointed out, this type of interrelationship also suggests a closed system; that is, change on any level or in any context has the potential to stimulate response and/or change at all other levels within the model. For example, adopting or changing cultural norms about the relative status of humans and animals (e.g., beliefs in a hierarchical relationship) affect humans' treatment of animals (e.g., as "good stewards"). However, change on the individual level can similarly affect the cultural level. Individuals who gather together to advocate for changes in their community about the treatment of abused animals might take additional steps to facilitate further transformation. These changes in local policies might lead to state, regional, or national changes, as well as stimulate countrywide dialogue on the cultural and/or international levels. In the sections that follow, we outline in more detail the proposed levels of context.

However, before we outline these contextual levels, a note about professional context: We challenge researchers and clinicians to be aware of our own unique experiences and the resulting of these on our perceptions of the human–animal bond. That is, for those within the field, we have a *professional context* to consider. Professional context includes our overall outlook toward our work as researchers and clinicians. This point of view is informed not only by our unique experiences across the full range of the proposed contextual levels, but also by our training as mental health practitioners and the culture of mental health professionals. For instance, we have our own individual contexts regarding the human–animal bond. Many may follow a line of inquiry that focuses on the significance to people–pet attachments because of their own personal, interpersonal, and cultural experiences. Yet these experiences do not exist in a vacuum; they intersect, perhaps clash, and ultimately are, to some extent, integrated with our training, participation in professional organizations, reading of (and publishing in) professional scientific journals, and our interaction with the world in our roles as mental health professionals. Our professional perspective might be considered a synthesis related to these different contextual influences shaping our knowledge, skills, and practice. In the best of situations, professional context can provide motivation, if not inspiration, for the work that is done; at other times, it has the potential to skew our perceptions by not integrating the various divergent experiences in a meaningful and objective way.

Individual Contextual Considerations

We suggest that an investigation focused at the individual contextual level is of special importance. We propose that the seat of phenomenological experience regarding the perception and meaning of the bond is ultimately at this personal level. While we may have various important influences and exchanges at other levels of context, the individual, in the end, ultimately perceives and constructs his or her own experience of the bond. With that said, the actual process of defining the bond at the individual level may vary across individuals in terms of actual deliberate involvement. For instance, in some cases, input at the family or cultural level determines one's whole attitude toward the bond. Some may even accept in a tacit manner what has been conveyed or experienced in the context of others as one's own personal truth in regard to the bond. Until defined differently, the resulting perception of the bond in this case is significantly fashioned, if not adopted, from others. Other individuals may experience a barrage of influences at various contextual levels, and yet rely most heavily on internal dialogue to create an indelible set of beliefs regarding what the bond means. It is expected that there will be a great deal of variability in terms of the way the bond is determined within families, culture, and across societies. We argue below one of the main goals of the therapist (and researcher) is to assist with a growing sense of individual agency regarding one's perception of the bond.

While the special emphasis is upon individual level as the seat of awareness may seem more consistent within individualistic societies, we also suggest that even in societies in which group and cultural perceptions may be more heavily weighted, the personal view of the bond is still a crucial level to conceptualize for researchers and clinicians. Regardless of the type of culture being studied, the individual may occupy different places on a continuum. Across cultures, individuals may attribute significantly different levels of importance to the beliefs, values, and actions to which one has been exposed at the family, cultural, and cross-cultural levels in regard to the bond. In practical terms, this may mean that a client is at odds with family or culture when it comes to the meaning of the bond, which in turn may lead to a lack of social support during the life of a pet companion as well as disen-franchised grief upon its death. By helping the individual sort through the various influences that either support or contradict his or her experience of the bond, the person stands on firmer ground regarding the meaning of the bond.

Several individual contextual factors may be of particular relevance in our dis-cussion. For instance, one may consider attachment history; an ability to form and maintain meaningful relationships with others (e.g., human or nonhuman compan-ions); personal history of loss, abuse, and neglect; and demographic factors such as age and living conditions (e.g., living alone versus living with others). Each of these aspects as well as many others may shape an individual's ability to connect with animal companions, as well as impact how one responds to the eventual loss. These various influences are significant in their own right, and shed additional light when interfaced with other factors in the larger context of the bond. For instance, is the human–animal bond the first reliable attachment, or one of many that are held as significant? Likewise, how have various losses impacted the individual, his or her response to loss of a pet, and the establishment of future attachments? Was a pet seen as a source of comfort upon the loss of another, or to what degree was the breaking of the human–animal bond considered significant in its own right? These are some of areas explored in this book.

On the individual contextual level, exploring various areas will broaden readers' understanding of the various influential dynamics and variations in meaning people attribute to their relationships with companion animals. For example, the sections on psychological issues of attachment well-being include theoretical discussions on multiple factors that contribute to the human–animal bond (e.g., attachment), provide review of the empirical findings regarding the human–animal bond and its effects on individual's well-being, and present an overview of animal-assisted therapies. These discussions not only will help readers to develop understanding of the individual factors that shape the human–animal bond, but will also increase their understanding of how the human–animal bond can alter personal factors in an individual's life. For example, readers will consider that an individual's relational history affects the way they relate to animals; at the same time, an individual's relationship with a companion animal, which may be perceived as based on unconditional love, can influence one's perception of himself or herself and relations with others.

To aid clinicians' and researchers' exploration with clients and research subjects across the proposed layers of context, we provide a short list of queries under each section that follows. We offer these questions as a means to begin a dialogue and develop a contextual perspective from various vantage points. For example, on the individual level, clinicians (or researchers) might consider:

1. What is the individual's personal history of making and sustaining attachments (with people and pets)? Does one category of connection (e.g., with pets or with people) seem more secure and reliable, or is it the case that both may be easily incorporated within one's relational network?

2. What type of attachment style does the individual predominately rely upon for constructing models of self, others, and the world (e.g., secure, anxious, avoidant)? How does the attachment style of the individual affect his or her relationship with companion animals and/or his or her response to loss of a companion animal?

3. What is the meaning and significance of an individual's relationship with his/her pet? In what role(s) does one envision current or past pets (e.g., child substitute, companion, filling the void left by loss of others)?

4. What is one's personal history concerning losses (with both people and pets)? Has one had successful resolution(s) regarding former losses? How does an individual's personal history of loss affect his or her response to loss of a pet and the forming of new relationships with pets?

5. Does the client (or clinician) operate from the perspective that a *continuing bonds* approach is warranted with the loss of significant relations one has (people and pets)? Or is it the case the individual operates from the perspective that detachment and withdrawal is the goal for grief work?

6. How do aspects of humans' identity, such as race, ethnicity, social class, age, nationality, sexual orientation, religion, and level of physical and mental ability, shape perceptions of the human–animal bond?

7. What is one's perspective on issues of speciesism and a perceived hierarchy between mankind and nonhuman animals? To what extent is the client anthropomorphizing her or his companion animal, and to what degree is that process useful in clinical or research applications? How might the clinician challenge anthropomorphic tendencies? How might the researcher address or include anthropomorphism during the research process?

8. Turning our attention inward, what models is one using (in the clinician or researcher role) to explore the human–animal bond in session (e.g., attachment

theory, evolutionary biology, veterinary medicine, social construction, feminism)? What is the intersection between this model and one's own personal or professional experience?

9. What are the personal-professional aims of clinician and researcher in terms of studying the human–animal bond?

10. What has been the role of the human–animal bond in terms of advancement of the individual's physical and/or mental health? In what ways (specific to the individual) would connection with an animal be beneficial?

Interpersonal Contextual Considerations

A complex contextual investigation of the human–animal bond should continue with attention to interpersonal and familial levels within any single cultural framework. As clinicians and researchers, we can strive to understand the various dynamics that influence the various relational and familial contexts. For instance, what were the prevailing family attitudes toward the bond and how have we integrated or rejected them? The interpersonal context allows us to gain access to needed vantage points regarding the significance of the bond. To be most effective as clinicians and researchers, we consider how the factors at play on the individual contextual level develop, are also potentially reinforced, and create change in various interpersonal contexts. For example, attachment styles, by definition, develop in interpersonal contexts. Exploring how those styles affect adult relationships that may influence one's experience of the human–animal bond (e.g., in terms of the perceived legitimacy of making "sacrifices" for one's pet, among others, in one's support system—or support for the grief one might experience at the loss of a pet) can add a great deal to the clinical picture. Similarly, looking to explore how the loss of a pet due to the actions of a parental figure can influence other family dynamics as well as a child's relational attachments to other pets in the house can help clinicians design an intervention plan that accounts for these and other multiple interpersonal realities. Also, considering the relative importance of the human–animal bond in determining relationships with other humans can add complexity to the clinical picture. Clinicians might consider how a client's relational approach to animals affects interpersonal relationships in their lives—for example, does one's dog serve as a litmus test for potential friends or romantic partners? Are decisions based on initial reactions or changes over time, or attempts to form relationships with the pet?

On another level, interpersonal context is also of importance for the clinician and researcher in terms of professional context. The professional models by which one was trained (e.g., social work, psychology) ultimately informs our understanding of the bond. Not only the specific profession, but also the kinds of attention that our professional training includes in terms of the salience of different types of relational bonds (e.g., family, society, animals) will affect the types and styles of relational realities that we examine. For instance, those trained in attachment theory will likely be predisposed to explore how clients form and sustain connections with others, and perhaps to consider the role that the relational context plays within the therapeutic dyad. For some who may be so trained—or involved in networks of professionals with such emphases—the relational and attachment components may also be expanded to include animal-assisted therapies. Some additional questions to consider include:

1. What was the prevailing attitude(s) toward the human–animal bond in one's family of origin (e.g., a pet was a family member, a pet was a protector, animals were chattel, beliefs about animal sentience)? How were those attitudes expressed and experienced in terms of daily life? How did the client (or research participant) incorporate or reject those attitudes?
2. Were there pivotal events in the family of origin or adult family (e.g., attachment, loss, abuse, neglect, relinquishment of the pet under difficult circumstances) that illustrate how prevailing altitude(s) toward the human–animal bond were transmitted in an interpersonal context?
3. In the construction of one's own family in adulthood, what aspects are retained from the family of origin, and what new perspectives have been added? How does one's relational approach to animals affect other interpersonal relationships?
4. Who (and what) are the current major interpersonal influences that shape one's attitudes and behaviors about how to interact with animals in their life? What are the mechanisms (e.g., interpersonal interactions, Internet forums, social clubs) by which these influences form and are continued?
5. Have there been important interpersonal events that shape one's newer perception(s) of the human–animal bond (e.g., is the pet seen by a couple as being integral to their first experience with "parenting," is a pet experienced as a significant relationship in its own right, and/or as a family member, is the loss of a pet experienced as a familial occurrence that was important)?
6. Does one affiliate with social networks and organizations in which the experience of the human–animal bond is pertinent (e.g., frequenting dog parks or horse stables, participating with animals in a competitive or pro-social format, participating in local and/or national pet-fostering organizations, or organizations involved with pet rescue)? How do these social networks provide support, encouragement, or other influence on the human–animal bond as present in the therapy or research setting?
7. How is the interpersonal context viewed within a therapeutic relationship? Is the relational aspect viewed as a curative aspect(s) of therapy? Is the relational context seen as a means to help the client feel understood, negotiate the potential of disenfranchised grief, and form new relations? What are the clinician's beliefs about pet loss and related grief, and how are those beliefs affecting the therapeutic relationship? Is there room for animal assistance in therapy, and, if so, how will that affect the interpersonal dynamic?
8. What is the personal/family/interpersonal context of the clinician or researcher with regard to the above questions? In what ways is that context shaping the work with clients or participants?
9. How does the clinician or researcher manage any pertinent but potentially conflicting roles evoked either in the helping environment or conducting research?

For instance, how does one manage one's roles as scholar, social advocate, leader of organization, trainer of students in relation to the human–animal bond? How do the interpersonal factors converge with one's beliefs about matters salient to human–animal relationships?

Cultural Contextual Considerations

We operate on the assumption that events that occur on the national and/or cultural scale permeate our thoughts, attitudes, and behaviors as clients, clinicians, and researchers in various degrees. Attention to the cultural level can provide meaningful information about diverse, but cumulative, beliefs and actions in regard to the bond that are evident in individual, interpersonal, and family and group interactions. For instance, a sociohistorical perspective allows us to chronicle how certain contextual events, such as social movements for both human and nonhuman animals, influence our perceptions of the bond. As noted above, Endenburg (2005) has suggested that demographic and social shifts in family size, increased longevity, and incidences of relationship breakdown can have ripple effects into the human–animal bond. We might turn our attention also to how the changing human–animal bond may foster continued cultural shifts. For example, individuals with strong connections to their pets may live longer, or be more thoughtful about the health choices that they make. Similarly, the animal rights movement (e.g., Singer, 1975) has certainly had an impact on the consciousness of many, and has arguably changed the landscape of perceptions of the human–animal bond in dramatic ways.

An anthropological approach similarly adds to our knowledge of the human–animal bond, and to our understanding of individual and interpersonal contexts by adding the unique dimension of the prehistoric contexts in which humans and nonhuman animals were first forming bonds, as well as the shaping of ensuing relationships over the millennia (e.g., Chapter 4). We may also witness context at the cultural level through analysis of how aspects of the bond are treated in popular and literary writings across history. For example, are pets seen as substitutes for human companionship, as in the context of Victorian era, or more recently with the rise of the pet memoir, as unique relationships in their own right (e.g., Chapter 5)? Likewise, how do cultural phenomena, such as classism, sexism, racism, homophobia, and other forms of discrimination, play out in beliefs about the human–animal bond (e.g., Chapter 16)? In what ways are social ills enacted in perceptions of the bond? How do widespread cultural themes that nonhuman animals are in a subservient position or even considered as chattel affect perceptions and lived experiences of the bond? Attention to these various threads can reveal the dialectic between individual and society on these matters that construct cultural perception(s) of the bond.

Similarly, as professionals we do not think or act within a culture-free vacuum. We must consider how culture shapes the lines of inquiry and methods by which we study the bond. Are there certain risks or benefits for staying in step with current cultural or professional foci regarding the human–animal bond? Do professionals face any potential benefit or backlash by not being in step with the norm within a culture or the professional field? How do the biases and assumptions of other professionals affect realities of the profession such as funding and employment opportunities, depending on what one believes about the importance of the human–animal bond? Similarly, how do our training and professional commitments affect our work related to the human–animal bond? In addition, we pose the following questions as examples of topics to consider:

1. What are the specific prevailing perceptions of the human–animal bond within one's immediate culture? Which key contextual factors, such as religion, prevailing ethical models, philosophies, education, shifting familial structure, socioeconomic status, and financial opportunities, significantly shape perceptions of the human–animal bond?
2. What images are made available through movies, news media, and other forms of mass communication that support the various perceptions of the bond?
3. What are common roles of animals in one's local community? For instance, do most families in a given culture have pets? Are pets considered differently than other nonhuman animals such as cattle? Are nonhuman animals portrayed as sentient beings? Are certain animals given favored status or acceptance? Why? Are animals involved in the professional sector (e.g., police, fire departments)? In what ways?
4. Are there financial incentives (e.g., the creation of jobs at a meat-packing plant, work on farms or ranches) that influence the immediate perception(s) of the bond? How are commitments of civic monies for shelters, animal control, dog parks, etc., viewed by the citizenry?
5. What crucial (recent or past) sociopolitical events have shaped the present climate of human–animal bond (locally or nationally)?
6. What is the current dominant perception of the human–animal bond within the larger state, or regional culture? How do local perceptions differ with those found in other adjoining settings and cultural subgroups? This might include differences in perception of the bond across rural versus urban settings, differences based on ethnicity or gender, as well as multiple attitudes that exists within one locale. What are the meanings of similarities and/or differences around the experience of the human–animal bond across the cultures?
7. To what extent is there political consonance between local and national cultural messages about the bond (e.g., federal versus local regulations or attitudes)? Do differences that exist between local and national messages create dissenting points of view or political tension between various factions? In what ways?
8. How entrenched are local attitudes and are there possibilities of change? For instance, does the social or political power of a group such as ASPCA (American Society for Prevention of Cruelty to Animals) or PETA (People for the Ethical Treatment of Animals) affect the roles of animals at the local level? In what ways does the power of animal rights organizations affect these roles

and resulting perception of the bond? How about on a farm, ranch, or in a lab where animals are used?

9. How do cultural expectations at the local, regional, and national levels concerning roles as clinicians or researchers affect the work being done on the individual and interpersonal levels? Is clinicians' or researchers' work valued within the society or viewed as a cultural fringe?

10. How do the APA ethical guidelines about research with animals affect decisions about study design and development? What is the current cultural zeitgeist that may be affecting those guidelines or how they are interpreted? Similarly, how do other organizational demands (e.g., public deliberation about the responsibility of mental health professionals to make a stand regarding torture situations—some of which include the use or misuse of animals in torture of humans) or media events (e.g., talk show topics) affect one's work with clients?

11. For the clinician or researcher, are there risks for not conforming to expected norms either on the local, regional, or national cultural levels? Likewise, are there distinct benefits?

12. What is the current role of professional societies, organizations, and peer-reviewed publications on how professionals and trainees conceptualize the human–animal bond? To what degree do these influences shape the research and clinical practice within the field?

Cross-Cultural Contextual Considerations

Any singular contextual analysis of the human–animal bond at the individual, interpersonal, and cultural levels can prove meaningful. However, adopting a cross-cultural perspective can increase the scope of our investigations significantly. To accomplish this task we can explore individual, interpersonal, and societal contexts from various countries and regions of the world. Clients potentially reap the benefits of such cultural exchanges through exposure to alternative perceptions of the bond and different treatment methods from around the world. Clinicians could consider whether such treatments—or elements of treatments—are workable within our own cultural contexts, and researchers can similarly consider whether the types of questions asked would have similar or different answers in local cultural contexts. In addition, another way to uncover one's own assumptions about the human–animal bond is through the study of other cultures' beliefs, attitudes, and assumptions—doing so can call our own beliefs, attitudes, and assumptions into sharp relief.

This type of cross-cultural dialogue can spur a wealth of investigation. However, it is not without accompanying challenges. For instance, what are the goals of such exploration for the professional? Is it to document similarities and differences that help inform research and practice in our own cultural context? What are the risks of doing so? Do the goals of the professional include homogenizing perceptions of the human–animal bond from one international context to another? What is the response of the professional when other cultural perceptions of the bond are different from our own perspectives? In what ways do the roles of social advocate and scholar converge when the study of cross-cultural differences uncovers attitudes and behaviors that significantly and palpably conflict with one's own cultural beliefs and values? How are those responses affected when issues of animal welfare intersect with differences in beliefs about animal sentience or the value of the human–animal bond (e.g., Chapter 15)? How does the mental health professional manage such conflicts and potentially competing responsibilities? There are no easy answers to these questions. Rather, the aim of this work is to provide a means to develop contextual awareness and sensitivity that encourages travel across various academic, clinical, cultural, and national borders, and fosters understanding through the convergence of diverse voices. Some questions to consider include:

1. How are experiences of the human–animal bond different and similar across cultures?
2. What does it mean to find similarities and/or differences regarding the experience of the human–animal bond across cultures? Is this the result of differences among the key contextual factors (e.g., religion, prevailing ethical models, philosophies, shifting familial structure) that significantly shape perceptions of the human–animal bond in various places in the world? What does the discovery of these differences mean with regards to notions of cultural relativism versus absolute truths about the bond?
3. Can one culture adopt and/or modify some theoretical and clinical notions from another country's approach toward the human–animal bond? If so, what makes this exchange possible? Is it desirable to share notions across cultures? In what ways?
4. To what extent do clinicians and/or researchers import their own cultural notions of the human–animal bond when working with individuals from another culture? How can one best be attuned to this process? From a clinical perspective, what are the hazards associated with remaining unaware (or less aware) of importing one's cultural notions? Is it worthwhile to talk about these in a clinical session? In what ways?
5. How do cross-cultural differences that might not seem related to the human–animal bond on the surface (e.g., differences in gender role expectations) affect the bond? What are the ways that these might be called to a client's attention? How about a therapist's attention? How do cross-cultural exchanges (in the therapy hour, or across a research project) affect, shape, and reform one's notions about aspects of the human–animal bond as part of the larger clinical picture?
6. Will there be some cultural barriers that prevent an exchange of theoretical and clinical notions on contextual grounds? If so, what are those?
7. What are the aims of clinicians and researchers at the international level in terms of the human–animal bond? Does one work toward influencing the perception of the bond across cultures? What values and beliefs affect one's actions in such instances?

Mapping Context

We can learn to map the influence and convergence of various individual, interpersonal, cultural, and cross-cultural dynamics. A contextual approach simultaneously broadens and deepens the perspectives of clinicians, researchers, and clients. We advocate for the continued articulation of the holistic, conceptual model suggested in this volume as a means for studying the psychology of the human–animal bond. It is crucial for those in mental health–related fields to obtain a clear perspective of the multiple dynamics that can interface in forming one's experience of the bond. Adopting a contextual stance will aid mental health professionals in appreciating why the human–animal connection has become a significant part of everyday life for many. Ultimately, using context to deepen one's understanding will enable practitioners to provide more effective treatment and extend their research and practice in new ways.

A brief case example can illustrate some of the various contextual vantage points. Let's discuss for a moment the contextual backdrop of how dogs came to play a significant role in the life of Sigmund Freud. As mentioned previously, Freud coined the "pure love" phrase that he associated with his canine companions. An example of the feeling of this type of unqualified love in the context of a pet relationship is present in a letter Freud wrote to Marie Bonaparte about her Chow Topsy:

> It really explains why one can love an animal like Topsy with such an extraordinary intensity: affection without ambivalence, the simplicity of life free from the almost unbearable conflicts of civilization, the beauty of an existence complete in itself... Often when stroking Topsy, I have caught myself humming a melody which unmusical as I am I can't help recognizing as the aria from Don Giovanni... (Sigmund Freud, 1964 pp. 434–435).

Such sentiments highlight the personal importance of Freud's human–animal bond. However, to better understand the important role the human–animal bond played in Freud's life one must appreciate further his own individual, interpersonal, cultural, and cross-cultural contexts. In this case, international context informs us of the influence Nazism and German nationalism had on Freud's eventual departure from his home country and his eventual arrival in England, both of which might have affected feelings of belonging, loss, and related emotions. There was also relevant cultural zeitgeist regarding the places of animals in society; pets were increasingly seen in some parts of Europe as suitable personal companions. Adding additional complexity to this shifting dynamic involves taking social class into account; pet ownership among the upper class carried certain significance, if not a symbol of status. If we continue to construct the context on the individual and interpersonal levels, the development of Freud's attachments and subsequent reactions to the loss of his dogs is clearer. Many years after first writing about loss in his seminal 1917 work, *Mourning and Melancholia*, Freud would later revisit his earlier work on grief after many painful personal losses in his own life. Freud had undergone more than thirty cancer-related operations, he had seen the passing of his closest daughter and grandson, and suffered the estrangement of a number of heirs apparent within the psychoanalytic inner circle. His remaining daughter, Anna, whom he had come to rely upon heavily, was growing more independent professionally and personally. Through pre–World War II period, he temporarily relied upon others, such as Marie Bonaparte, for financial assistance. In fact, he was involved in translating the book about her dog Topsy into German as a way of earning his keep. In the midst of these various losses, Freud confided to a friend that he believed himself incapable of loving again. It was into this void that his pet companions would appear. Freud was able to find some comfort and relief from the company of his dogs. Michael Molnar, the Research Director of the Freud Museum in London, noted the man–canine relationship manifested in a number of ways (1996). In the latter years of his life, Freud was frequently photographed with one of his chows. They even accompanied him during the analytic hour with his patients. Also, Freud, who now wore a prosthetic jaw as the result of the cancer, made good use of his dog's canine teeth on his behalf, allowing her to masticate his meat so he could eat it.

Conclusion

There have been dramatic increases in the financial, emotional, and psychological investment in the human–animal bond over the past four decades within the United States and in many places abroad. The increasing significance of animal companions in people's lives has resulted in a growing emphasis within academic literature, with a rising number of books and scholarly articles published in recent years. Works such as these have generally focused upon one of a number of pertinent topics, including issues of attachment, developmental life span considerations in forming a bond, ethics, animal-assisted therapies, and bereavement. Or when a multidisciplinary approach has been pursued, oftentimes there is further need of a unifying theme to aid integration of the diverse topics. While the existing literature is essential in increasing our understanding of the nature and impact of the human–animal bond, the next step is to further psychological perspectives informed by interdisciplinary contextual work. This approach is a part of the larger gestalt of the human–animal bond. The purpose of this book is to provide both a contextual understanding of the psychology of the human–animal bond, as well as present to the reader a sampling of the specific ways that these themes emerge both within and across disciplines.

In keeping with the contextual theme, the anthology begins with *PART I: Contextual and Cultural Issues.* Chapters within this part provide various multidisciplinary views on the human–animal bond that include religion, ethics, anthropology, history, and literature. Although this sampling should not be considered an exhaustive list of disciplines or topics to explore within each field, the various approaches orient the reader toward the multifaceted ways that the human–animal bond is experienced and explored. At the beginning of the text, we highlight the importance of adopting a multidisciplinary perspective. The multidisciplinary approach sets the tone for the importance of convergence and integration of contextual factors in exploring the human–animal bond. Such integration will foster readers' understanding of the nature and benefits of the human–animal bond, which will be the focus of the following parts of the book.

PART II: Psychological Issues of Attachment and Well-Being; PART III: Bereavement, Loss, and Disenfranchised Grief; and PART IV: Animal Rights, Abuse, and Neglect will help readers develop a knowledge base concerning fundamental issues and contemporary approaches to the nature and the benefits of the human–animal bond. In these sections, authors discuss cutting-edge research and theoretical conceptualizations about the bond and its effects on human's well-being. Developing appreciation of the attachment between humans and animals will also help readers comprehend issues related to grief and loss. These sections make up the clinical core of the book, which provides scientifically informed topics related to practice and research.

The final part (*PART V: Tests, Measurements, and Current Research Issues*) includes discussion of methodological issues and challenges (e.g., theoretical issues, study design, and sampling issues) related to conducting human–animal bond research as well as recommendations for future research. This section also includes a review of previous instruments used in human–animal research, including an overview of the psychometric characteristics and strengths and weaknesses of these instruments. This section is intended as a valuable resource for clinicians and researchers interested in conducting research in this area.

Explaining the psychological significance of the human–animal bond is a complex endeavor. As with any other important clinical dynamic, training and preparation are needed to gain competence for professional practice and research. To this end, an ensemble of international scholars across the fields of psychology and mental health explore topics that will help both new and established clinicians increase their skills and understanding of the various ways the human–animal bond manifests itself. Perspectives from beyond the scope of psychology and mental health, such as anthropology, philosophy, literature, religion, and history, provide a sampling of the significant interdisciplinary perspectives in which the human–animal bond appears. Taken together, these chapters provide readers with an understanding of some of the more significant and diverse contexts that underlie working with human–animal concerns. The reader thus gains access to a much broader picture of why the human–animal bond is an important issue on an individual, interpersonal, cultural, cross-cultural, and professional levels. What brings these divergent topics together in a meaningful way is their relevance and centrality to the contextual bonds that underlie the psychology of the human–animal connection. When viewed within this larger contextual framework, each chapter can add to the unique mosaic of our understanding.

References

Allen, K., Blascovich, J., & Mendes, W. B. (2002). Cardiovascular reactivity and the presence of pets, friends, and spouses: The truth about cats and dogs. *Psychosomatic Medicine, 64,* 727–739.

American Pet Products Association (2005). http://www.americanpetproducts.org/press_industrytrends.asp

Arnett, J. J. (2008). The neglected 95%: Why American psychology needs to become less American. *American Psychologist, 63*, 602–614.

Blazina, C. (2003). *The cultural myth of masculinity*. Westport, CT: Praeger.

Blazina, C., & Shen-Miller, D. (2011). *An international psychology of men: Advances, case studies, and clinician innovations*. New York: Routledge.

Bonaparte, M. (1994/1940). *The story of a golden haired chow* (pp. 1–26). New Brunswick, NJ: Transaction Publishers.

Bowlby, J. (1982/1969). *Attachment and loss: Vol 1. Attachment* (2nd Ed.). New York: Basic. (Original work published 1969).

Bronfenbrenner, U. (1979). *The ecology of human development*. Cambridge: Harvard University Press.

Brown, S. E. (2004). The human-animal bond and self psychology: Toward a new understanding. *Society & Animals, 12*, 67–86.

Cain, A. O. (1983). A study of pets in the family system. In A. H. Katcher & A. M. Beck (Eds.), *New perspectives on our lives with companion animals* (pp. 72–81). Philadelphia: University of Pennsylvania Press.

Cass, V. C. (1984). Homosexual identity formation: Testing a theoretical model. *Journal of Sex Research, 20*, 143–167.

Connell, R. W. (1995). *Masculinities*. Berkeley: University of California Press.

Connell, R. W., & Messerschmidt, J. W. (2005). Hegemonic masculinity: Rethinking the concept. *Gender and Society, 19*, 829–859.

Corson, S. A., & Corson, E. (1981). Companion animals as bonding catalysts in geriatric institutions. In B. Fogle (Ed.), *Interrelations between people and pets* (pp. 146–174). Springfield, IL: Tomas.

Doka, K. J. (1989). *Disenfranchised grief: Recognizing hidden sorrow*. Lexington, MA: Lexington.

Endenburg, N. (2005). The death of a companion animal and bereavement. In F. H. de Jonge & R. van den Bos (Eds.), *The human-animal relationship: Forever and a day* (pp. 110–122). Assen, Netherlands: Royal Van Gorcum.

Enns, C. Z. (2008). Toward a complexity paradigm for understanding gender role conflict. *The Counseling Psychologist, 36*, 446–454.

Falmagne, R. J. (2000). Positionality and thought: On the gendered foundations of thought, culture, and development. In P. H. Miller & E. Kofsky Scholnick (Eds.), *Toward a feminist developmental psychology* (pp. 191–213). New York: Routledge.

Fischer, A. R., Jome, L. M., & Atkinson, D. R. (1998). Reconceptualizing multicultural counseling: Universal healing conditions in a culturally specific context. *The Counseling Psychologist, 26*, 525–588.

Freud, S. (1964). *The letters of Sigmund Freud* (E. L. Freud, Trans.). New York: McGraw-Hill.

Garrity, T. F., Stallones, L., Marx, M. B., & Johnson, T. P. (1989). Pet ownership and attachment as supportive factors in the health of elderly. *Anthrozoos, 3*, 35–44.

Genosko, G. (1994). Introduction to the transaction Edition. In *Topsy: The story of a golden haired chow* (pp. 1–26). New Brunswick, NJ: Transaction Publishers.

Goldmeier, J. (1986). Pets or people: Another research note. *Gerontologist, 26*, 203–206.

Gosse, G. H., & Barnes, M. J. (1994). Human grief resulting from the death of a pet. *Anthrozoos, 7*, 103–112.

Helms, J. E. (1990). *Black and white racial identity: Theory, research, and practice*. Westport, CT: Greenwood Press.

Heppner, P. P., & Heppner, M. J. (2008). The gender role conflict literature: Fruits of sustained commitment. *The Counseling Psychologist, 36*, 455–461.

Leong, F. T. L., & Savickas, M. L. (2007). Introduction to special issue on international perspectives on counseling psychology. *Applied Psychology: An International Review, 56*, 1–6.

Lewin, K. (1935). *A dynamic theory of personality*. New York: McGraw-Hill.

Liu, W. M., Ali, S. R., Soleck, G., Hopps, J., Dunston, K., & Pickett, T., Jr. (2004). Using social class in counseling psychology research. *Journal of Counseling Psychology, 51*, 3–18.

Marks, S. G., Koepke, J. E., & Bradley, C. L. (1995). Pet attachment and generativity among young adults. *The Journal of Psychology, 128*, 641–650.

Meyers, B. (2002). Disenfranchised grief and the loss of an animal companion. In J. K. Doka (Ed.), *Disenfranchised grief: New directions, challenges, and strategies for practice* (pp. 251–264). Lexington, MA: Lexington Books.

Molnar, M. (1996). Of dogs and doggerel. *American Imago, 53*, 269–280.

Nieburg, H. A., & Fischer, A. (1982). *Pet loss: A thoughtful guide for adults and children.* New York: Harper & Row.

Planchon, L. A., & Templer, D. I. (1996). The correlates of grief after death of a pet. *Anthrozoos, 4*, 107–113.

Sharkin, B. S., & Bahrick, A. S. (1990). Pet loss: Implications for counselors. *Journal of Counseling and Development, 68*, 306–308.

Sharkin, B. S., & Knox, D. (2003). Pet loss: Issues and implications for the psychologist. *Professional Psychology: Research and Practice, 34*, 414–421.

Siegel, J. M. (1993). Companion animals: In sickness and in health. *Journal of Social Work, 49*, 157–167.

Singer, P. (1975). *Animal liberation.* New York: Harper Perennial.

Stevens, M. J., & Wedding, D. (2004). International psychology: An overview. In M. J. Stevens & D. Wedding (Eds.), *Handbook of international psychology* (pp. 1–21). New York: Brunner-Routledge.

Stewart, A. J., & McDermott, C. (2004). Gender in psychology. *Annual Review of Psychology, 55*, 519–544.

Stewart, C. S., Thrush, J. C., & Paulus, G. (1989). Disenfranchised bereavement and loss of a companion animal: Implications for a caring communities. In J. K. Doka (Ed.), *Disenfranchised grief: New directions, challenges, and strategies for practice* (pp. 251–264). Lexington, MA: Lexington Books.

Sue, D. W., Arredondo, P., & McDavis, R. J. (1992). Multicultural counseling competencies and standards: A call to the profession. *Journal of Counseling and Development, 70*, 477–486.

Sue, D. W., Bingham, R. P., Borche-Burke, L., & Vasquez, M. (1999). The diversification of psychology: A multicultural revolution. *American Psychologist, 54*, 1061–1069.

Voith, V. L. (1985). Attachment of people to companion animals. *Veterinary Clinics of North America: Small Animal Practice, 15*, 289–295.

Wester, S. R. (2008). Thinking complexly about men, gender role conflict, and counselling psychology. *The Counseling Psychologist, 36*, 462–468.

Winnicott, D. W. (1971). *Playing and reality.* Middlesex, England: Penguin Books.

Wrobel, T. A., & Dye, A. L. (2003). Grieving pet death: Normative, gender, and attachment issues. *Omega, 47*, 385–393.

Chapter 2
British Animal Behaviour Studies in the Twentieth Century: Some Interdisciplinary Perspectives

David A.H. Wilson

An understanding of our relationship with animals, and of the uncertain boundary between our dependence on them and our exploitation of them, demands an awareness of the historical extent of the purposes of our interaction. An examination of this past relationship provides a context for a better assessment of the present-day importance many of us place on animals as other beings who ultimately have independent interests and a discreet power over our own human behaviour: they have become agents who affect the quality of our own lives. Our study, knowledge and manipulation of animal behaviour lie at the centre of the human–animal relationship, as demonstrated by the variety of situations in which attempts have been made to acquire a better understanding of animal behaviour in order to secure human interests. From the standpoint of the historian, this variety demands much interdisciplinary analysis concentrating on the late-nineteenth and the twentieth centuries. In this chapter, some British examples will be discussed in relation to developments in the United States, where scientific studies of animal behaviour soon stole the lead from Britain at the beginning of the last century.

The interdisciplinary potential of the historical study of British comparative (animal) psychology and ethology straddles many aspects of the arts and sciences; and the same is true of studies of animal behaviour that have been undertaken on a less scientific basis. It is perhaps surprising to find that a relatively new and ostensibly narrow research area (the history of studies of animal behaviour) has links with so many centres of thought and activity beyond its immediate academic boundaries. The history of comparative psychology and other studies of animal behaviour (pure and applied) in Britain offers interdisciplinary links with institutional, professional, ethical, recreational, literary and military histories. We will identify some of these links, most of which continue to offer opportunities for research across disciplines and subject areas. In doing so, we may perhaps also be able to understand the extent to which our attitudes to non-human animals have altered since the dissemination of Darwinian evolutionary theory.

D.A.H. Wilson (✉)
School of Historical Studies, University of Leicester, Leicester, UK
e-mail: dw149@le.ac.uk

C. Blazina et al. (eds.), *The Psychology of the Human–Animal Bond*,
DOI 10.1007/978-1-4419-9761-6_2, © Springer Science+Business Media, LLC 2011

Some of the special themes discussed here were identified during the preparation of a doctoral dissertation on the historical development of comparative psychology in Britain since the late nineteenth century (Wilson, 1999). It soon became clear that comparative psychology could serve as a representative vehicle for an investigation of such interdisciplinary themes, many of which were also applicable to aspects of general science history; and that this investigation would be particularly dependent on an examination of a range of primary sources which revealed influences on the progress of the discipline itself. Because the development of comparative psychology as an academic specialism was significantly affected by certain pioneering figures, in order to illuminate these thematic areas it was necessary to locate and analyse personal and departmental papers in institutions and organizations whose staff had made a historic contribution to the subject and had influenced the environment in which it evolved. These sources, mainly within British universities' archives and the National Archives (formerly the Public Record Office), were subsequently able to throw light on associated areas, such as national and institutional support for science; the role of "markets" which encouraged professionalization; the efforts of women in the early twentieth century to establish a foothold in scientific research; experimental military applications of novel ideas (including a strange alliance between science and the performing arts, Wilson, 2001b); international cooperation both in research programmes and in theoretical debates (especially concerning learning theory); the emerging concept of ethical cost, and interest in the human–animal relationship; and the nature and effect on scientific activity of public opinion, pressure groups and the media.

New Contexts of Understanding

The scientific study of animal behaviour had first been made possible by the original theoretical frameworks of Darwin (1872) who proposed that the instincts, emotions and intelligence of non-human animals differed from those of man only in degree and not in kind. Darwin's evolutionary theories are popularly associated with the explanation of the development of physical characteristics in animals (human and non-human) reflecting the influence of heredity and the environment. During the nineteenth century, his demonstration of human kinship with the animal world through the apes provoked controversy. Assumptions about human uniqueness and the religious beliefs that humans were separate and entirely different from the rest of creation were brought into question. But Darwin's work was significant not just for its attempt to explain the evolution of those physical attributes in all animals that made them fit and able to compete and survive in their environments; he also suggested that behaviour had evolved, and that in this evolution there were again links between humans and other animals.

There soon followed, as a result, some pioneering experimental work in Britain by Douglas Spalding, John Lubbock, George Romanes, Conwy Lloyd Morgan and Leonard Hobhouse, and at the end of the nineteenth century it seemed as though there was a domestic tradition of comparative psychology in the making. This "anecdotal" phase predominated in Britain before more procedurally exact scientific enquiries shifted via Lloyd Morgan and Hobhouse to the United States of America, leaving a lull in Britain. The work that was carried out was described as anecdotal because it was not subject to the controls of laboratory method. However, it represented the first attempts to find behavioural links between human and non-human animals, to learn more of the effect on this behaviour of the relationship between heredity and the pressures of the environment, and even to show that animal behaviour could serve as examples for the development of human society. This was indeed pioneering work, and as a consequence we have become much more ready to attribute qualities of loyalty, affection and even altruism to non-human animals (see, for example, Hamilton, 1964). Over the years since the late nineteenth century, therefore, our developing knowledge of the behaviour of animals has led to an awareness of their interests and of the importance of our relationship with them. However, in the meantime, human self-interest has continued to pull in the other direction, and very often we restrict our generosity to our pets. A paradox lies in the fact that the more we know of animals, the more we can also exploit them for economic or medical reasons. Our relationship with them is, therefore, characterized by another Darwinian theory, that of competition and fitness for survival in species—a theory that leaves little room for morality or sympathy. That is why we continue to restrict most of our generosity to animals we are close to, such as pets, or, to a lesser extent, to threatened animals brought into our living rooms by those television documentaries that remind us of their interests.

Pioneers of Interpretation

The first British investigator to employ experimental techniques to investigate animal behaviour was Douglas Spalding, a Scottish slater who became interested in Darwinian implications of mental continuity between animals and man. He set out to examine the relationship between instinct and the environment as factors affecting the behaviour of newly born animals such as chicks and piglets. In a short series of experiments conducted in the early 1870s, he established the existence of inborn or instinctive behaviour. His experiments were not carried out in any laboratory, but his careful measures to cause temporary sensory deprivation in his subjects until several hours after birth provided convincing scientific evidence (Spalding, 1872, 1873). Like the later field-oriented ethologists, he believed it important to study animals in as natural conditions as possible in order to achieve reliable results. His own view had been that instinct and learning were closely linked, instinct guiding learning rather than suppressing it (Gray, 1967). He also developed materialist interpretations of human and animal behaviour, leading to the idea of "conscious automatism", when the organism interacts as if automatically with its environment, and when the mind does not direct the body: consciousness accompanies but does not cause behaviour. Such a materialistic psychology did not catch hold in England, but helped to prepare the ground for John Watson's behaviourism in the new century (Gray, 1968).

Darwin claimed that he relied especially on the opinions of another British investigator of the late nineteenth century, John Lubbock, politician and banker, whose analysis and explanation of insect societies, as in his *Ants, bees, and wasps* (1882), was set before the public so that lessons might be learned from insects about social organization, and so that the achievement of science in gleaning this information could be properly acknowledged (Fig. 2.1).[1] George Romanes also published accounts of animal behaviour that were often popular or anecdotal (G.J. Romanes, 1878, 1882, 1883, 1885; E.G. Romanes, 1896), but the rigour of his scientific work has lately been re-assessed, and Darwin had bequeathed much of his unpublished writing on animal behaviour to him, some of this material on instinct being incorporated into Romanes's *Mental Evolution in Animals* (1883) (Gottlieb, 1979, p. 149). From 1884, Lloyd Morgan engaged Romanes in a controversy centred on the possibility of a comparative science of psychology and the definition of instinct (Gray, 1963).

As one of T. H. Huxley's disciples, Lloyd Morgan was a strong advocate of an evolutionary approach in comparative psychology, and later in retirement set out a doctrine of the emergent evolution of consciousness (1923).[2] Of his many experiments, most have been described as informal studies of animals in natural surroundings outside the laboratory, but he recognized the limitations of anecdotes (Dewsbury, 1984, p. 315). He had stressed the need for the precise operational definition of terms and for the replication of experiments, and later asked: "Did one get out of the animal mind aught else than that which one put into it?" (1930, p. 248). He established some universal terminology that remains current, including "trial and error", "reinforcement" and "inhibition." Notwithstanding Spalding's contribution, he has been described as the real founder of experimental animal psychology (Thorpe, 1956), and his Canon, later to be excessively applied by the American Behaviourists, required the judicious application of a law of parsimony in experiment and observation: "In no case may we interpret an action as the outcome of the exercise of a higher psychical faculty, if it can be interpreted as the

---

[1] He was nevertheless "aware of the collectivist ideological uses of social insects", and "employed 'disinterested' experimentation to cast doubts upon the utopian depictions of co-operative, altruistic communities of ants and bees" (Clark, 1997).

[2] Lloyd Morgan's desk became a forum for most of those involved in psychological research with animals in Britain until the 1930s. All types of investigators as well as some foreign workers corresponded with him. New publications were exchanged and admired, and points of disagreement discussed. The following correspondence is preserved in the Bristol University History Collection (as referenced). Charles Sherrington wrote in 1901 in appreciation of his newly received copy of *Animal Behaviour* (DM 612); and much later both he (in 1923) and, via his wife, an infirm Henry Head (in 1929) expressed great interest in Lloyd Morgan's published studies of "emergent evolution" (DM 128/346 and DM 128/415). In 1913, Margaret Washburn referred to Lloyd Morgan's criticisms of her *The Animal Mind*, to her misgivings about Watsonian behaviourism and to her appreciation of Lloyd Morgan's *Instinct and Experience* (DM 128/290). Much further correspondence on each other's work took place between Lloyd Morgan and C. S. Myers, E. B. Poulton (Hope Professor of Zoology at Oxford), William McDougall, J. A. Thomson and others (DM 128/various numbers and DM 612). Lloyd Morgan remained at the centre of a network of correspondence on matters concerning animal behaviour long after he ceased his own experiments.

Fig. 2.1 A cartoon of 19 August 1882 satirizing John Lubbock and his work with insects. Reproduced with permission of Punch Ltd, www.punch.co.uk

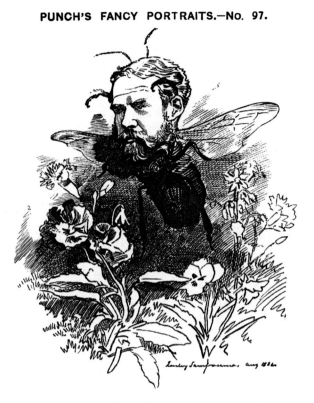

PUNCH'S FANCY PORTRAITS.—No. 97.

SIR JOHN LUBBOCK, M.P., F.R.S.

How doth the Banking Busy Bee
Improve his shining Hours
By studying on Bank Holidays
Strange Insects and Wild Flowers !

outcome of one which stands lower in the psychological scale" (Lloyd Morgan, 1894, p. 53). In other words, we should not offer elaborate explanations of animal behaviour or of the mental attributes of animals if simple ones are equally valid. Dewsbury (1984, p. 188) notes that the Canon has often been misinterpreted. It was not written in an effort to eliminate the attribution of consciousness to nonhuman animals but rather to counteract casual anthropomorphism in comparative psychology. Since its enunciation, continues Dewsbury, many scientists have acknowledged that rampant application of it can lead to a denial of the existence of complex processes where complex processes exist. Lloyd Morgan himself found this problem in Edward Thorndike's puzzle-box experiments with cats.

The experimental work described in Lloyd Morgan's *Habit and Instinct* (1896) illustrated his theory of imitation and also approached the problem of habit formation and learning in birds by "trial and error." His studies were an important contribution in the application of laboratory methods to the behaviour of higher vertebrates. This work was explained in the spring of 1896 in his Lowell Lectures at Harvard University. The lectures, and a further series at other places in the United States soon afterwards, have been credited with triggering the outburst of American work that followed (Warden, 1928). Linus Kline began similar work on the chick at Clark University in 1897, and Willard Small introduced the rat-maze there in 1899, but already by the autumn of 1896 Thorndike had begun his work on instinct and habit formation in the chick at Harvard. The strong influence of British theory, as evolved by this time, and the sudden American capture of the lead in the new work that resulted from it are especially represented in the pioneering experiments of Thorndike. Lloyd Morgan's lectures directly influenced Thorndike in his initiation of animal experimentation, and also led him to form his "connectionist" theory, which he later retained in the face of Behaviourism. He set out to develop the theories of Lloyd Morgan by subjecting them to systematic laboratory experiments that would yield quantitative results, and he thereby changed the standards for studies of animal behaviour (Boakes, 1984, p. 181; Mackenzie, 1977, pp. 68–80).

Just as Thorndike's work had been inspired by Lloyd Morgan, so its publication in 1898 encouraged a reciprocal phase of experimental activity in Britain carried out by the last investigator of this early series of influential British comparative psychologists. L. T. Hobhouse believed that the design of Thorndike's experiment did not permit the animals to display their full imitative and problem-solving capacities, or their capacity to learn quickly, since their state of agitation and natural histories had not been taken into account (Hobhouse, 1915, pp. 176–185, 236). He found it especially easy to criticize Thorndike's work because the latter's procedure and findings were so well recorded. His experimental design was better than Thorndike's (Weiskrantz, 1985), but his arrangement of methods, procedure, analysis and recording failed to match the new rigorous scientific standards of the American (Boakes, 1984, pp. 181–182), whose work is often considered to mark the beginning of controlled animal experimentation in psychology (Singer, 1981, p. 268). Hobhouse studied perceptual learning in cats, dogs and monkeys, and he incorporated his findings into an evolutionary theoretical structure that was both parsimonious and comprehensive (Mackenzie, 1977, p. 72); his analysis was, according to Gottlieb (1979, p. 162), "the most comprehensive theoretical exposition of the evolution of learning of its time." He identified what the later ethologists termed "releasing stimuli" as the mechanism of instinct. Organisms themselves were not passive or mechanical, but active, assertive, plastic and self-determining, while remaining subject to general requirements of homeostasis. Hobhouse accepted perceptual (rather than merely imitative) learning in animals, which Thorndike's "law of effect" had rejected; and he also identified the principle of stimulus generalization and learning sets (Hearnshaw, 1966). He presented an extraordinary variety of problems to a wide range of animals, including an otter and an elephant, and influenced both Robert Yerkes (an American who untypically developed his investigations outside mainstream behaviourism) and the Gestalt psychologist Wolfgang Koehler in the creation of discrimination apparatus and tasks for chimpanzees (Hearnshaw, 1964, p. 103). Much of the material in *Mind in Evolution* (1901) touched on issues that would later be widely considered in the study of animal behaviour, such as the

possible purposive nature of animal activity as well as the animal's ability to experience (later Gestalt-type) perceptual relationships (Boakes, 1984, pp. 182–184).
Dewsbury notes of him: "Hobhouse proposed that apes and monkeys have a near-
human capacity for mastering concrete perceptual relationships", which he called
"practical judgment"; and he proposed that "the capacity for reasoning can be seen
even in Thorndike's own data—as in the sudden improvements. . . in the learning
curves of individual animals". He also originated the tasks of box-stacking and
raking-in of food and other objects with sticks and ropes (Dewsbury, 1984, p. 303).

In common with other students of animal behaviour in Britain at the turn of
the century, Hobhouse supplemented his book-writing with articles in the popular press. He contributed a series called "The diversions of a psychologist" to *The
Pilot* in which, apart from frequent references to his *Mind in Evolution*, he warns
of the unreliability of anecdotal evidence but describes experiments that readers can
try for themselves (1902). In these articles, Hobhouse analyses his own work and
that of Thorndike, and refers to his studies in learning and imitation carried out
at home with his cat and dog, and to his comparison of different species' abilities
through work with circus and zoo animals such as elephant, rhesus monkey and
chimpanzee, by arrangement with Messrs Jennison, proprietors of the Belle Vue
Gardens in Manchester. Although Hobhouse's short-lived experimental work represented the most highly developed phase of British comparative psychology and
inspired several later foreign workers, his influence in Britain had no material effect,
and he was not remembered for his animal work once the First World War had got
under way and he had turned to sociology at the London School of Economics.

A Change in Direction, and the Role of "Markets"

In spite of this British activity, very little experimental comparative psychology survived in Britain immediately beyond the turn of the century (Wilson, 2001a). The
lead was then lost to the United States where, following earlier British influence
largely through Lloyd Morgan, new, procedurally precise, laboratory-based experimental investigations began with Edward Thorndike, Willard Small, John Watson
and others, but soon led to a neglect of the role of evolutionary theories in favour
of the experimental study of short-term, observable learning behaviour, mainly in
the rat and under various artificial environmental conditions. Thorndike began to
encourage the belief that, in the words of Jenkins (1979, p. 183), "an intensive
experimental analysis of the effects of reward and punishment in a few species could
yield the laws for a general psychology of learning. In this way he contributed to the
virtual disappearance for many years of the evolutionary comparative framework."
O'Donnell (1985, p. 165) notes that "the need to find an experimental basis for an
educational psychology underwritten by the genetic viewpoint led paradoxically to
an abandonment of that viewpoint." In this way, the expected influence of individuals' inherited characteristics (their "nature") on learning behaviour was supplanted
by a belief in the exclusive role of external environmental influences: learning was
attributed only to the effect of experience, which could be controlled and quantified,

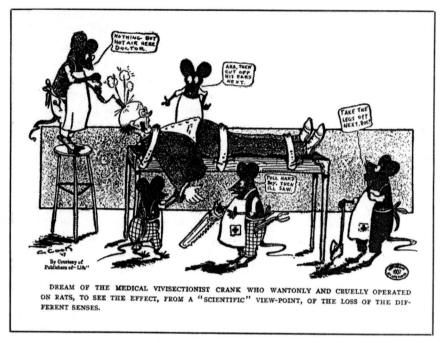

Fig. 2.2 A cartoon attributed to *Life*, aimed at the work of John Watson and published in the *Journal of Zoophily*, 1907, 16 (6), 65. The author has endeavoured to trace the copyright holder of this cartoon. If he has unwittingly infringed copyright, please contact him

and "nurture" eclipsed "nature." The experimental study of instinct became unfashionable, and the discursive approach of the earlier British anecdotalists was frowned upon as the American workers set about the task of creating a hard, objective science free of those nineteenth-century embellishments so characteristic also of much general Victorian culture (Fig. 2.2).[3]

It was not long before American development of animal psychology within the laboratory, especially under Watson and then B. F. Skinner, resulted in a new movement, Behaviourism, which set out to explain all human and animal activity as learned and exclusively dependent on environmental influences, being, therefore, controllable and predictable. Although this materialistic interpretation of behaviour had no time for subjectivity, intuition, instinct or spiritual feeling, it acquired for itself, ironically, almost religious status, and perhaps it was able to make headway because new American society was so cosmopolitan and was not hidebound with innate conservative outlooks. It is perhaps less significant that comparative psychology failed to develop in Britain than that it succeeded in developing in the

---

[3]Rollin (1989, pp. 67–68) observes: "One can indeed find elements of this reductionistic, 'no frills' philosophy throughout European culture. By the end of the nineteenth century, art, architecture, design, music, and literature had become extremely extravagant. . ... Much early twentieth-century culture can be seen as an attempt to eliminate or trim away that excess."

United States, where the new science was employed to serve objectivist theories favoured by what was essentially a new, cosmopolitan and more materialistic society willing to consider scientific contributions to social development and control, as within establishment educational provision or in child-rearing. Meanwhile Pavlov's conditioning work with his dogs continued after the Russian Revolution, when he was accepted as someone whose findings might fit well with contemporary political ideology concerning the education, control and "shaping" of another new and even more materialistic society. In America and Russia new markets for experimental psychology therefore grew rapidly in the first decades of the last century, but not in Britain, which was less open to such bold new social applications of scientific theory.

Not much happened in Britain until after the Second World War, but in the meantime, among limited numbers of laboratory workers in animal psychology, the key part in keeping a British grasp on the subject was played by women, including E. M. Smith (who later married Frederic Bartlett, first Professor of Experimental Psychology at Cambridge) at the Cambridge Psychological Laboratory, and Victoria Hazlitt, on the staff of Beatrice Edgell at Bedford College for Women (Valentine, 2006). A reason for this is suggested in Wilson (2003), where it is proposed that because in Britain at the time there was a preponderance of female workers in experimental animal psychology, this novel activity might have been regarded by them as a route into the scientific world from which women had been excluded.

As for the original, overall loss of lead by Britain, experimental work in comparative psychology came to depend on markets such as the educational establishment in the United States (Danziger, 1987; Wilson, 2002b), but no market appeared in Britain until the time of the Second World War. Moreover, other nations like France, Germany and the United States were more generally inclined than Britain to support scientific research and application.[4] The only earlier attempt scientifically to apply understanding of animal behaviour consisted of the efforts of the Admiralty's Board of Invention and Research to train sea lions and gulls to detect submarines, as a desperate, top-secret measure to counter the U-boat threat in 1916 and 1917 (Allen, 1917; Wilson, 2001b, 2006). This was not an encouraging experience for the official authorities, resulting in failure, and did nothing to convince the armed services that civilian science of this kind was indispensable to them. In any case, a marine biologist and music-hall trainer were in charge of the sea lion programme, not a psychologist; and advice on the use of gulls was entrusted to a naturalist. As far as can be established, no British comparative psychologist was consulted, although at the same time it was thought appropriate to invite an American naval surgeon to attend some of the trials, after the United States had entered the war in April 1917 and established a naval headquarters in Britain.[5]

---

[4]See, for example, "Report by Professor Sir Ernest Rutherford FRS and Commander Cyprian Bridge RN, on Visit to the USA in company with French Scientific Mission, May 19th to July 9th, 1917." BIR 28208/17. Public Record Office ADM 293/10.

[5]The Admiralty's use a little later of Cambridge University staff for hydrophone personnel selection and training, staff who were themselves responsible for overseeing animal work in

Pure and Applied Research After the Second World War

Soon after the close of hostilities in the Second World War, there was a sudden and spectacular change in the way scientific studies of animal behaviour were undertaken in Britain. A recognition of the importance of international links and cooperation began to emerge. The Dutch ethologist Nikolaas Tinbergen had written to the British ornithologist David Lack in 1940: "There are so few really serious students of animal behaviour and yet there is so much to do. When the war is over, it will be highly necessary to reconstruct international cooperation in our science as soon as possible" (Tinbergen, 1940). Of course, having taken up a lectureship at Oxford in 1949, Tinbergen later shared the Nobel Prize with Konrad Lorenz and Karl von Frisch in 1973, so illustrating the international status of the subject by then. The thoroughgoing establishment of ethology in Britain after the war was based on the earlier work of E. S. Russell and Julian Huxley, but was then greatly assisted by W. H. Thorpe as well as by Tinbergen's arrival in Oxford. Field-oriented ethology came to represent the zoological study of animal behaviour both for its own sake and as a possible means of interpreting human behaviour, while laboratory-based, often invasive, animal psychology began to serve rather more as an applied science (or even technique) assisting related, primary research programmes in pharmacology, psychiatry and agriculture: these represented the new markets which had so far been lacking. For example, Hans Eysenck at the Maudsley Hospital used strains of rats developed for their differing emotionality to serve as human models in his psychiatric research (Gwynne Jones, 1969), while in 1946 Glaxo had sponsored Michael Chance's work at Birmingham University on the effects of drugs on rodent behaviour. British laboratories after the Second World War were used as much for applied animal psychology as for that American-style comparative psychology which had never, in any case, been fully accepted as an adequate substitute in Britain for evolution-based research.

The relationship between ethology and animal psychology was sometimes competitive and difficult, especially concerning disagreements over the validity of research methodologies, but a reconciliation took place as some, like Thorpe and Tinbergen, began to combine field and laboratory-based research. Cambridge University's Sub-Department of Animal Behaviour, established at Madingley in 1950, encouraged this. After the war, certain key figures of the academic establishment, whose interests dictated the nature of research programmes, had changed. For example, the highly influential Frederic Bartlett had not shared those interests of his wife as mentioned above, and did little to encourage animal psychology at Cambridge before the war. Then Oliver Zangwill took over in 1952 and transformed research priorities so that they included much more experimental animal work.

---

the Cambridge Psychological Laboratory, demonstrates that a sufficient network existed for the employment of animal psychologists, had that been preferred. But the application of psychological expertise did not extend into this area, and in another, concerned with the identification, acceptance and treatment of what later came to be known as "shell shock", the psychologists' analysis was resisted.

The war itself had inevitably encouraged applied science, and studies of animal behaviour provided both economic and military advantages in such areas as the development of pest control and camouflage. Opportunities were taken much more seriously then than they had been at the time of the First World War. In this way, Solly Zuckerman (1988, pp. 150–153) was asked from 1948 to 1956 to study the capacity of dogs to be trained reliably to detect buried explosives in non-metallic casings, as they did buried bones, and his findings were found to be of use much later, in the aftermath of the Falklands War in the 1980s. During these post-war developments, new societies appeared, accompanied by new journals: the Experimental Psychology Society (EPS) and the Association for the Study of Animal Behaviour (ASAB, founded just before the war as an institute). These soon largely replaced the limited academic involvement in animal behaviour of the British Psychological Society (BPS). There was growing collaboration among psychologists, ethologists, zoologists, physiologists and neuroendocrinologists, and some came to think that psychology was becoming entirely dependent on neurophysiology, as others later wondered whether it was not mortally threatened by sociobiology. In the 1960s, British behaviour genetics contributed to forthcoming sociobiological theories and discussions of biological altruism (Hamilton, 1964), with the ironic consequence that in a period of highly sophisticated, objective and complex scientific analysis, non-scientific philosophical commentary on psychological interests and the old questions about the moral basis of the human–animal relationship began to reappear.

The Emerging Ethical Dimension

The expansion in British higher education in the 1960s following the Robbins Report (1963) was an encouragement for all aspects of behaviour study and psychology.[6] From the 1950s, public interest in animal behaviour had also grown, assisted by a range of popular or explanatory works as from Tinbergen and Desmond Morris, and also from P. L. Broadhurst (1963), who at the time foresaw a point in the future when whole crops might be harvested by ape labour and when industry might employ pigeon pilots and chimpanzee engine-drivers.[7] But expanding television coverage, notably through the work of David Attenborough, led to better public understanding of the lives and interests of animals in their natural environment. This resulted in greater respect and sympathy for their prospects in the threatening

---

[6]L. C. Robbins (later Baron Robbins of Clare Market) was Chairman of the Committee on Higher Education (1961–1964), which was partly responsible for the major expansion and reforms of British university education in the 1960s.

[7]Meanwhile, in the United States, attempts had been made during the Second World War to train pigeons to guide missiles: "The pigeon—an organism—is essentially an extremely reliable instrument, rugged in construction, simple and economical to obtain, and easily conditioned to be entirely predictable in behaviour [and which could] be made into a machine, from all practical points of view" (B.F. Skinner cited by Capshew, 1993, pp. 850–851).

conditions of the modern world, and at the same time contributed to the growing concern about the human–animal relationship.

The 1970s saw the re-establishment of the role of evolution in the interpretation of behaviour by extending and modifying Darwin's theories, making the gene, rather than the individual organism, the unit of evolution in studies of social behaviour. The renewed evolutionary emphasis of animal behaviour studies of the 1970s that coincided with a revival of interests in the moral aspects of the human–animal relationship was set against the background of the environmental ethics of the 1960s and 1970s in Westernized societies, and the tendency to question the establishment and conservative viewpoints. It came to be argued that if an animal were psychologically like us, there might be more scientific reason to experiment, but less moral justification to do so (Fox, 1981). It was, therefore, not possible to avoid anthropomorphism altogether, and some aspects of it were recognized as acceptable. Ethical considerations arose as a consequence of the acceptance of the legitimacy of comparability, a consequence with, therefore, a scientific basis rather than one resulting only from philosophical arguments, or from emotive and subjective traditions of common-sense morality (Wilson, 2002a). As British public interest in these matters, insofar as they threatened psychological work, grew for the first time (Wilson, 2004), the specialist societies undertook some overt self-regulation.[8] Psychologists had, in fact, come to work within the spirit of the 1876 Cruelty to Animals Act, although it was intended to regulate vivisection and not experimentation, and was therefore often inappropriate for animal psychology.

Lloyd Morgan had referred sympathetically to the cat "victims" of "utter hunger" of Thorndike's [too] "strained and straitened" puzzle-box experiments (1900, pp. 147 and 151). Nevertheless, concern and discussion about experimental psychology and the treatment of its animals had received little attention before the 1970s: there had been no public involvement, because the limited experimental psychological experimentation with animals was not readily associated with the long-standing physiological vivisection that attracted public concern. But after the Second World War, as the Universities Federation for Animal Welfare decided to begin to turn its attention to animals and experimentation, some links with psychological work were created for it through Frederic Bartlett at Cambridge and through the ASAB (Hume, 1959). Julian Huxley and W. H. Thorpe also developed a special interest in the humane treatment of farm animals, when knowledge of the behaviour of animals kept in artificial environments could most readily be applied by people like them (Thorpe, 1927–1984). In the 1970s, experimental animal psychology became a new, special and, perhaps, a rather soft target for those members of the public, philosophers and indeed psychologists (especially, it turned out, clinical psychologists) who espoused the newly expressed concepts of animal rights. Heated correspondence began in the *Bulletin of the British Psychological Society* from late 1975. The BPS set up a working party in 1977 to investigate the nature of animal work in

---

[8]This involved the issue of guidelines for the use of animals in research to members and correspondents of the ASAB (1981 and 1986), BPS (1985) and EPS (1986).

psychology in Britain, and a Psychobiological Section was soon established to represent the interests of animal researchers. Not long after, the controlling legislation was revised in the form of the Animals (Scientific Procedures) Act of 1986, but the tensions caused by some aspects of animal research both within psychology and in its public relations have not disappeared.

The Scientific Milieu and Beyond

An examination of the history of animal behaviour studies in Britain, whether those based in the field, the laboratory or another professional environment, provides fertile ground for research into associated areas. A general approach to the subject might at first attempt to produce an "internal" account of its academic development as a new subject that led, in due course, to the creation of university departments and the inauguration of specialist societies and journals; then, secondly, one might study the development of its applied form within society, resulting much later in professional recognition and consultation,[9] as it responded to newly available markets. Such investigations would soon reveal a historic lack of government and institutional support (representing "external" influences), not just for this evolving discipline, but also for those other, longer-established ones which were competing for funds at the same time, such as physics and biology. The evolution of the modern study of comparative psychology therefore invites a linked assessment of general twentieth-century science policy in Britain (as also related to the state of the nation's social traditions and contemporary outlooks), right up to the publication of the Robbins Report on British higher education provision in 1963.

Endeavour in this scientific area became internationalized and more cooperative after the Second World War, especially in the study of ethology within Western societies. Although experimental psychology had succeeded in shaking itself free from association with philosophy and philosophers at the end of the nineteenth century (in order to strengthen its claim to be a new and independent science), ironically in Britain, philosophical and ethical debates (now about principles, methods and procedures) began to take the stage once more in the 1970s, in paradoxical contrast with the highly objective methods which laboratory psychology was using routinely by that time; these debates were very soon accompanied by concerted responses from pressure groups. There is a wide field of research connected with the history and tactics of these groups, their objectives, the basis of their concerns, their programmes of action and the nature of their publications and communications with the public (e.g., Ryder, 2000).

Of course, studies of animal behaviour have not been confined to the academic environment. An earlier modern example of the role of pressure groups and the

---

[9]For example, following pressure from its membership, a leading ethologist, Patrick Bateson, was commissioned by the British landowning conservation charity, the National Trust, to assess the suffering occasioned by hunting stags with hounds on its land, so that Trust policy could be informed and decided upon (Bateson, 1997).

media in focussing and sustaining attention on the application and exploitation of knowledge of animal behaviour for the purposes of commercial entertainment is represented by the performing animals controversy in Britain, which came to a head in the early 1920s with the appointment of a parliamentary Select Committee of inquiry. Perhaps it was inevitable that the scale of public and press interest guaranteed the interest of politicians, and soon the trade began to organize its defences through its professional associations and specialist journals. The controversy concerned the use of animals in the circus, fairground, music hall or vaudeville, and, later, in film. The Select Committee's brief was "to inquire into the conditions under which performing animals are trained and exhibited, and to consider whether legislation is desirable to prohibit or regulate such training and exhibition, and, if so, what lines such legislation should follow" (United Kingdom Parliament, 1921). The findings of the Select Committee were published as reports, proceedings and extensive minutes of evidence (United Kingdom Parliament, 1921 and 1922), and were the basis of the Performing Animals (Regulation) Act, passed in 1925. An examination of the controversy lends itself to an interdisciplinary analysis also of the associated history of specialist pressure groups, the press, trade organizations and politics (Wilson, 2008, 2009a) (Fig. 2.3). During the arguments around this issue

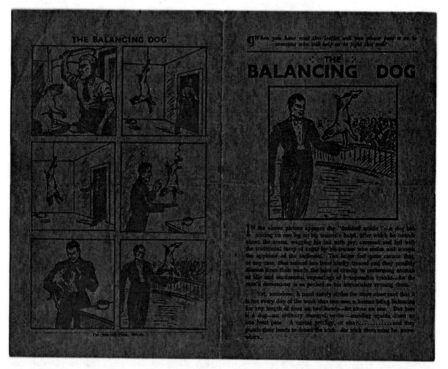

Fig. 2.3 Part of a pamphlet circulated in the 1930s by the Performing Animals' Defence League, showing the alleged methods of a trainer and his assistant. © National Fairground Archive, University of Sheffield Library

after the First World War, there was even evidence of the use of tactical racial prejudice. British trainers told the Select Committee that any previous shortcomings in the treatment of performing animals were attributable to the methods of German trainers, referred to as the "alien enemy" and now boycotted by the Variety Artistes' Federation so that they could not appear in Britain in the early 1920s. Nevertheless, before the war they had been praised as the most effective trainers (Wilson, 2009b).

A further effect of the performing animals controversy was to draw attention to a related problem which thereafter received growing attention: the close confinement of animals in unnatural conditions. Concern about this aspect of the human treatment of non-human animals entered debates about the cruelty of intensive "factory farming" and of the standards of many zoos and laboratories, and it remains a predominant argument of critics (Fig. 2.4). Such concerns can be placed in wider discussions about agricultural production and policies, the role of zoos in education and species preservation, and the use of animals for scientific research. For example, as secretary of the Zoological Society of London from 1935, Julian Huxley had become concerned by the cramped conditions and boredom of the animals at the London Zoo, but after the Second World War, close confinement was systematically extended to agricultural processes so that food production could be industrialized. By 1977, 45 million birds were kept in battery cages. In a later review of the

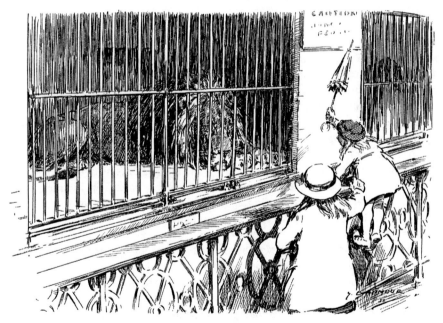

Elder Sister. "Don't frighten the poor animal. It isn't fair."

Fig. 2.4 A cartoon of 9 May 1923, when the confinement of animals and the symbolism of the British lion had come under public scrutiny as a result of the performing animals controversy. Reproduced with permission of Punch Ltd, www.punch.co.uk

publication of the Royal Society for the Prevention of Cruelty to Animals symposium on animal rights (Patterson & Ryder, 1979), the ethologist William Thorpe complained:

> I am... convinced of the cruelty of "factory farming". Sir Julian Huxley was right in saying when he and others wrote to *The Times* concerning the new and disgracefully feeble "Codes of Practice", issued in 1968 by the then Minister of Agriculture, "It is obvious to us that behavioural distress to animals has been completely ignored. Yet it is the frustration of activities natural to the animal which may well be the worst form of cruelty" (Thorpe, 1927–1984).

Knowledge and Responsibility

Throughout the history of the developments in comparative psychology, ethology and applied studies of animal behaviour in Britain since the late nineteenth century, other special, related areas for research have therefore suggested themselves. These include the role of women in furthering their academic standing by sustaining such subjects in times of uncertainty at the beginning of the twentieth century; the comparative development of learning theory and educational policies at home and abroad; the opportunities presented by special potential markets like defence research in times of national emergency; and the significance of the use made by other disciplines of behavioural work to serve their own primary purposes, as in the pharmaceutical industry and in agriculture. Then there is the opportunity to study the roles of politicians and of various types of media in educating and focussing public interest and opinion on controversial and emotive aspects, both of scientific activity and the commercial exploitation of the understanding of animal behaviour. This leads to consideration of ethical questions in the human–animal relationship, enhanced by our improved knowledge of animals and their behaviour, knowledge which is only quite recent.

Until well into the Industrial Revolution, the natural environment was often regarded as an inconvenience to be feared, challenged and overcome, and within that environment the status of animals was closely related to the degree to which they could be exploited. Early improvements in communications through road and rail ushered in a different view of a now-less-threatening natural environment, and, alongside romantic reactions to industrialization, it became subject to changing views in nineteenth-century society. This confident society, relatively secure and comfortable in its technological achievement, could now afford to reflect on its impact on nature and animals as well as on itself. The parallel interest in educational and moral improvement gave rise to social reforms and also to new organizations concerned with animal welfare and, shortly afterwards, with conservation. Many of these organizations were supported by the emergent middle classes of the nineteenth century, and on their letterheads they gave their activities social respectability by listing aristocrats as patrons—today, celebrities often fulfil this role. This change of outlook in the nineteenth century was characteristic, mainly, of the Western world, and took place as religious and doctrinal influences continued to be questioned as a result of the effects of the Enlightenment of the previous century. But we must remember that changes in human–animal relationships have varied around the world according to geographical and cultural contexts, and continue also to be affected by economic conditions. Human poverty relegates animal interests, but where there is wealth, greed and human self-indulgence, these interests can also be set back.

For less than 150 years, and especially as global communications have developed, the size of Earth has effectively reduced, and concern for the interests of the pet has in the meantime extended—at least in enlightened nations—to those of all animals, as experience of our relationship with them has become more easily shared. In that time, we have finally come to confront and articulate the problems of our exploitation of animals of every kind, of the extent of our attachment to them, of our effect on their well-being, and of the loss (literal and moral) that would result from continued neglect of their separate interests as cohabiters of our world. In promoting these ideas, the animal rights movement has not hesitated to draw analogies between the situation of, for example, laboratory animals and the inhumane and tyrannical treatment of large numbers of helpless human victims in the concentration camps, or between the treatment of the vulnerable animal and the vulnerability of the child or the mentally impaired. The "might is right" assumption and the biblical assertion of human dominion have also come under increasing scrutiny as the public is asked to consider, as in the light of our policies concerning laboratory animals, its expectations in the event (not now so incredible) of links with a more powerful and equally exploitative alien civilization.

An understanding of the psychology of the human–animal bond can only be enhanced by a better understanding of animal behaviour. Some of the historic attempts to achieve this understanding have been dealt with here, although the purposes of such understanding have been various, at first with limited involvement of society at large. However, within the past 50 years, an enthusiastic general public has been brought into this area of interest, especially through the televised natural history documentary. Public attitudes to animals and the natural environment have changed dramatically in line with the communications revolution of the twentieth century. Because most of us now feel confident, rightly or wrongly, that we can interpret behaviour as a result of our own experience and imagination (psychology and behaviour analysis are less forbidding to the lay person than, say, physics or chemistry), and because we remain in close personal contact at least with domesticated animals, interest in the human–animal bond is increasing apace. That is a good thing and it may even be crucial to our human destiny. Nature in the present century is more vulnerable than ever, and because we are a part of nature we agree that we share that vulnerability, especially if we accept the idea that the Earth survives as a kind of organism in its own right (Lovelock, 1979). Our relationship with animals is the most visible and emotive example of that vulnerability.

References

Allen, E. J. (1917). *Report upon experiments on the hearing powers of sea-lions under water, and on the possibility of training these animals as submarine trackers*. B.I.R. 30051/17. London: Admiralty Board of Invention and Research. Public Record Office ADM 293/5, 450–69.

Bateson, P. P. G. (1997). *The behavioural and physiological effects of culling red deer*. London: Council of the National Trust.

Boakes, R. A. (1984). *From Darwin to behaviourism: Psychology and the minds of animals*. Cambridge: Cambridge University Press.

Broadhurst, P. L. (1963). *The science of animal behaviour*. Harmondsworth: Pelican Books.

Capshew, J. H. (1993). Engineering behaviour: Project Pigeon, World War II, and the conditioning of B.F. Skinner. *Technology and Culture, 34*, 835–857.

Clark, J. F. M. (1997). 'The ants were duly visited': Making sense of John Lubbock, scientific naturalism and the senses of social insects. *British Journal for the History of Science, 30*, 151–176.

Danziger, K. (1987). Social context and investigative practice in early twentieth-century psychology. In M. G. Ash & W. R. Woodward (Eds.), *Psychology in twentieth-century thought and society*. Cambridge: Cambridge University Press.

Darwin, C. R. (1872). *The expression of the emotions in man and animals*. London: John Murray.

Dewsbury, D. A. (1984). *Comparative psychology in the twentieth century*. Stroudsburg: Hutchinson Ross.

Fox, M. W. (1981). Experimental psychology, animal rights, welfare and ethics. *Psychopharmacology Bulletin, 17*, 80–84.

Gottlieb, G. (1979). Comparative psychology and ethology. In E. Hearst (Ed.), *The first century of experimental psychology*. Hillsdale, IN: Lawrence Erlbaum.

Gray, P. H. (1963). The Morgan–Romanes controversy: A contradiction in the history of comparative psychology. *Proceedings of the Montana Academy of Sciences, 23*, 225–230.

Gray, P. H. (1967). Spalding and his influence on research in developmental behaviour. *Journal of the History of the Behavioral Sciences, 3*, 168–179.

Gray, P. H. (1968). Prerequisite to an analysis of behaviorism: The conscious automaton theory from Spalding to William James. *Journal of the History of the Behavioral Sciences, 4*, 365–376.

Gwynne Jones, H. (1969). Clinical psychology. *Supplement to the Bulletin of the British Psychological Society, 22*, 21–23.

Hamilton, W. D. (1964). The genetical evolution of social behaviour, I, II. *Journal of Theoretical Biology, 7*, 1–52.

Hearnshaw, L. S. (1964). *A short history of British psychology 1840–1940*. London: Methuen.

Hearnshaw, L. S. (1966, 5 May). *The comparative psychology of mental development* (L. T. Hobhouse Memorial Trust Lecture no. 36). London: Bedford College, University of London.

Hobhouse, L. T. (1902). Articles under the title "The diversions of a psychologist". *The Pilot: a weekly review of politics, literature, and learning, 5*.

Hobhouse, L. T. (1915). *Mind in evolution* (2nd Ed.). London: Macmillan.

Hume, C. W. (1959). In praise of anthropomorphism. *The UFAW Courier, 1*, 1–13.

Jenkins, H. M. (1979). Animal learning and behavior theory. In E. Hearst (Ed.), *The first century of experimental psychology*. Hillsdale, IN: Lawrence Erlbaum.

Lloyd Morgan, C. (1894). *Introduction to comparative psychology*. London: Scott.

Lloyd Morgan, C. (1896). *Habit and instinct*. London: Arnold.

Lloyd Morgan, C. (1900). *Animal behaviour*. London: Arnold.

Lloyd Morgan, C. (1923). *Emergent evolution*. London: Williams and Norgate.

Lloyd Morgan, C. (1930). *The animal mind*. London: Arnold.

Lovelock, J. (1979). *Gaia: A new look at life on Earth*. Oxford: Oxford University Press.

Lubbock, J. A. (1882). *Ants, bees, and wasps*. New York: Appleton.

Mackenzie, B. D. (1977). *Behaviourism and the limits of scientific method*. London: Routledge and Kegan Paul.

O'Donnell, J. M. (1985). *The origins of behaviorism: American psychology, 1870–1920*. New York: New York University Press.

Patterson, D. and Ryder, R. D. (Eds.) (1979). *Animals' rights – a symposium*. Fontwell: Centaur.

Robbins, L. C. (1963). (chairman) *Report of the Committee on Higher Education*. Cmnd 2154. London: HMSO.

Rollin, B. E. (1989). *The unheeded cry: Animal consciousness, animal pain and science.* Oxford: Oxford University Press.

Romanes, G. J. (1878). *Evening discourse delivered before the British Association, Dublin.* London: Taylor and Francis.

Romanes, G. J. (1882). *Animal intelligence.* London: Kegan Paul, Trench.

Romanes, G. J. (1883). *Mental evolution in animals.* London: Kegan Paul, Trench.

Romanes, G. J. (1885). *Jelly-fish, star-fish and sea-urchins. Being a research on primitive nervous systems.* London: Kegan Paul, Trench.

Romanes, E. G. (1896). *The life and letters of George John Romanes.* London: Longmans, Green.

Ryder, R. D. (2000). *Animal revolution: Changing attitudes towards speciesism.* Oxford: Berg.

Singer, B. (1981). History of animal behaviour. In D. MacFarland (Ed.), *Oxford companion to animal behaviour.* Oxford: Oxford University Press.

Spalding, D. A. (1872). On instinct. *Nature, 6*(154), 485–486.

Spalding, D. A. (1873). Instinct; with original observations on young animals. *Macmillan's Magazine, 27,* 282–293.

Thorpe, W. H. (1927-1984). William Homan Thorpe: Papers. Add. MS 8784/M13. Cambridge: Cambridge University Library Department of Manuscripts and University Archives.

Thorpe, W. H. (1956). Some implications of the study of animal behaviour. *The Advancement of Science, 13,* 42–55.

Tinbergen, N. (1940). Correspondence with D. Lack, 26 February 1940. In the David Lack Papers, Edward Grey Institute, Oxford, item 155. Cited by Durant, J.R. in The making of ethology: the Association for the Study of Animal Behaviour, 1936 to 1986. *Animal Behaviour* 1986, *34,* 1601–1616.

United Kingdom Parliament. (1921). *Parliamentary Debates (Commons),* 144, column 1243. London: HMSO.

United Kingdom Parliament. (1921 and 1922). *Report from the select committee on performing animals, together with the proceedings of the committee and minutes of evidence.* London: HMSO.

Valentine, E. R. (2006). *Beatrice Edgell: Pioneer woman psychologist.* New York: Nova.

Warden, C. J. (1928). The development of modern comparative psychology. *Quarterly Review of Biology, 3,* 486–522.

Weiskrantz, L. (1985). Categorization, cleverness and consciousness. *Philosophical Transactions of The Royal Society, B, 308,* 3–19.

Wilson, D. A. H. (1999). *Encouragements and constraints in the development of experimental animal behaviour studies in Great Britain since the late nineteenth century.* Unpublished Ph.D. thesis, University of Leicester, Leicester, England.

Wilson, D. A. H. (2001a). A 'precipitous dégringolade'? The uncertain progress of British comparative psychology in the twentieth century. In G. C. Bunn, A. D. Lovie, & G. D. Richards (Eds.), *Psychology in Britain: Historical essays and personal reflections.* Leicester: British Psychological Society, in association with the Science Museum, London.

Wilson, D. A. H. (2001b). Sea lions, greasepaint and the U-boat threat: Admiralty scientists turn to the music hall in 1916. *Notes and Records of The Royal Society, 55,* 425–455.

Wilson, D. A. H. (2002a). Animal psychology and ethology in Britain and the emergence of professional concern for the concept of ethical cost. *Studies in History and Philosophy of Biological and Biomedical Sciences, 33,* 235–261.

Wilson, D. A. H. (2002b). Experimental animal behaviour studies: The loss of initiative in Britain 100 years ago. *History of Science, 40,* 291–320.

Wilson, D. A. H. (2003). British female academics and comparative psychology: Attempts to establish a research niche in the early twentieth century. *History of Psychology, 6,* 89–109.

Wilson, D. A. H. (2004). The public relations of experimental animal psychology in Britain in the 1970s. *Contemporary British History, 18,* 27–46.

Wilson, D. A. H. (2006). Avian anti-submarine warfare proposals in Britain, 1915-18: The Admiralty and Thomas Mills. *International Journal of Naval History, 5,* 1–25.

Wilson, D. A. H. (2008). Politics, press and the performing animals controversy in early twentieth-century Britain. *Anthrozoös, 21*, 317–337.

Wilson, D. A. H. (2009a). 'Crank legislators', 'faddists' and professionals' defence of animal performance in 1920s Britain. *Early Popular Visual Culture, 7*, 83–101.

Wilson, D. A. H. (2009b). Racial prejudice and the performing animals controversy in early twentieth-century Britain. *Society and Animals. Journal of Human-Animal Studies, 17*, 149–165.

Zuckerman, S. (1988). *Monkeys, men and missiles. An autobiography 1946-1988*. London: Collins.

Chapter 3
The History of Animal Ethics in Western Culture

Rod Preece

This chapter is intended as an overview of the major trends of the development of Western attitudes to animals from early biblical times to the present. Although Western culture, in its subservience to commercial, industrial and technological innovation, has scarcely been what is commonly called "at one with nature," a concern with the status of our fellow animal relatives has never been entirely absent from Western consciousness. The history of animal ethics in Western culture is not, however, a story of a consistent ethic in any one era developing into a different ethic in a succeeding era. Rather, it is the evolution of an unresolved debate in which adversaries offer alternative conceptions of the human–animal relationship and alternative conceptions of our obligation to our fellow animals.

Biblical Origins and Animal Souls

The symbolic beginning of the debate may be traced to the Book of Genesis, a parable of the origins and early condition of humanity. In the King James version of the Bible, God allowed humans as their food: "every herb bearing seed and every tree, in which is the fruit of a tree yielding seed" (Genesis 1: 29). Their diet was to be vegetables and fruit. All other animals were likewise prescribed a vegan diet. Perhaps somewhat surprisingly, the notion of humans and other animals as uniformly vegetarian in origin is common throughout cultural history. It is present, for example, in the myths of the Cheyenne and of the Makritare of the Orinoco. Following the vegan beginning in the Bible, the deity relented from the restricted diet originally imposed and permitted Noah and his successors the corpses of animals as food: "Every moving thing that liveth shall be meat for you...But the flesh with the life thereof... shall ye not eat" (Genesis 9: 3-4). The stage for the dispute was being set.

In Genesis 4: 3-8, Cain, son of Adam and Eve, sacrificed the "fruit of the ground" to the deity, while his brother Abel sacrificed an animal. A vehement dispute between Cain and Abel erupted over whose sacrifice was more appropriate—on

R. Preece (✉)
Faculty of Arts, Wilfrid Laurier University, Waterloo, ON, Canada
e-mail: rodpreece@rogers.com

C. Blazina et al. (eds.), *The Psychology of the Human–Animal Bond*,
DOI 10.1007/978-1-4419-9761-6_3, © Springer Science+Business Media, LLC 2011

what precise grounds and in what precise manner the Bible does not mention. But that the dispute was heated and acrimonious was beyond question, resulting in Cain slaying Abel in apparent rage. That the first murder was occasioned by a quarrel over the appropriateness of animal sacrifice reflects the significance accorded the issue in the culture of the period in which Genesis was written, several centuries before the Christian era; that it remained so is evidenced by the frequency with which the matter was raised in the Old Testament, sometimes in favour of animal sacrifice, as in Leviticus 17.6, for example, where the proper procedure for animal sacrifice pleasing to God is ordained, sometimes against, as in Psalms 66, 3-4, where God's disgust at the practice of sacrifice is expressed. In Genesis, the ground had been laid for the debate that continued thereafter: are we sufficiently like other animals that we owe them a measure of obligation, and, if so, how much; or are we sufficiently dissimilar from other animals that we have minimal, or no, obligations to them?

In early Western history for which we have adequate records, the possession or absence of a rational soul was often deemed the relevant criterion of obligation. Those who thought animals deserving of ethical consideration frequently maintained that animals had such a soul, while those who dismissed animal interests denied species other than human the relevant soul. Today, many scholars would consider the question of whether animals, or even humans, possessed a soul—an archaic question devoid of relevance, or even meaning, in the modern world. But whether so or not, the question of an animal's possession of a soul, and, if so, what kind of soul, was the manner in which issues of animal ethics were customarily formulated from the time of the classical Greeks until at least well into the nineteenth century.

While the followers of René Descartes treated animals as automata and denied them souls, and the radical materialists, such as Julien Offray de La Mettrie, denied souls to humans as well, if not always consistently, almost all others ascribed some kind of soul to animals. However, most gave them sentient rather than rational souls, the latter of which was considered the exclusive human prerogative, rationality being considered the prerequisite of immortality. Sentience, the capacity for possessing feelings, was deemed to be common to all animals but absent from other entities. Nonetheless, a small but significant minority ascribed immortal souls to animals—including the moralist Abraham Tucker, the vegetarian physician George Cheyne, the poet Anna Seward, the parliamentarian Soame Jenyns, the revolutionary leveller Richard Overton, the academic Thomas Brown, the Anglican bishop Joseph Butler, the Swiss naturalist Charles Bonnet, the evangelist John Wesley, and the philosophers Leibniz and Pierre Bayle. The core of the argument appears to have been that there were no relevant differences between humans and other animals, all significant human attributes being deemed to be present in other animals, even if in lesser degree. If humans had the capacity for an immortal afterlife, so too had other animals. A greater portion of those who respected animal interests acknowledged that the animals' sentient souls warranted a considerable obligation on the part of humans not to harm them. And, from the sixteenth to eighteenth centuries, a stalwart few even argued—the Italian cardinal Robert Bellarmine, the Catholic poet Alexander Pope and the Anglican cleric Humphry Primatt, among them—that the very fact of the exclusion of animals from heaven by their lack of an immortal soul, whereby they could not be compensated in the afterlife for ills done to them in their earthly life, required an even greater duty to accord animals moral consideration in the here and now.

The fact that animals were accorded sentient souls, that is, sentience being their defining essence, a fact taken as self-evident from common observation, proved of considerable benefit to their cause in the long term, for, increasingly, it came to be recognized that the possession of sentience, rather than reason or speech or some other attribute, was the relevant criterion of ethical consideration. Already in early Jewish legal commentary it had been observed that:"It is forbidden according to the law of Torah to inflict pain on any living creature. On the contrary, it is our duty to relieve the pain of any creature" (Ganzfried, 1977). Throughout the medieval era and the Renaissance such varied thinkers as Moses Maimonides, Ambroise Paré and Leonardo da Vinci, from Spain, France and Italy, respectively, recognized the moral worth of animals and the relevance of their sentience. In 1641, a recent immigrant from Ireland to the Massachusetts Bay Colony, the Reverend Nathaniel Ward, drew up *The Bodies of Liberties* in which, ostensibly on account of animal sentience, it was stated (Liberty 92) that: "No man shall exercise any Tyranny or Cruelty toward any creature which [is] usually kept for man's use."[1] By the eighteenth century, the recognition of the paramountcy of sentience was common. The English cleric Richard Dean, for example, wrote *An Essay on the Future Life of Brutes* (1767) in which we read: "Brutes have sensibility; they are capable of pain; feel every bang, and cut or stab, as much as man himself, some of them perhaps more, and therefore they should not be treated as stocks or stones...Surely the sensibility of brutes entitles them to a milder treatment than they usually meet."[2]

Cartesianism

The greatest potential foe to the development of a consistent animal ethic lay in Cartesianism, which had a profound effect on seventeenth-century and later thought, especially with regard to the dualism of mind and body. With reference to animals, Descartes argued, with just a touch of ambivalence, that they were not sentient but were complex machines like watches. Descartes' disciples, notably Nicolas Malebranche, were decidedly unambiguous and preached the insentience of animals unequivocally. The implication of their deliberations was that animals could be treated without any ethical consideration. However, the court physician Marin Cureau de la Chambre and the abbot and mathematician Pierre Gassendi concurred in finding the idea repellent, the former declaring animals rational and ingenious as well as sentient, while the latter was appalled at Decscartes' blindness as to the similarity of human and other animals' senses. The Cambridge Platonist Henry More

---

[1] Quoted in Whitlock and Westerlund (1975), p. 36. Spelling modernized.
[2] Quoted in Nicholson and Preece (1999), p. 72.

denounced the unwarranted dismissal of animal sensibility. The German philosopher Immanuel Kant found the mechanist idea of animals wholly untenable. A number of notables from Samuel Johnson through Alexander Pope and John Locke to Jonathan Swift, and many more, were loud in their denunciations. A certain John Norris was convinced by Descartes' reasoning, but found it safer to disregard the practical implications and to continue to treat the animals "with as much tenderness and pitiful regard, as if they had all that Sense and Perception which is commonly. . .attributed to them."[3]

The French poet Bernard Fontenelle and the English Tory essayist Lord Bolingbroke were contenders for the wittiest rebuttal of Descartes. Fontenelle's rebuke was the most fulsome:

> "You say that the animals are both machines and watches, don't you? But if you put a male dog machine in close proximity with a female dog machine, a third little machine may be the consequence. In their place, you may put two watches in close proximity with each other for the whole of their lifetimes without ever producing a third watch. Now, according to our philosophy, all those things that have the capacity to render three out of two possess a greater nobility which elevates them above the machine."[4]

Bolingbroke's quip was equally persuasive, claiming that the plain man would persist in believing that there was a difference between the town bull and the parish clock (Bolingbroke, 1754, p. 344). In fact, very few outside France, and not many there, could be found to side with Descartes on the question of animal sentience even though his rationalist philosophy, in general, was widely acclaimed. If animals were treated far less well than they deserved, nonetheless animal Cartesianism was in itself largely without effect. Had it been widely subscribed to, it would have made animal lives, already deplorable, immeasurably worse.

Animals for Human Use

We should be careful not to infer from the relative failure of animal Cartesianism that the treatment of animals was benevolent or that there was a widespread subscription to the inclusion of animals within ethical discourse. The idea that animals "were intended for human use" had a lengthy and respected history and continued pervasively to be believed. Beginning with Xenophon and Aristotle in classical Greece, the idea of animals being created for human advantage had come to dominate Western culture for centuries, even though there had been some in the classical world, such as Plutarch, Lucretius and Pliny the Elder, who were of the decidedly contrary opinion—Plutarch, for example, observing that animals possessed intelligence, probity, ardour and courage, and suggesting their lives were in many respects superior to those of humans. Having described what he thought the superior

---

[3] Quoted in Harwood (1928), p. 104.
[4] Quoted in the original French in Boas (1932), p. 141.

characteristics of humans, while ignoring the superior capacities of other animals, Xenophon announced: "the beasts are born and bred for man's sake" (*Memorabilia*, IV, ii, 9–12). After discussing the relationship of plants to animals and some distinctions between wild and domesticated species, Aristotle concluded: "as nature makes nothing purposeless or in vain, all animals must have been made by nature for the sake of man" (*Politics*, 1, VIII, 11–12). Although Aristotle himself was respectful of animal capacities and interests when his mind was directed to matters zoological, as it sometimes was, when his attention was turned to more immediately human concerns such as politics, poetics, ethics and metaphysics, as it more commonly was, his focus was exclusively anthropocentric. If there was occasional nuance and some degree of inconsistency in Aristotle's perceptions, there was little among the Peripatetics, Stoics, Augustinians and Thomists who followed him. Their orientation was more or less uniformly in favour of the unquestioned superiority and exclusivity of the human species. And so were most of those from the succeeding centuries. As late as the mid-nineteenth century, we find Anne Brontë in her novel *Agnes Grey* depicting her heroine as being constrained to oppose the view of her employer that "the creatures were all created for our convenience" (Brontë, 1847, p. 106).

Once again, however, there was no inerrant orthodoxy in the development of animal ethics, for we find numerous scholars arrayed in opposition to the conception of animals as appropriate objects of human use. Thus, Aristotle's students and successors in the Lyceum, Dicaerchus and Theophrastus, were alive to the perception of animals as self-directed with their own purposes, wants and needs.

The seventeenth-century naturalist and taxonomist John Ray observed that the view of animals as intended for human use had been superseded: "Wise men nowadays think otherwise" (Ray, 1691, p. 127). On seeing the stars through a telescope, the celebrated seventeenth-century natural philosopher (and vivisectionist!) Robert Boyle felt compelled to reject the view that everything had been made for human ends. Even René Descartes was moved to remark that it "is not at all probable that all things have been made for us."[5] The cantankerous antiquarian Joseph Ritson stated at the opening of the nineteenth century that the "*sheep* is not so much 'design'd' for the *man*, as the *man* is for the *tyger*...If god made *man*, or there be any *intention* in *nature*, the life of the *louse*, which is as natural to him as his frame of body, is equally sacred and inviolable with his own" (Ritson, 1803, p. 231). The twentieth-century doyen of the study of the history of ideas, Arthur Lovejoy, declared that it was a general provision of the great chain of being—the dominant concept with regard to relative species value from medieval times to the nineteenth century and with considerable influence even beyond—that every link in the chain existed for its own sake and not primarily for the benefit of any other link.[6]

---

[5] Quoted in Lovejoy (1933), p. 124.
[6] A. O. Lovejoy. *The Great Chain of Being*, p. 186.

Animals as Ends in Themselves

It was only toward the end of the eighteenth century that the idea of each individual as an end in him or herself was first formulated. In what became known as the categorical imperative, Immanuel Kant declared that you should "act in such a manner that you always treat humanity, both in your own person and that of any other, always as an end and never solely as a means" (Kant, 1785, p. 52). However, since in Kant's view, animals lacked self-consciousness and were accordingly not moral agents, we do not owe ethical consideration to the animals in their own selves. Our duty to the animals is indirect. Virtuous action toward animals was still necessary, but it was a requirement of our moral duty to ourselves to improve our character. By and large, Kant's principle meant that the behaviour required of us toward non-human animals was no different from that recommended by the moderate animal advocates who believed we owed the animals our moral responsibility directly. It did, however, emphasize the conception of the animals as essentially different from and inferior to humans.

In an obscure minor poem on evolution, *Metamorphose der Tiere* (metamorphoses of the animals) of 1803, the polymath Johann Wolfgang Goethe borrowed the Kantian language and formulation directly, but announced the contrary conclusion: *Zweck sein selbst ist jegliches Tier* (i.e., each animal is an end in itself). Goethe's formulation had little impact and its importance went unrecognized. But slowly the notion of each animal being an end in itself became the underlying implied premise of the animal ethics of the more thoroughgoing animal advocates. No animal was to be treated as a mere means to human satisfaction.

Early Legislation and the Institution of Animal Protection Societies

The beginning of the nineteenth century was witness, in Britain, to the first efforts to legislate nationally on behalf of animals since the short-lived Protectorate of the seventeenth century. In general, the nineteenth century was a time of abysmal cruelty to animals in unregulated vivisection; family pets being stolen for sale to the vivisectors willing to buy them to conduct their next experiment on with no questions asked; the skinning of cats alive for their fur; the stealing of cats to provide the source of pet food on the carts trundled around the cities; the trapping of birds for their plumage; the stuffing of animals for display, often killed expressly for the purpose; the theft and subsequent sale of valuable dogs to those wanting an inexpensive high-status companion; and even a brisk and profitable trade in the kidnapping and ransom of favoured family pets. There were bull- and bear-baiting; dog-, badger-, cock- and rat-fighting; the callous treatment of food animals in slaughterhouses, where the pole-axe was still in use for some animals; the radical misuse of horses in the pulling of barges, public conveyances and private coaches; and sundry other vices such as the blinding of songbirds to make them sing more sweetly, as well, of course, as the continuation of so-called field sports (i.e., combats against animals conducted on natural open terrain rather than in confined spaces according to the lusts of human diversions).

On the other hand, there was a growing recognition of the need for legislation to curtail the worst of these evils. Already in the mid-eighteenth century, the novelist and magistrate Henry Fielding had proposed the idea, but it came to naught. Beginning in 1800, remedial legislation was introduced in the British Parliament but was defeated, as were other successive efforts. However, in 1822 the first legislation was successfully passed, followed by further legislation on seven occasions during the century. In 1824 the Society for the Prevention of Cruelty to Animals (SPCA) was founded with the express purpose of enforcing the legislation through its inspectorate and educating the public on animal welfare issues. By the grace of Queen Victoria, the society became the Royal SPCA in 1840. It is doubtful that there was any previous period in which so much legislation was devoted to one particular area of public concern. This innovation reflected both the fact that legislation had not in the past been thought appropriate to apply directly on behalf of animals and that there was a growing awareness that we had a legislative responsibility toward our fellow animals, limited in scope though it initially was. It reflected too that, in general, interference in the private rights and liberties of citizens which were not a threat to public order had been traditionally deemed beyond the province of legitimate legislation.

The legislation was not always as progressive as it appeared on the surface. For example, the Animal Cruelty Acts of 1835 and 1849 divided animals into the categories of "domestic" and "wild." The Acts offered some protection to domesticated animals but allowed for the unregulated continuance of field sports. Domestic animals were property and property was thought to be more deserving of respect and protection than the unowned. In practice, the distinction amounted to curtailing drastically what were regarded as the "entertainments" of the working class while those of "gentlemen" and men of property went unscathed. Until at least the middle of the nineteenth century, animal protection laws were the consequence more, but not entirely, of the desire to produce civility in the population, to elevate rather than brutalize the human mind, and to promote the nineteenth-century obsession with "civilization," rather than as a consequence of a concern for animal well-being in itself.

Field sports, such as fox- and deer-hunting took place in the open and on "natural" courses. They were exempt from legislation which controlled bull- and bear-baiting, cock- and dog-fighting, and the like. Fox- and deer-hunting were the province of the privileged and were seen as "manly" and "moral" pursuits. Field sports were deemed to contribute to virtue while cock- and dog-fighting smacked of public disorder. Nonetheless there was popular support for cock- and dog-fighting beyond the lower classes, and not all from the bloodthirsty. It was considerably easier to arouse indignation against bull- or bear-baiting than against cock- and dog-fighting because the former were seen as essentially unfair combative activities while cocks and dogs were regarded as natural fighters of their own volition. The contests were regarded as sporting events governed by strict and fair rules as written down in rigorous codes of conduct. Those who owned the fighting animals and those who were enthusiastic supporters at these organized events regarded themselves as engaged in legitimate sporting activities, much as would boxing or wrestling fans today. Notwithstanding their popularity, the fact that they were predominantly lower-class activities made it easier to outlaw them and for the RSPCA to prosecute infractions of the law.

Returning from a diplomatic post in Russia in 1865, where he had been appalled at the treatment of transport horses, Henry Bergh of New York stopped en route to confer with John Cotlam, Secretary of the RSPCA, and his previous acquaintance the Earl of Harrowby, President of the Society. Persuaded that the existence of such an organization was overdue in the United States, Bergh succeeded in having the American Society for the Prevention of Cruelty to Animals (ASPCA), based on the British model, incorporated by the state of New York legislature in 1866. Its charter contained a "declaration of the Rights of Animals" which Bergh described as a "a species of Declaration of Independence," believing it would eventually receive similar recognition and reverence as had Jefferson's monumental pronouncement. Bergh moved quickly to have animal cruelty legislation passed by the state legislature, which provided a degree of protection for both domesticated and wild animals. The New York SPCA was followed in short order by the founding of societies in Pennsylvania, Massachusetts, New Jersey, San Francisco and Minnesota, the last two including the protection of children in their remit. Like the Royal Society for the Prevention of Cruelty to Animals, the American Society for the Prevention of Cruelty to Animals became, in large measure, an organization devoted to public education and the enforcement of protective legislation. A second outstanding contributor to early animal welfare in the United States was wealthy Bostonian lawyer and anti-slavery campaigner George Angell. In outraged response to an infamous horse race in which both equine competitors died as a consequence of being overridden, he helped found the Massachusetts SPCA and became its first president on the society being granted a state charter in 1876. Like Bergh, Angell was an advocate of humane education, founding the Bands of Mercy in 1882 and the American Humane Education Society in 1889, thereafter devoting his life to the reform of an education system he found remiss in its lack of emphasis on compassion.

Animal Experimentation

Along with evolution, the *cause célèbre* of the later nineteenth century was vivisection. In fact, vivisection had long been a bone of contention with several major literary figures trumpeting in unison against the practice. They ranged from Shakespeare through the seventeenth-century diarist Samuel Pepys, the poet Alexander Pope, and the doyen of eighteenth-century literature Dr. Samuel Johnson to the consummate radical Percy Bysshe Shelley. At the turn of the nineteenth century we find the revolutionary John Oswald, the printer George Nicholson and the wayward Joseph Ritson writing caustic books that were in part diatribes against animal experimentation. In the mid-century, Charles Dickens and Robert Browning were fulsome in their distaste toward vivisection. Robert Louis Stevenson, Lewis

Carroll (i.e., the Oxford University mathematician Charles Dodgson) and the poet Christina Rossetti followed them. Despite the protests, the practice continued unregulated until 1876, and then without satisfying the concerns of its opponents. Still, the stinging rebukes appear to have had effect; by the 1850s British physiologists often restricted themselves to the use of reptiles rather than employing mammals in their experiments.

On the whole (but certainly not completely), they left what was commonly regarded as the unacceptable practice of experimenting on mammals without anaesthesia—which became generally available in the early 1850s—to the French and Italian vivisectors. Once anaesthesia was available it was often not used, for it was thought to make the experiments unreliable. At this time, the research of François Magendie, the reputed founder of experimental physiology; Louis Pasteur, expert on the effect of germs; Claude Bernard, Magendie's successor at the Collège de France; and Moritz Schiff, who conducted research on the thyroid gland in Florence, produced what were undoubted advances in knowledge unavailable to British physiologists. Envious of continental successes and desiring to emulate their European counterparts, the British scientists were constrained to adopt their methods. These European scientists had, in fact, relied on the demonstrable supposition, a supposition which they had previously denied, claiming humankind to be *sui generis* (i.e., unique unto itself), that the structure and function of human and other animals followed from their being of the same biological template. Ironically, in light of their neo-Cartesian stance of human exclusivity, a very premise of their work was that the suffering and pain of humans would be replicated in the more complex mammals.[7] Consequently, the conflict about vivisection came to revolve around whether scientific knowledge was more or less important than the value of the lives and the pain and suffering endured by the animals who were sacrificed. As Wilkie Collins observed in exasperated dismay in his novel *Heart and Science:* "All for knowledge! All for knowledge!" (Collins, 1883, p. 191). It was the view of the opponents of vivisection that there were moral limits to the legitimate acquisition of knowledge, even if for a beneficial purpose, and the vivisectors had exceeded them. If other animals were unlike us, there was no validity in the science. If they were like us, there was no moral justification for the research method.

The long-brewing issue of the ethics of vivisection came to a head in 1865 with the publication of *Introduction to the Study of Experimental Medicine* by the Parisian physiologist Claude Bernard. The revolutionary text established the principle of the laboratory, rather than medical practice, as the foundation for medical knowledge. Bernard convinced most of the medical profession and research scientists of the benefit of the artificial production of disease by chemical means through reliance on live animal models. According to Bernard, such models were "very useful and entirely conclusive of the toxicity and hygiene of man from the therapeutic

---

[7]This does not invalidate the earlier statement on the failure of Cartesianism in its animal sentience dimensions. These neo-Cartesians did not doubt the sentience of animals, indeed they relied on it, but still regarded the human as a being on an entirely different plane from other animals.

point of view."[8] Prior to Bernard, the argument that vivisection was cruel and inhumane, *and* that nothing beneficial ever came from it, was powerful and persuasive. After Bernard, the utility of animal experimentation became increasingly evident, especially to scientific observers, and for many in the medical and physiological fraternities, utility overrode moral considerations regarding the intrinsic value of animal life. If human health could be improved by vivisection at the expense of animals that was, for them, adequate justification in itself. After Bernard, those who opposed vivisection found increasingly that their arguments bore far more weight if they could also argue that the medical benefits derived from vivisection could be achieved at least as effectively as by non-invasive methods.

After some preliminary sniping, the opening salvo in the vivisection conflagration was fired by George Hoggan, a reluctant former vivisector who had first-hand experience of Bernard's work. In a letter to the *Morning Post* early in 1875, later reprinted in the *Spectator*, he accused Bernard of "monstrous abuses" that "were neither justified nor necessary." The battle lines were immediately drawn and a rancorous public debate ensued that prompted swift parliamentary reaction. The debate was bitter and hard fought and lingered into the early 1920s. The growing Victorian public distaste for what many saw as the barbarism of vivisection encouraged the cooperation of Unitarian preacher and Kant scholar Frances Power Cobbe, who had inspired the initial sniping, editor of the *Spectator* Richard Hutton, who had been deeply disturbed by Hoggan's letter, and George Hoggan himself, to join forces in founding the Victoria Street Society for Protection of Animals from Vivisection. The society's early membership was impressive, consisting, in part, of a considerable variety of establishment figures, including an Anglican archbishop, a Roman Catholic cardinal, the Lord Chief Justice, the poet laureate, and prominent artist and literary figures. The society was presided over by the evangelical Tory humanitarian reformer Lord Shaftesbury.

Arrayed against them were the discoverer of evolution by natural selection, Charles Darwin; T. H. Huxley, popularly known as Darwin's bulldog for his stalwart defence of Darwinism; and many prominent members of the medical profession. The opponents of vivisection declared they would be satisfied by nothing less than total abolition. The supporters of vivisection aimed for animal experimentation without formal regulation, the decision on suitability being left to the discretion and judgment of the vivisectors themselves as to what was and what was not appropriate.

In response to the public clamour aroused by the Hoggan letter and the consequent countervailing response in defence of what the vivisectionists saw as the public value of their research, two competing Bills were presented to Parliament, whereupon the Home Secretary announced in May of 1875 the establishment of an evenly balanced Royal Commission to investigate the issue. The majority report of the Royal Commission rejected total abolition but recommended strict controls.

Each side set to work on the preparation of new Bills, with the anti-vivisectionists being better organized and bringing forward their revised Bill first. The Bill included

---

[8]Quoted in Sharpe (1989), p. 89.

the licencing of practitioners, the strict supervision of those licenced, the use of anaesthesia for all laboratory animals and the prohibition of all vivisection on horses, dogs, cats, asses and mules. The measure was introduced in Parliament by Lord Carnarvon and would almost certainly have carried had he not been called away by the severe illness, and subsequent death, of his wife. The ensuing respite allowed the medical and scientific lobby to gather its forces and persuade the Home Secretary of the necessity for a Bill far more favourable to medical practitioners. Such a measure was introduced by the Home Secretary and speedily passed in a sparsely attended chamber. Hurriedly put together, the Act proved quite unsatisfactory, full of loopholes and effectively almost impossible to enforce. It was, the anti-vivisectors complained, an Act to defend the medical profession rather than to protect the interests of animals, being stimulated by the unjustified awe in which science and medicine were held. It was, however, rather less than the vivisectors had initially hoped for. Each of the adversarial sides vowed the fight would continue. Each was determined to fight on behalf of its respective cause to secure the passage, in the near future, of legislative provisions more favourable to itself. But neither achieved its goal.

In the United States, the ASPCA "made an unsuccessful attempt" in the winter of 1879–1880 "to secure the passage of a law [against vivisection] which would entirely abolish the practise as now in vogue in our medical schools, or cause it to be secretly carried on, in defiance of legal enactments."[9] The goals of the American and British anti-vivisectionists were essentially in accord. The Anti-Vivisectionist Society was formed in 1883, thereafter followed by the Vivisection Reform Society, which sought drastically to reform vivisection, having learned from the British experience that route was more likely of success. It was incorporated in 1903, and in 1907 included among its officers a US Senator, a cardinal, a bishop, two former college presidents and a former judge as well as a smattering of surgeons, professors and journalists, a complement no less impressive than that of the Victoria Street Society. The most prominent American anti-vivisectionist was the surgeon Dr. Albert Leffingwell who argued that "our moral duty to all living creatures, from the highest to the lowest form of life, is to treat them precisely as we ourselves should be willing to be treated for the same objects in view, were we instantly to exchange with them every limitation and circumstance of their condition and form" (Leffingwell, 1907, p. 80).

The Humanitarian League

The principle Leffingwell enunciated may be said to have been the implicit basis on which the Humanitarian League was established in England by the former Eton teacher and prolific author Henry S. Salt in 1891, having first been mooted by Salt at a Fabian Society meeting in 1889. The League proved to be the

---

[9] Albert Leffingwell, "Does Vivisection Pay?", *Scribner's Monthly*, July 1880, 1.

organization which went the furthest in the history of animal protection in drawing a corresponding parallel between human and other animal considerations, and, at least in terms of explicit agenda, has not been surpassed since, perhaps not even matched.

The novelty of the Humanitarian League lay in its concern with pain and suffering of all species, including the human species. It saw the human moral task as the elimination of pain and suffering, whether committed against human or animal. The first sentence of the programme of the League ran: "The Humanitarian League has been established on the basis of an intelligible and consistent principle of humaneness - that it is iniquitous to inflict suffering directly or indirectly on any sentient being, except when self-defence can justly be pleaded."[10] He elaborated the doctrine of "humanitarianism" as "not merely an expression of sympathy with pain, it is a protest against all tyranny and desecration, whether such wrong be done by the infliction of suffering on sentient beings, or by the Vandalism which can ruthlessly destroy the natural grace of the earth."[11] In his last book *The Creed of Kinship,* he advanced the principle that "the basis of any real morality must be the sense of kinship between all living beings" (Salt, 1935, p. viii). Humanitarianism, Salt wrote, "must aim at the redress of *all* needless suffering, human and animal alike - the stupid cruelties of social tyranny, of the criminal code, of fashion, of science, of flesh-eating."[12] By "social tyranny" he was referring to class, gender and racial prejudice. Uppermost in his mind with regard to the abuses contained in "the criminal code" were flogging and capital punishment. His concerns with "fashion. . .science [and]. . .flesh-eating" were, respectively, the killing of animals and birds for their fur and plumage, the horrors of the science laboratories, and the moral necessity of vegetarianism.

For Salt and the Humanitarian League, persons of refined sensibilities would be equally concerned with human and animal suffering. Such persons would not compartmentalize themselves and become animal advocates alone, or even supremely, or be solely concerned with justice for the human population, but would treat humans and animals as intrinsically inseparable victims of the same type of social problem. The more eminent supporters of the League included the playwright George Bernard Shaw, the renowned theosophist leader Annie Besant, the primitivist Edward Carpenter, the historian of the ethics of diet Howard Williams and Sidney Olivier, destined to become Governor of Jamaica.

Salt found the most accomplished proponent of the doctrine he promoted not among the members of the League but across the Atlantic in the person of Chicago science teacher J. Howard Moore, of whose writings he observed: "I have long thought Moore's chief book *The Universal Kinship*. . .is the best book ever written

---

[10] *The Manifesto of the Humanitarian League*, excerpted in G. Hendrick and W. Hendrick (1989), p. 43.

[11] Quoted from *Seventy Years Among Savages* in G. Hendrick and W. Hendrick (1989), p. 113.

[12] Quoted in Hendrick (1977), p. 193.

in the humanitarian cause."[13] The opening lines of Moore's book show that, indeed, Salt had found a truly kindred spirit:

> *The Universal Kinship* means the kinship of all the inhabitants of planet Earth. Whether they came into existence among the water or desert sands, in a hole in the earth, in the hollow of a tree, or in a palace; whether they build nests or empires; and whether they realize it or not, they are all related, physically, mentally, morally - this is the thesis of this book. . .The chief purpose of these pages is to prove and interpret the kinship of the human species with the other species of animals.[14]

Salt recognized, as Moore demonstrated in the body of the book, that his unswerving goal was "to put science and humanitarianism in place of tradition and savagery."[15]

Emblematic of the vastly increased role played by women in the animal protection movement was the prominence of the science-educated Louise Lind-af-Hageby. It was not that women had not voiced their concerns before, from the poets Margaret Cavendish, Anne Finch and Anna Sewell, to the essayists Sarah Trimmer, Mary Wollestoncraft and Priscilla Wakefield, but now societal conditions were changing and women could play a more direct and influential role. Of Swedish descent, but resident in England and a member of the Humanitarian League, Lind-af-Hageby had come to prominence in 1903 through her book, *The Shambles of Science,* an exposé which revealed the abjectly cruel vivisection practices conducted at University College, London. Later, she played a role in the women's suffrage movement and promoted the state regulation of prostitution and vice. At the outset of the First World War she was in the forefront of united human–animal endeavours. She threw herself into the establishment of services to alleviate the sufferings of both soldiers and animals, predominantly warhorses, on the battlefield. Her work exemplified in practice the principle of inclusive justice which the Humanitarian League promoted and of which women were in the vanguard of promotion.

The Twentieth-Century Hiatus

Following the death of his wife, Kate, Henry Salt disbanded the Humanitarian League in September 1919, many members finding a home in other animal welfare organizations. However, the time was not propitious for rebuilding inclusive humanitarian sentiments. The Victorian and Edwardian optimism that practical solutions to ethical and social problems were imminent was dealt a mortal blow by the miseries and deprivations of the war and the loss of confidence that ensued. Those few who continued in their seemingly utopian endeavours were usually deemed eccentric, if not bordering on outright lunacy. Both World Wars provided not only increased

---

[13]Quoted from Salt (1905), p. ix.

[14]J. Howard Moore, *The Universal Kinship*, xxxv.

[15]Quoted from *Seventy Years Among Savages* in *The Savour of Salt,* ed. Hendrick and Hendrick, 55.

opportunities for vivisection research, but also a more readily accepted justification for engaging in it because of the widespread mutilations suffered by those in the armed forces. And that research was designed to alleviate those sufferings. In both World Wars, and in the ensuing decades, concerns with animal suffering and well-being were displaced by almost solely human concerns as a consequence of the prevalence of human suffering and deprivation occasioned by the conflicts.

With the demise of the Humanitarian League in 1919, the period of the all-embracing approach of inclusive justice—justice for humans and animals in tandem and simultaneously—came to an end. In fact, with a few exceptions, the concern with animal well-being sank into a serious decline, not to be revived until some two decades after the Second World War had ended. Among the exceptions were the institution of the Pit Ponies' Protection Society in 1927, Our Dumb Friends' League campaigning against poor zoo and slaughterhouse conditions, and the strenuous efforts of the League for the Prohibition of Cruel Sports against fox- and deer-hunting in particular.

Though not himself a member of the Humanitarian League and not even an animal advocate, the philosopher and mathematician Bertrand Russell had the most telling observation on the animal rights' issue in the years between the wars. He was amused by a certain mountaineer's bizarre belief the deity had designed the mountains with the pleasure of the rock climber in mind. "It seems to me," Russell mused,

> that the mountain goat, the ibex and the chamois might have other views on this subject. If they had a parliament, they would congratulate each other on the clumsiness of this horrid creature Man, and would render thanks that his cunning is impeded by such a clumsy body. Where they skip, he crawls; where they bound freely, he clings to a rope. Their evidence of beneficence in nature would be the opposite of the mountain climber's and every bit as convincing. There is no impersonal reason for regarding the interests of human beings as more important than those of animals. We can destroy animals more easily than they can destroy us; that is the only solid basis of our claim to superiority. We value art and science, because these are things in which we excel. But whales might value spouting and donkeys might maintain a good bray is more exquisite than the music of Bach. We cannot prove them wrong except by the exercise of arbitrary power (Russell, 1931, pp. 91–92).

The implication of Russell's argument was far reaching: if we value art and science for no better reason than because we excel in art and science, then the basis on which we give preference to human rights over the rights of other animals on account of our superior reason and more refined moral sense is no more valid. It is because these are attributes in which we surpass other animals that they are chosen. We choose these categories as the criteria of eminence for no better reason than that we are doing the choosing and opt for the criteria which it is in the human interest to select.

Reason, speech, moral sense and the dexterity provided by opposable thumbs have no impartial priority over the unaided flight of birds; the echolocation capacities of whales, dolphins, and bats; or the direction-finding of the honeyguides. They are as important to these animals in fulfilling their needs, wants and purposes as reason or opposable thumbs in fulfilling human needs, wants and purposes. Our superiority lies in nothing other, the Russellian argument implies, than might and we can justly claim priority over the rights of other animals only if might makes right. We have, on this reasoning, no impartial rights to use animals for human purposes, whether it is in using a horse to pull a cart, in employing a cow for milk and sustenance, or a pig for its hide.

The Renaissance of Animal Ethics

Animal welfare protection having been largely out of the public mind since the close of the Edwardian era, its resurrection in the 1960s was a startling revelation to many. It was as though a fundamental concern for the rights and well-being of animals was a wholly new phenomenon rather than a renaissance of past glories. In fact, the idea of "animal rights" that now came into vogue had a venerable history. Its first apparent use was by the seventeenth-century anabaptist vegetarian Thomas Tryon and came shortly after the idea of "natural rights" had first been promoted as legitimate human possessions. Confronted by human wholesale destruction of birds, Tryon asked, under the pseudonym of Philotheus Physiologus, whence humans derived their authority to destroy " the natural rights and privileges" of other species.[16] At least two nineteenth-century books referred to the rights of animals in their titles, one by the Irish Unitarian William H. Drummond under the title of *The Rights of Animals, and Man's Obligation to Treat Them with Humanity* (1838) (Drummond, 2005) and the other by the aforementioned Henry Salt—his most popular book— *Animals' Rights Considered in Relation to Social Progress* (1892) (Salt, 1892). But if the term "animal rights" was not new, the importance attributed to the idea of "animal rights" and what those rights were took on new meaning with the advent of scholarly concerns in the 1960s. Philosophers, historians, theologians and psychologists now began to address the questions of animal rights in a direct and often controversial manner.

When Rachel Carson wrote her inspiring yet ominous *Silent Spring* in 1962, her attention was devoted almost entirely to impending environmental devastation, but she was still able to warn also of the prevalent anthropocentrism of Western thought. "We cannot have peace among men," she advised, "whose hearts delight in killing any living creature." The Quaker Ruth Harrison wrote *Animal Machines* in 1964, an acerbic critique of intensive farming, in which she advocated legislation to ensure adequate conditions for battery hens and veal calves. In 1965, the Shavian Brigid Brophy wrote an article for the London *Sunday Times* on "The Rights of Animals," which attracted significant public attention.

In 1969, Oxford University became the centre of a group of young intellectuals devoted to promoting the rights of animals; among their number were Stanley and

---

[16]Quoted from "The Complaints of the Birds and Fowls of Heaven to their Creator for the Oppressions and Violences Most Nations on Earth do Offer Them" in *The Country-man's Companion* (1683) in Preece and Chamberlain (1993), p. 73.

Roslind Godlovich, John Harris and Richard D. Ryder, soon to be joined by Stephen Clark, Andrew Linzey and the Australian Peter Singer. In the United States, Bernard Rollin, Tom Regan, Steve F. Sapontzis, Daniel Dombrowski and Carol Adams shortly thereafter had a profound impact and continue to do so. Peter Singer's *Animal Liberation* became the most popular early ambassador of this new thought. Animal welfare science was instituted as a recognized and reputable discipline which was increasingly effective in improving somewhat farm animal conditions in Europe, North America and the Antipodes. The renowned South African–born Australian J. M. Coetzee, eminent literary figure and Nobel Prize winner, gave the promotion of animal rights a new prominence and far greater respectability.

In the late nineteenth century, the literary critic Matthew Arnold had described Oxford famously as "the home of lost causes, and forsaken beliefs, and unpopular names, and impossible loyalties!" It became instead, in this instance, the ever outward-branching home of resurrected beliefs, appealing names and loyalties to all of animalkind. Whether these loyalties are possible to sustain in the long term only time will tell, but they are certainly far less impossible than they would have been thought to be a half-century ago.

In the twenty-first century, more attention is being devoted to issues of animal ethics and by far more people than at any time in the past. Increasingly, the media give significantly more space and time to animal-related issues. Throughout Western cultural history there have always been a significant minority who addressed questions of animal ethics, and some in a decidedly radical manner, but never before has there been a more general recognition that questions of animal ethics deserve serious and prolonged discussion and consideration.

References

Boas, G. (1932). *The Happy Beast in French Thought of the Seventeenth Century*. Baltimore: Johns Hopkins Press.

Bolingbroke, L. (1754). *The Works of Henry St. John, Lord Viscount Bolingbroke* (Vol. 5). (Reprint London: D. Mallet, 1809).

Brontë, A. (1847). *Agnes Grey*. (Reprint, London: Penguin, 1988).

Collins, W. (1883). *Heart and Science: A Story of the Present Time*. (Reprint, Peterborough: Broadview, 1996).

Drummond, W. H. (2005). *The Rights of Animals, and Man's Obligation to Treat them with Humanity (1838)*. (Reprint; ed. Rod Preece and Chien-hui Li (Lampeter: Mellen Press)).

Ganzfried, R. S. (1977). *Code of Jewish Law* (bk. 4, ch. 19, 184). New York: Hebrew Publishing Company.

Harwood, D. (1928). *Love for Animals and How it Developed in Great Britain*. (Reprint, ed. Rod Preece and David Fraser, Lampeter: Mellen, 2003).

Hendrick, G. (1977). *Henry Salt: Humanitarian Reformer and Man of Letters*. Urbana: University of Illinois Press.

G. Hendrick, & W. Hendrick (Eds.). (1989). *The Savour of Salt: A Henry Salt Anthology*. Fontwell: Centaur.

Kant, I. (1785). *Grundlagen zur Metaphysik der Sitten*. (Reprint, Hamburg: Meiner, 1994).

Leffingwell, A. (1907). *The Vivisection Question* (2nd ed.). Chicago: The Vivisection Reform Society.

Lovejoy, A. O. (1933). *The Great Chain of Being: A Study in the History of Ideas*. Cambridge: Harvard University Press.

Nicholson, G., & Preece, R. (Ed.). (1999). *On the Primeval Diet of Man (1801)*. Lampeter: Mellen.

Preece, R., & Chamberlain, L. (1993). *Animal Welfare and Human Values*. Waterloo: Wilfrid Laurier University Press.

Ray, J. (1691). *The Wisdom of God Manifested in the Works of Creation*. (Reprint, New York: Garland, 1979).

Ritson, J. (1803). *An Essay on Abstinence from Animal Food as a Moral Duty*. London: Richard Phillips.

Russell, B. (1931). "If animals could talk." In H. Ruja (Ed.), *Morals and others: Bertrand Russell's American essays 1931–1935*. Excerpted in Paul A. B. Clarke & A. Linzey (eds.), *Political theory and animal rights*. London: Pluto Press, 1990.

Salt, H. (1892). *Animals' Rights Considered in Relation to Social Progress*. (Reprint, preface by Peter Singer, Society for Animal Rights, Inc.: Clark Summit, Pa., 1980).

Salt, H. (1905). *Company I Have Kept*. In C. Magel (Ed.), Introduction to J. Howard Moore, *The Universal Kinship*. (Reprint, Fontwell: Centuar, 1992).

Salt, H. (1935). *The Creed of Kinship*. London: Constable.

Sharpe, R. (1989). Animal Experiments - A Failed Technology. In G. Langley (Ed.), *Animal Experimentation: The Consensus Changes*. New York: Chapman and Hall.

Whitlock, E., & Westerlund, S. R. (1975). *Humane Education: An Overview*. Tulsa, OK: The National association for the Advancement of Humane Education.

Chapter 4
The Human–Animal Experience in Deep Historical Perspective

Todd J. Braje

Introduction: Qualifying the "Natural"

A variety of academics, including archaeologists, geographers, ecologists, historians, political scientists, philosophers, and others, have been critical of the notion of "pristine, natural, or wild" areas, arguing that human impacts on environments have been widespread over millennia (Frazier, 2009). While study of human impacts on the environment is vast and extends back to the nineteenth century (see Grayson, 1984), over the last several decades it has become increasingly apparent that ancient human populations exerted a significant influence on local environments, including impacts to a wide array of plant and animal communities (e.g., Grayson, 2001; Krech, 1999, 2005; Redman, 1999; Rick & Erlandson, 2009). Debates over the nature and scale of these impacts and whether prehistoric groups acted as conservationists (see Alcorn, 1993, 1996; Krech, 2005) or with little regard for preservation and sustainability (see Kay & Simmons, 2002a; Sluyter, 2001; Smith & Wishnie, 2000) have been hotly contested. Regardless, it has become clear, to archaeologists at least, that as Europeans expanded around the globe, the indigenous landscapes and plant and animal communities they encountered were the result of millennia of human manipulations.

A growing body of research on the historical ecology of terrestrial and marine ecosystems has demonstrated that ancient human populations were significant agents in shaping local ecologies. Historical ecology is a broad field focused on understanding how people have interacted with, and altered, their environments over time. Through collaboration and the integration of a variety of disciplines, historical ecologists trace the evolution of land- and seascapes over deep time, recognizing that humans play a critical role in structuring local floral and faunal communities (e.g., Balée, 1998; Balée & Erickson, 2006; Crumley, 1994; Dean, 2009; Egan & Howell, 2001; Rick & Erlandson, 2008). These studies demonstrate that many

T.J. Braje (✉)
Department of Anthropology, San Diego State University, 5500 Campanile Drive, San Diego, CA 92182-6040, USA
e-mail: tjb50@humboldt.edu

C. Blazina et al. (eds.), *The Psychology of the Human–Animal Bond*,
DOI 10.1007/978-1-4419-9761-6_4, © Springer Science+Business Media, LLC 2011

modern environmental problems have parallels to those faced in the ancient past, positioning historical ecology to become an essential framework for addressing modern environmental crises (e.g., Diamond, 2003, 2005; Redman, 1999; Redman, James, Fish, & Rogers, 2004). To understand and manage modern-day ecosystems, we must investigate contemporary and ancient human activities. As Crumley (1994, p. 9) noted:

> Past and present human use of the earth must be understood in order to frame effective environmental policies for the future; this necessitates deft integration of both environmental and cultural information at a variety of temporal and spatial scales.

Archaeology, then, is uniquely positioned to offer a variety of insights on the long history of human–environmental interactions that have helped shape the structure of modern ecosystems around the globe.

Studies of the impacts of ancient human populations on faunal populations have been undertaken for over a century, but in the last several decades an increasingly sophisticated set of data and methods have demonstrated a broad range of impacts that extend into the deep past. While the invention and spread of agriculture and pastoralism after about 12,000 years ago is often seen as a crossroads in the relationship between humans and animals, archaeological research is demonstrating that hunter-gatherer populations significantly influenced animal communities, distinct from, and long before, the rise of agrarian, state-level societies (Rick & Erlandson, 2009). In the same vein, agricultural populations transported and influenced domesticated and wild animals. Megafaunal extinctions and aboriginal overkill have posited continental wide impacts on prehistoric fauna that extend back tens of thousands of years (e.g., Alroy, 2001; Grayson, 2007; Grayson & Meltzer, 2003; Martin & Klein, 1984). Island fauna in the Caribbean, Mediterranean, and Pacific were permanently altered by human colonization (e.g., Kirch, 1996; Nagaoka, 2005; Sonddar, 2000; Steadman, Pregill, & Burley, 2002). Work in the last decade even extends these impacts to a wide range of marine and aquatic fauna, including sea mammals, fish, and shellfish (e.g., Braje, 2010; Braje, Erlandson, Rick, Dayton, & Hatch, 2009; Erlandson, Rick, Braje, Steinberg, & Vellanoweth, 2008; Nagaoka, 2005; Rick & Erlandson, 2008, 2009; Simenstad, Estes, & Kenyon, 1978; Springer et al., 2003).

In this chapter, I highlight recent research concerning ancient human impacts on faunal communities around the world. While a comprehensive review is beyond the scope of this chapter, I cover some of the most striking examples of human–animal interactions by preindustrial hunter-gatherer-fisher populations, highlighting the dynamic relationship between humans and animals beginning 50,000 years ago in the Old World. My purpose is to demonstrate that complex relationships between humans and wild animals extend into deep antiquity. The following case studies reveal that the adaptive success of anatomically modern humans (AMHs) was inextricably tied to the human–animal experience long before large-scale agriculture and pastoralism. I conclude by suggesting how a better understanding of the long-term interactions between humans, animal communities, and the environment can help address modern environmental crises and conservation biology, and is relevant to clinical psychologists and researchers interested in the human–animal bond.

Modern Human Behavior in the Middle Stone Age and the Human–Animal Genesis

While our early human ancestors certainly engaged in hunting, scavenging, and interactions with a variety of animals, the transition between the Middle and Upper Paleolithic, between about 50,000 and 40,000 years ago, may mark a turning point in human evolution (Klein, 2000). For an as-of-yet unclear set of reasons, AMHs began to intensively engage in a variety of symbolic, artistic, and innovative behaviors—activities that first appear between about 160,000–125,000 years ago. Much of this art and iconography involves animal depictions in some form. The stunning 17,000-year-old polychrome rock art of Lascaux Cave in France depicts Pleistocene aurochs, for example, running across the cave walls, playing with one another, or being hunted by humans. Cave art at Chauvet Cave in southern France, dated between 30,000 and 26,000 years ago, includes at least 13 different animal species engaged in a variety of movements and actions (Chauvet, Deschamps, & Hillaire, 1996). A 35,000-year-old necklace of animal teeth from a variety of Pleistocene carnivores was unearthed southeast of Paris. Scores of examples like these, that date back tens of thousands of years, suggest that the relationship between humans and animals began to dramatically change during this interval. Although debates continue to rage over whether earlier humans obtained animals more by scavenging than hunting (see Binford, 1985; Chase, 1988), there is little evidence to suggest that people were very successful at obtaining large animals prior to about 50,000 years ago (Klein, 1994). After that time, an explosion in symbolic representations of a variety of animal species across the Old World suggests that humans were developing a deep connection with animal communities that not only permeated their subsistence economies, but also their social, cultural, and cosmological systems (Klein, 1989).

Archaeologists and paleoanthropologists have used the products of this "Creative Explosion" (cave paintings, sophisticated hunting techniques, portable art, and personal ornamentation) to track the spread of AMHs out of Africa. Shell beads and other typically Upper Paleolithic technologies from Blombos Cave in South Africa, Grotte de Pigeons in Morocco, and Skhul in Israel suggest that the antecedents of this "modern human behavior" may date to the Middle Stone Age as much as 100,000–120,000 years ago (Bouzouggar et al., 2007; d'Errico, Henshilwood, Vanhaeren, & van Niekerk, 2005; Henshilwood, d'Errico, Vanhaeren, van Niekerk, & Jacobs, 2004; Henshilwood & Marean, 2003; Mcbrearty & Brooks, 2000; Vanhaeren et al., 2006). Regardless of the exact timing, this moment in human history signals the genesis of a "modern" human–animal experience, where humans began exerting significant influences on the shape and structure of not only animal communities, but also local and regional ecosystems around the globe. While early AMHs and ancestral hominins certainly influenced animal communities, it is during this time period that we see the first definitive evidence of symbolic animal representations, a clear understanding of animal behavior, and, possibly, the extinction of animal species by humans (see below). This process has continued and accelerated through time, resulting in the anthropogenically modified sea- and landscapes we know today.

The Spread of Anatomically Modern Humans:
Animal Extinctions and Translocations

The literature concerning human impacts on terrestrial ecosystems and animal populations is vast. Studies have clearly demonstrated that AMHs exerted a strong influence on terrestrial animal populations almost immediately as they spread across the globe. In many cases, archaeologists have employed evolutionary theory to quantify these impacts, demonstrating the potential and realized effects of small-scale hunter-gatherer groups as they colonized new areas (see Grayson, 2001 for a review). Foraging theory has been a particularly useful tool and has demonstrated, in a number of cases, that sustained human hunting of faunal landscapes results in resource depletion, declining faunal abundances, changing prey age and size structures, and associated behavioral changes in animals and humans.

A review of foraging theory and resource depletion, and the numerous documented case studies of these, is outside the scope of this chapter. Instead, I focus on, potentially, the first wide-scale impact of humans on animal populations—continental megafaunal extinctions during the Pleistocene (see Table 4.1)—and on the long-distance transport of wild vertebrate terrestrial animals. These are powerful examples of the deep history of the human–animal experience and the significant role humans have played in shaping faunal landscapes around the world.

Continental Megafaunal Extinctions

While animal extinctions are clearly a natural part of the evolutionary process, just as clear is that humans have accelerated and, in many cases, directly caused the extinction of numerous species around the globe. This has been especially pervasive in delicate island ecosystems where human burning, landscape clearing, hunting, and the introduction of new plants and animals often have resulted in wide-scale and rapid extinctions of native species (see Grayson, 2001; Rick & Erlandson,

Table 4.1 The geological time scale and major evolutionary events mentioned in the text

Era	Period	Epoch	Stage	Million Years Ago	Major Event
Cenozoic		Holocene		0.012	Invention of agriculture
	Quaternary	Pleistocene	Late	0.012–0.126	Modern human behavior
			Middle	0.126–0.78	Anatomically modern humans
			Lower	0.78–2.6	
	Tertiary	Pliocene		5	First hominins
		Miocene		22	
		Oligocene		35	First ape-like forms
		Eocene		55	
		Paleocene		65	First primates

2009). The largest human-induced animal extinction event may be linked, however, to continental extinctions of megafauna (traditionally defined as animals weighing more than 45 kg) in North America and Australia during the Late Pleistocene.

In North America, approximately 35 genera of mostly large mammals went extinct between about 13,000 and 10,500 years ago, including mammoths, mastodons, giant ground sloths, horses, tapirs, camels, bears, cats, and a variety of other animals (Alroy, 1999; Grayson, 1991). In Australia, some 28 genera of large mammals, birds, and reptiles went extinct approximately 50,000 years ago, including giant kangaroos, wombats, and snakes. Much of the current evidence suggests that initial human colonization of Australia and North America at about 55,000–50,000 and 15,000–13,000 years ago, respectively, played an integral role in the extinction of these animals, although the influence of humans is much debated (e.g., Brook & Bowman, 2002, 2004; Grayson, 2001; Roberts et al., 2001; Surovell, Waguespack, & Brantingham, 2005; Wroe, Field, Fullagar, & Jermin, 2004).

A number of scholars have implicated climate change as the prime mover in megafaunal extinctions (see Wroe, Field, & Grayson, 2006) and new research has even suggested that an extraterrestrial impact (i.e., comet) that struck North America at about 12,900 years ago triggered biomass burning and food shortages that resulted in the North American extinctions (Firestone et al., 2007). In both North America and Australia, there are very few archaeological sites with the remains of megafauna hunted by humans, the proverbial smoking gun of the human "overkill" hypothesis (see Fiedel & Haynes, 2004; Grayson, 2001; Grayson & Meltzer, 2003). Proponents of an anthropogenic role in these extinctions counter that many African megafauna survived due to their co-evolution with humans and megafauna in North America and Australia survived major climatic fluctuations through the Ice Age Epoch with initial human colonization correlated with extinction events (Martin, 2005). In addition, Steadman and colleagues (2005) found that the extinction of giant sloths on the West Indian islands corresponds with the arrival of humans and not glacial–interglacial climate change.

It seems likely to me that both climate and humans contributed to continental megafaunal extinctions in both North America and Australia (see Barnosky, Koch, Feranec, Wing, & Shabel, 2004). Warming at the end of the Last Glacial Maximum (LGM, ca. 18,000 years ago) in North America and a stepwise progression of aridification over the last 400,000 years in Australia (Wroe et al., 2006) combined with anthropogenic impacts in the form of landscape burning (Miller et al., 1999) or hunting of keystone herbivores (Owen-Smith, 1988) resulted in the greatest loss of vertebrate species diversity in the Cenozoic Era. Megafaunal extinctions in North America and Australia, then, constitute the first wide-scale impacts of pre-agriculturalists on wild animal populations. These events signaled a fundamental change in the role of humans in shaping local and regional animal communities, the results of which have played a powerful role in shaping modern history. Prior to this, there is no evidence for human driven extinction events as a result of anthropogenic ecosystem modification or direct human hunting. Rather, humans operated largely as a part, rather than a modifier, of nature, a role that has dramatically accelerated through time. The extinction of large animals such as horses, camels, and other herbivores in North America, for example, left Native Americans with few options for animal domestication and beasts of burden that could be used to plow agricultural fields. In the Old World, on the other hand, cattle, sheep, and pigs were prized domesticates that allowed for food surpluses, increased agricultural production, and resistance to many deadly diseases. These advantages ultimately provided Europeans with a head start in agriculture and state building and armed them with infectious diseases that devastated indigenous populations around the globe (see Diamond, 1997). The modern, globalized world, characterized by the haves and have nots, then, began to take shape millennia ago with the human–megafauna experience.

Animal Translocations and Island Colonizers

Conservation biologists and applied ecologists often define translocation as "... the intentional release of animals to the wild in an attempt to establish, reestablish, or augment a population..." (Griffith, Scott, Carpenter, & Reed, 1989, p. 477). Archaeologists and other historical scientists extend this definition to include the introduction of new fauna to a variety of landscapes, regardless of whether these introductions are intentional or not (see Flannery & White, 1991; Grayson, 2001). Clearly such introductions and translocations occurred after ca. 12,000 years ago and the domestication of plants and animals with, for example, pigs, goats, sheep, barley, and wheat spreading out of Mesopotamia into Africa and Europe and, eventually, around the globe. Less widely recognized is the translocation of wild animals by hunter-gather and small-scale agricultural populations.

The number and variety of these wild animal translocations are astounding, including rodents like agoutis and hutias in the Caribbean (de France, Keegan, & Newsom, 1996; Wing, 1993); macaques in island Indonesia (Flannery et al., 1998); shrews, deer, foxes, and cats across Mediterranean islands (Reese, 1996; Vigne & Valladas, 1996); and, likely, foxes to California's Channel Islands (Collins, 1991; Rick, n.d.; Rick, Erlandson, et al., 2009). In addition to a diverse set of invertebrates, including land snails, beetles, and (human and animal) lice (Grayson, 2001), mice and rats were common stowaways on maritime voyages to new islands, including during the colonization of islands in the Mediterranean (Zeder, 2008), North Atlantic (McGovern et al., 2008), Pacific Ocean (Anderson, 2009; Johnson, 1983; Kirch, 1996, 2004; Matisoo-Smith, 2009; Rick, n.d.), and Indian Ocean (Blench, 2007).

Recent research suggests that the earliest wild animal translocation may date back to the Late Pleistocene, some 20,000 years ago, with the human-assisted introduction of the gray cuscus (*Phalanger orientalis*) by hunter-gatherers to New Ireland in Melanesia (White, 2004). These translocations are not restricted to oceanic islands, however, and have been identified archaeologically in a number of continental settings. The clearest examples come from south Asia with the spread of the house rat (*Rattus rattus*) and the southwestern United States with trading of the scarlet macaw by agricultural populations (*Ara macoa*; Armitage, 1994; Grayson, 2001; Minnis, Whalen, Kelley, & Stewart, 1993). Such continental translocations were probably quite frequent, but are often difficult to distinguish from natural biogeographic events.

Human-assisted translocations to islands are much easier to identify archaeologically, and there is considerable evidence that the ancient transport of wild animals has, in many cases, fundamentally altered native flora and fauna. For example, the introduction of the Polynesian rat from mainland southeast Asia, along with human land clearing and anthropogenic changes in delicate island ecosystems, has been implicated in the extinction of snails, frogs, and lizards in New Zealand (Brook, 1999), giant iguanas and bats in the Kingdom of Tonga (Koopman & Steadman, 1995; Pregill & Dye, 1989), and an incredible diversity of birds across the Pacific (Kirch, 1997; Kirch, Steadman, Butler, Hather, & Weisler, 1995; Steadman, 1989; Steadman & Kirch, 1990). The staggering story of deforestation, competitive statue building, and environmental deterioration on Easter Island (Rapa Nui), often used as a cautionary tale about the dangers of overexploitation (Bahn & Flenley, 1992), may be as much a story about rats as it is humans. Flenley (1993; Flenley, King, Jackson, & Chew, 1991) identified Polynesian rat gnaw-marks on the seeds of the now-extinct Easter Island palm, suggesting that these rodents played a powerful role in the extinction of this species, the decreased richness of island biotas, and subsequent lack of construction material for ocean-going canoes, housing timber, and beams and rollers for transporting and erecting the colossal statue effigies (Moai).

In total, archaeological work over the years has demonstrated that human populations have transported wild animals great distances, both intentionally and unintentionally, for thousands of years. Often, their motivations remain mysterious but the consequences have been considerable for native flora and fauna and the structure of local ecosystems. For biogeographers and other scientists, the challenge becomes detecting such human translocations and not confusing them with other kinds of "natural" dispersal events (Grayson, 2001). We can no longer afford to ignore the significant role of humans in shaping local landscapes and faunal communities around the world for millennia, an issue I return to later.

The Human–Animal Experience on the Margins: Coastal Interactions

Over the last decade, incredible strides have been made in understanding the long-term and often pervasive effects humans have had on a variety of marine ecosystems, including a diverse range of marine animals (Braje, 2010; Braje & Rick, 2011; Jackson et al., 2001; Rick & Erlandson, 2009; Starkey, Holm, & Barnard, 2008). Recent archaeological studies have demonstrated, for example, that humans have engaged in fishing for tens of thousands of years. The archaeological record of shellfish gathering extends back at least 700,000 years (see Erlandson, 2001, 2010) and the earliest evidence of fishing technology and finfishing (the capture of finfish that required specialized technology such as boats, fishhooks, harpoons, or nets or traps) comes from the banks of the Congo River with Middle Stone Age bone harpoons dated to about 90,000 years ago (Yellen, Brooks, Cornelissen, Mehlman, & Stewart, 1995).

Archaeological evidence also suggests that predation by early agriculturalists on wild aquatic fauna has been associated with reductions in biodiversity, average body size, and abundances. Desse and Desse-Berset (1994) demonstrated, for example, an overall reduction in average body size of large groupers and other fish captured off Cyprus beginning about 8,000 years ago. Morales, Rosello, and Canas (1994) documented a decrease in fish diversity and average size over 12,000 years ago at Andalusian Cave, Spain. Wing (1994) found decreases in the mean trophic level of coral reef fish (3.78 in 1500 cal BP to 3.6 in 600 cal BP) from shell middens on St. Thomas, Virgin Islands. Bourque, Johnson, and Steneck (2008) found compelling evidence for hunter-gatherers fishing down marine food webs in the Gulf of Maine beginning over 4,000 years ago, where cod and other apex predators decline in abundance through time. Rick and Erlandson (2008) recently edited an entire volume dedicated to worldwide case studies of human interactions with marine ecosystems, demonstrating that humans have played a significant role in shaping nearshore marine fauna for millennia.

Below, I review three cases of such human manipulations of marine fauna. While examples from terrestrial animals have been more widely recognized, the seas have long been considered too vast and diverse and offering enough hidden recesses, crack and crevasses, that ancient hunter-gatherer-fishers could never have induced measurable impacts to marine animals. Additionally, it has long been assumed that after considerable impacts to a variety of marine mammals, fish, and shellfish by modern commercial overfishing, reducing predation pressure would allow marine organisms to recover along a "natural" trajectory (see Ellis, 2003 for a review of the scale of historic and modern commercial overfishing). The following case studies illustrate the fallacy of these assumptions; the first demonstrates that sea mammals of the northeastern Pacific have undergone considerable changes in their biogeography as they have repopulated the Pacific after historic overhunting and the second and third illustrate that ancient people have had a heavy hand in shaping local marine animal compositions and the structure and function of nearshore and kelp forest ecosystems for thousands of years.

Seals, Sea Lions, and Ancient Phase Shifts

From about the mid-seventeenth to early twentieth centuries, the North Pacific could be adequately described as a "sea of slaughter." During this interval, Spanish, Russian, British, and American traders competed in a frantic race to harvest the luxuriant fur of the sea otter (*Enhydra lutris*), a commodity fetching exorbitant prices in overseas Chinese markets (Ellis, 2003). With the emergence of the first truly global industrialized economies, the sea mammal hunting industry expanded to include many pinnipeds—seals, sea lions, and similar animals with finlike flippers—and cetaceans. Marine mammals were relentlessly hunted to (or beyond) the brink of extinction for their blubber, furs, ivory, and other products or purposes.

Nearly extinct as recently as 50 years ago, North Pacific seal and sea lion populations now number in the hundreds of thousands. The northern elephant seal, for example, has made a remarkable recovery during the past 100 years, expanding from a small relict population on Isla de Guadalupe, Baja California, Mexico, in AD 1892 to a current population of approximately 150,000 animals (see Busch, 1985; Ellis, 2003). Although still extirpated from much of its prehistoric range, estimates of the current North Pacific sea otter population exceed 150,000, rebounded from only 13 colonies, composed of about 1,000–2,000 individuals, in the early twentieth century (Ellis, 2003). Similar population growth has been documented among northern elephant seals and Guadalupe fur seals, while others like Alaskan populations of Steller sea lions are in a state of decline.

Federal protection beginning in the early twentieth century and the passage of the 1972 Marine Mammal Protection Act have resulted in the recovery of many species to levels that may be comparable to those prior to intensive historical predation (Jefferson, Weber, & Pitman, 2008). Given an adequate food base, most pinnipeds are assumed to be repopulating Pacific Coast waters, establishing rookeries, and, perhaps, recovering to "prehistoric levels," the product of deeply engrained evolutionary forces. Nowhere is the success of marine mammal management and recovery more obvious than on California's Channel Islands. Today, this group of eight offshore islands shelter more than 200,000 seals and sea lions of six different species, including the California sea lion (*Zalophus californianus*), the northern elephant seal (*Mirounga angustirostris*), the northern fur seal (*Callorhinus ursinus*), the harbor seal (*Phoca vitulina*) and the relatively rare Steller sea lion (*Eumetopias jubatus*) and Guadalupe fur seal (*Arctocephalus townsendi*), and more than a dozen large and small cetacean species swim through or are seasonally resident in island waters (DeLong & Melin, 2002).

Since the historic blitzkrieg and the worldwide decimation of marine mammal populations occurred so quickly, there are very few historical records prior to the mid-nineteenth century to test whether or not the modern distributions of these animals are following "natural" trajectories. Archaeology, then, is one of the few sources of data for reconstructing pinniped biogeography. Recent syntheses from coastal North Pacific archaeological sites suggest, however, that there have been dramatic shifts in the biogeography of these animals as they have expanded their ranges and recolonized the Pacific over the last several decades. Guadalupe fur seals, for example, were considerably more common in California, especially in southern California, than they are today (Rick, DeLong, et al., 2009). Their remains are commonly identified in archaeological sites but they rarely venture outside of waters off Mexico today. Conversely, northern elephant seals are a common sight throughout California and the larger North Pacific; however, their remains are rarely found in archaeological sites in much of their present range (Rick et al., n.d.). An understanding of the long-term history of human–animal interactions, then, may be key to illuminating the biogeography, natural history, and management of marine (and terrestrial) organisms around the world.

Shellfish "Farming"

Humans have been harvesting abundant and easy-to-gather shellfish taxa for hundreds of thousands of years. It is not until about 23,000 years ago, however, that evidence for a human–shellfish experience emerges with hunter-gatherers influencing the size and structure of nearshore communities (Steele & Klein, 2008; Stiner, 2001; Rick & Erlandson, 2009). As humans migrated to new regions of the globe over the last 10,000 years, these influences expanded and intensified. Often times, this came in the form of direct predation pressure and a decline in the average size of prey shellfish over time (e.g., Anderson, 2001; deBoer, Pereira, & Guissamulo, 2000; Erlandson et al., 2008; Mannino & Thomas, 2002; Morrison & Hunt, 2007). Recent research has revealed cases of a much more intimate relationship between humans and shellfish communities, suggesting a long history of complex interactions.

On the Northwest Coast of North America, Williams (2006), with the help of a Klahoose elder, documented a series of terraced rock features in the intertidal zone of Waiatt Bay and Gorge Harbour on the northeast end of Vancouver Island, British Columbia. In total, Williams (2006) recorded over 400 relict rock-walled structures, visible only at the lowest tides. These "clam gardens" were used by indigenous peoples to promote butter clam growth, a process Williams (2006) calls "mariculture," or agriculture of the seas. Hunter-gatherers expanded and maintained these clam gardens, likely increasing clam yields, and although their antiquity is poorly known they probably span centuries or, perhaps, millennia. This is a powerful example of how hunter-gatherers intentionally managed marine ecosystems and local animal communities, akin to anthropogenic burning of terrestrial landscapes to promote the growth of seed-bearing plants that could be harvested for human consumption and to attract economically important game animals.

Research also has demonstrated that coastal hunter-foragers in the deep past, at times, played a significant role in shaping the structure and function of nearshore coastal communities. Incorporating a diverse set of archaeological, ecological, historical, and paleoclimatological data, researchers have found that Native American predation of sea otters in California beginning about 9,000 years ago and in the Aleutians about 3,000 years ago resulted in significant changes in Pacific food webs (see Braje et al., 2009; Corbett et al., 2008). Whether intentional or not, the reduction of sea otters, a keystone predator of many marine shellfish taxa, from local watersheds released abalone, sea urchins, and other shellfish from predation pressure and allowed for increased sizes and densities. This outcome would have been advantageous to local foragers who often relied on shellfish for their daily subsistence. Data suggest, however, that there also may have been unintended negative consequences. Zooarchaeological evidence from stratified shell midden deposits suggests that this trophic cascade may have created localized urchin barrens, where sea urchin populations are so large that they feed directly on kelp holdfasts and deforest the local seascape. Kelp provides much of the prime productivity for many nearshore ecosystems, and a deforested seascape would be an ecological disaster analogous to an unchecked terrestrial wildfire. Increased human predation on sea urchins likely kept urchin barrens to a short-lived phenomenon, but demonstrate the dramatic effects humans have long had on nearshore and kelp forest ecosystems for millennia.

Animal Conservation Biology, Archaeology, and the Myth of Pristine

In this chapter, I provided a set of themes and case studies, grounded in historical ecology, in an attempt to demonstrate that humans, and particularly AMHs, have not just adapted to local environments, rather, they have played a powerful role in shaping ecosystems and vertebrate faunal land- and seascapes. Through a constant dialectical interaction between humans, the environment, organisms, and natural climate systems (see Balée, 1998; Crumley, 1994), the anthropogenic world we know today has taken shape. Until recently, the basic assumption has been that humanity's influence on nature and faunal communities in the deep past was negligible. The notion that dramatic anthropogenic forcing on local and regional ecosystems did not begin until the advent of complex, state-level sociopolitical organization has been shown to severely underestimate the influence of humans (Grayson, 2001; Rick & Erlandson, 2008, 2009; Redman, 1999; Redman et al., 2004). In North America, for example, there are virtually no post-Pleistocene ecosystems, landscapes, or faunal communities (except perhaps far corners of the Arctic and some high elevations) that have not been influenced by human activity, and, thus, could be considered natural or pristine.

This stands in stark contrast to many concepts that currently underpin conservation biology and wildlife management. Concepts such as sustainability, conservation, preservation, and wilderness are heavily value laden, often dictated by a personal or policy vision of what is "natural" or "pristine" (Lyman & Cannon, 2004, p. 5). This vision is extremely fluid, influenced by a complex mix of ecological, social, political, and economic values. Kay and Simmons (2002b, pgs. xiv-xv) have referred to this phenomenon as "political ecology," where scientific data are selected (or manufactured) "to support preordained philosophical values or political agendas." As such, there are generally no agreed-upon definitions of many integral conservation concepts, such as what constitutes a wilderness area. Is this a location where no human presence is allowed? Or, is it an area that is actively managed by humans through culling animal populations, burning the landscape, and other similar influences known to have occurred before European arrival? These are common questions and concerns when looking at the management goals of national parks within the United States. Charles Kay (2002, pgs. 259–260) points out, for example, that Yellowstone National Park, ". . . now contains some of the worst overgrazed riparian areas in the nation. . . because park managers and environmentalists refuse to abandon misguided concepts of 'wilderness' and 'natural regulation,' while ignoring the fact that aboriginal people were once a critical component of that and other ecosystems." Kay (2002) suggests that the lack of management and culling of bison populations within the park has resulted in a severely degraded terrestrial ecosystem.

ar debate is currently playing itself out in Channel Islands National Park, see Levy, 2010). Here, biologists and park managers have undertaken decade-long captive breeding program to save the endangered island _ocyon littoralis_) and to reintroduce it to the wild. Part of the justification for this multimillion dollar project has been that island foxes are a "natural" part of the landscape, perhaps evolving from a single, pregnant mainland grey fox that unintentionally rafted out to the islands 14,000 or more years ago. Recent archaeological work has suggested, however, that mainland foxes may have been intentionally transported to the islands by Native Americans as little as 6,000 years ago (Rick, Erlandson, et al., 2009). While this may not change their right to federal protection and millions of dollars in recovery efforts, it certainly raises questions as to how we make management decisions. Should Native American dogs be reintroduced to the Channel Islands, for instance, since they also lived on the islands for millennia prior to European contact?

It is not my intention here to resolve these issues or to make policy decisions. As archaeologists and other scientists continue to engage in developing long-term histories of animal communities, controversies over wise management practices surely will arise. In some of these cases, major contradictions appear between what the archaeological record shows about the human–animal experience and what contemporary observers, the public, and interest groups would like to believe. In my view, the development of deep historical perspectives of the relationship between humans, animals, and the environment is the key to better understanding and managing animal populations around the world. Objective scientific data, free from political entanglement, with increasingly refined and sophisticated methodologies offers the best opportunity for resource managers, conservation biologists, politicians, and the public to determine the desired future condition of an ecosystem or species and how to best implement resource management strategies.

Summary: Contextualizing the Human–Animal Bond in the Longue Durée

Although the mechanisms and precise timing are poorly understood, beginning at least 50,000 years ago the relationship between AMHs and animals fundamentally changed. It is only after this time that art and ornaments depicting animals and, often, created from animal remains become commonplace (Klein, 2000). Animals, then, transform from more than sources of calories to symbols of nature, the cosmos, or mythology; that is, they are imbued with cultural meaning. Experts disagree on why this is, some arguing that these cognitive abilities were present but "weakly expressed" prior to 50,000 years ago and others that the "modern capacity for culture" only evolved after this time (Klein, 2000, p. 28).

Regardless, after this point, humans began to have far-reaching and accelerating effects on animal communities as they colonized the globe. Extinction events began in the Late Pleistocene, wild animals were transported across continents and to new islands, and even marine fauna were influenced by human action. These impacts are not necessarily coupled with agriculture and state-level societies, but rather to the rise of modern human behavioral traits—likely linked to biological changes in the human brain (Klein, 1989, 2000).

For psychologists and other researchers interested in the human–animal bond, it is essential to recognize that, while this connection has deepened and evolved over time, it began tens of thousands of years ago and was crucial to the adaptive success of AMHs. To understand the modern human–animal bond, it is essential to recognize that it is the product of deeply engrained evolutionary forces, and while malleable, it is not solely the product of contemporary cultural systems. Ultimately, there should be some commonalities linking the nature of the human–animal bond across cultures, time, and space.

Acknowledgments This paper was substantially improved by conversations with Robert DeLong, Jon Erlandson, Douglas Kennett, and Torben Rick. I thank Chris Blazina, David Shen-Miller, and Güler Boyraz for inviting me to participate in this volume and for their constructive comments on an earlier version of this chapter. Any error of fact or omissions, however, are solely my responsibility.

References

Alcorn, J. B. (1993). Indigenous peoples and conservation. *Conservation Biology, 7*, 424–426.

Alcorn, J. B. (1996). Is biodiversity conserved by indigenous peoples? In S. K. Jain (Ed.), *Ethnobiology in human welfare* (pp. 233–238). New Delhi: Deep Publications.

Alroy, J. (1999). Putting North America's end-pleistocene megafaunal extinction in context: Large-scale analyses of spatial patterns, extinction rates, and size distributions. In R. D. E. MacPhee (Ed.), *Extinctions in near time: Causes, contexts, and consequences* (pp. 105–143). New York: Kluwer Academic.

Alroy, J. (2001). A multispecies overkill simulation of the end-pleistocene megafaunal mass extinction. *Science, 292*, 1893–1896.

Anderson, A. (2001). No meat on that beautiful shore: The prehistoric abandonment of subtropical polynesian islands. *International Journal of Osteoarchaeology, 11*, 14–23.

Anderson, A. (2009). The rat and the octopus: Initial human colonization and the prehistoric introduction of domestic animals to Remote Oceania. *Biological Invasions, 11*, 1503–1519.

Armitage, P. L. (1994). Unwelcome companions: Ancient rats reviewed. *Antiquity, 68*, 231–240.

Bahn, P. G., & Flenley, J. (1992). *Easter island, earth island: A message from our past for the future of our planet.* New York: Thames & Hudson.

Balée, W. (Ed.) (1998). *Advances in historical ecology.* New York: Columbia University Press.

Balée, W., & Erickson, C. (Eds.) (2006). *Time and complexity in historical ecology: Studies in neotropical lowlands.* New York: Columbia University Press.

Barnosky, A. D., Koch, P. L., Feranec, R. S., Wing, S. L., & Shabel, A. B. (2004). Assessing the causes of late pleistocene extinctions on the continents. *Science, 306*, 70–75.

Binford, L. R. (1985). Human ancestors: Changing views of their behavior. *Journal of Anthropological Archaeology, 4*, 292–327.

Blench, R. (2007). New paleozoogeographical evidence for the settlement of madagascar. *Azania, 42*, 69–82.

Bourque, B. J., Johnson, B. J., & Steneck, R. S. (2008). Possible prehistoric fishing effects on coastal marine food webs in the Gulf of Maine. In T. C. Rick & J. M. Erlandson (Eds.), *Human impacts on ancient marine environments* (pp. 165–185). Santa Barbara: University of California Press.

Bouzouggar, A., Barton, N., Vanhaeren, M., d'Errico, F., Collcutt, S., Higham, T., et al. (2007). 82,000 year-old shell beads from North Africa and implications for the origins of modern human behavior. *Proceedings of the National Academy of Sciences, 104*, 9964–9969.

Braje, T. J. (2010). *Modern oceans, ancient sites: Archaeology and marine conservation on San Miguel Island, California.* Salt Lake City, UT: University of Utah Press.

Braje, T. J., Erlandson, J. M., Rick, T. C., Dayton, P. K., & Hatch, M. (2009). Fishing from past to present: Long-term continuity and resilience of red abalone fisheries on California's northern channel islands. *Ecological Applications, 19*, 906–919.

Braje, T. J. & Rick, T. C. (Eds.). (2011). *Human impacts on ancient seals, sea lions, and sea otters: Integrating archaeology, history, and ecology in the Northeast Pacific.* Berkeley, CA: The University of California Press.

Brook, F. J. (1999). Changes in the landsnail fauna of Lady Alice Island, northeastern New Zealand. *Journal of the Royal Society of New Zealand, 29*, 135–157.

Brook, B. W., & Bowman, D. M. J. S. (2002). Explaining the pleistocene megafaunal extinctions: Models, chronologies, and assumptions. *Proceedings of the National Academy of Sciences, 100*, 10800–10805.

Brook, B. W., & Bowman, D. M. J. S. (2004). The uncertain blitzkrieg of pleistocene megafauna. *Journal of Biogeography, 31*, 517–523.

Busch, B. C. (1985). *The war against the seals: A history of the North American seal fishery.* Kingston, ON: McGill-Queen's University Press.

Chase, P. G. (1988). Scavenging and hunting in the middle paleolithic: The evidence from Europe. In H. L. Dibble & A. Montet-White (Eds.), *Upper pleistocene prehistory of Western Asia* (pp. 225–232). Philadelphia: University Museum, University of Pennsylvania.

Chauvet, J. -M., Deschamps, E. B., & Hillaire, C. (1996). *The dawn of art: The chauvet cave, the oldest known paintings in the world.* New York: Abrams.

Collins, P. W. (1991). Interaction between island foxes (*Urocyon littoralis*) and Indians on islands off the coast of Southern California: I. Morphologic and archaeological evidence of human assisted dispersal. *Journal of Ethnobiology, 11*, 51–81.

Corbett, D. G., Causey, D., Clementz, M., Koch, P. L., Doroff, A., Lefèvre, C., et al. (2008). Aleut hunters, sea otters, and sea cows: Three thousand years of interactions in the Western Aleutian Islands, Alaska. In T. C. Rick & J. M. Erlandson (Eds.), *Human impacts on ancient marine ecosystems: A global perspective* (pp. 43–75). Berkeley, CA: University of California Press.

Crumley, C. (1994). Historical ecology: A multidimensional ecological orientation. In C. Crumley (Ed.), *Historical ecology: Cultural knowledge and changing landscapes* (pp. 1–16). Santa Fe, NM: School of American Research Press.

de France, S. D., Keegan, W. F., & Newsom, L. A. (1996). The archaeobotanical, bone isotope, and zooarchaeological records from Caribbean sites in comparative perspective. In E. J. Reitz, L. A. Newson, & S. J. Scudder (Eds.), *Case studies in environmental archaeology* (pp. 289–304). New York: Plenum Press.

Dean, R. M. (Ed.). (2009). *The Archaeology of Anthropogenic Environments.* Center for Archaeological Investigations, Occasional Paper No. 37, Southern Illinois University, Carbondale.

deBoer, W. F., Pereira, T., & Guissamulo, A. (2000). Comparing recent and abandoned shell middens to detect the impact of human exploitation on the intertidal ecosystem. *Aquatic Ecology, 34*, 287–297.

DeLong, R. L., & Melin, S. R. (2002). Thirty years of Pinniped research at San Miguel Island. In D. Brown, K. Mitchell, & H. Chaney (Eds.), *The fifth California islands symposium (CD publication)* (pp. 401–406). U.S. Department of the Interior Minerals Management Service, Pacific OCS Region.

Desse, J., & Desse-Berset, N. (1994). Osteometry and fishing strategies at Cape Andreas Kastos (Cyprus, 8th millenium BP). In W. van Neer (Ed.), *Fish exploitation in the past* (pp. 67–79). Tervuren, Belgium: Annales du Musee Royale pour L'Afrique Centrale.

Diamond, J. (1997). *Guns, germs, and steel: The fates of human societies.* New York: W. W. Norton & Company.

Diamond, J. (2003). The last Americans: Environmental collapse at the end of civilization. *Harper's Magazine, 306*, 43–51.

Diamond, J. (2005). *Collapse: How societies choose to fail or succeed*. New York: Viking Press.

d'Errico, F., Henshilwood, C., Vanhaeren, M., & van Niekerk, K. (2005). *Nassarius kraussianus* shell beads from blombos cave: evidence for symbolic behaviour in the middle stone age. *Journal of Human Evolution, 48*, 3–24.

Egan, D., & Howell, E. A. (Eds.). (2001). *The historical ecology handbook: A restorationist's guide to reference ecosystems*. Washington, DC: Island Press.

Ellis, R. (2003). *The empty ocean*. Washington, DC: Island Press/Shearwater Books.

Erlandson, J. M. (2001). The archaeology of aquatic adaptations: Paradigms for a new millennium. *Journal of Archaeological Research, 9*, 287–350.

Erlandson, J. M. (2010). Food for thought: The role of coastlines and aquatic resources in human evolution. In S. Cunnane & K. Steward (Eds.), *Environmental influences on human brain evolution.* (pp. 125–136). Hoboken, NJ: John Wiley & Sons, Inc.

Erlandson, J. M., Rick, T. C., Braje, T. J., Steinberg, A., & Vellanoweth, R. (2008). Human impacts on ancient shellfish: A 10,000 year record from San Miguel Island, California. *Journal of Archaeological Science, 35*, 2144–2152.

Fiedel, S., & Haynes, G. (2004). A premature burial: Comments on Grayson and Meltzer's "Requiem for Overkill". *Journal of Archaeological Science, 31*, 121–131.

Firestone, R. B., West, A., Kennett, J. P., Becker, L., Bunch, T. E., Revay, Z. S., et al. (2007). Evidence for an extraterrestrial impact 12,900 years ago that contributed to the megafaunal extinctions and the Younger Dryas cooling. *Proceedings of the National Academy of Sciences, 104*, 16016–16021.

Flannery, T. F., Bellwood, P., White, J. P., Ennis, T., Irwin, G., Schubert, K., et al. (1998). Mammals from Holocene archaeological deposits on Gebe and Morotai Islands, Northern Moluccas, Indonesia. *Australian Mammalogy, 20*, 391–400.

Flannery, T. F., & White, J. P. (1991). Animal translocation. *National Geographic Research and Exploration, 70*, 96–113.

Flenley, J. R. (1993). The paleoecology of Easter Island, and its ecological disaster. In S. R. Fischer (Ed.), *Easter Island studies: Contributions to the history of Rapanui in memory of William T. Mulloy* (Oxbow Monograph No. 32, pp. 27–45). Oxford: Oxbow Books.

Flenley, J. R., King, A. S. M., Jackson, J., & Chew, C. (1991). The late quaternary vegetational and climatic history of Easter Island. *Journal of Quaternary Science, 6*, 85–115.

Frazier, J. G. (2009). Call of the wild. In R. M. Dean (Ed.), *The archaeology of anthropogenic environments* (pp. 341–369). Center for Archaeological Investigations, Occasional Paper No. 37, Southern Illinois University, Carbondale.

Grayson, D. K. (1984). Explaining pleistocene extinctions: Thoughts on the structure of a debate. In P. S. Martin & R. G. Klein (Eds.), *Quaternary extinctions: A prehistoric revolution* (pp. 807–823). Tucson, AZ: University of Arizona Press.

Grayson, D. K. (1991). Late pleistocene extinctions in North America: Taxonomy, chronology, and explanations. *Journal of World Prehistory, 5*, 193–232.

Grayson, D. K. (2001). The archaeological record of human impacts on animal populations. *Journal of World Prehistory, 15*, 1–68.

Grayson, D. K. (2007). Deciphering North American pleistocene extinctions. *Journal of Anthropological Research, 63*, 185–213.

Grayson, D. K., & Meltzer, D. J. (2003). A requiem for North American overkill. *Journal of Archaeological Science, 30*, 585–993.

Griffith, B., Scott, J. M., Carpenter, J. W., & Reed, C. (1989). Translocation as a species conservation tool: Status and strategy. *Science, 245*, 477–480.

Henshilwood, C., d'Errico, F., Vanhaeren, M., van Niekerk, K., & Jacobs, Z. (2004). Middle stone age beads from South Africa. *Science, 304*, 404.

Henshilwood, C. S., & Marean, C. W. (2003). The origin of modern human behavior: Critique of the models and their test implications. *Current Anthropology, 44*, 627–651.

Jackson, J. B. C., Kirby, M. X., Berger, W. H., Bjorndal, K. A., Botsford, L. W., Bourque, B. J., et al. (2001). Historical overfishing and the recent collapse of coastal ecosystems. *Science, 293*, 561–748.

Jefferson, T. A., Weber, M. A., & Pitman, R. (2008). *Marine mammals of the world: A comprehensive guide to their identification*. San Diego, CA: Academic Press.

Johnson, D. L. (1983). The California continental borderland: Land bridges, watergaps, and biotic dispersals. In P. M. Masters & N. Flemming (Eds.), *Quaternary coastlines and marine archaeology: Towards the prehistory of land bridges and continental shelves* (pp. 481–527). London: Academic Press.

Kay, C. E. (2002). Afterward: False gods, ecological myths, and biological reality. In C. E. Kay & R. T. Simmons (Eds.), *Wilderness and political ecology* (pp. 238–261). Salt Lake City, UT: University of Utah Press.

Kay, C. E., & Simmons, R. T. (Eds.). (2002a). *Wilderness and political ecology: Aboriginal influences and the original state of nature*. Salt Lake City, UT: The University of Utah Press.

Kay, C. E., & Simmons, R. T. (2002b). Preface. In C. E. Kay & R. T. Simmons (Eds.), *Wilderness and political ecology: Aboriginal influences and the original state of nature* (pp. xi-xix). Salt Lake City, UT: The University of Utah Press.

Kirch, P. V. (1996). Late Holocene human–induced modifications to a central Polynesian island ecosystem. *Proceedings of the National Academy of Sciences, 93*, 5296–5300.

Kirch, P. V. (1997). Microcosmic histories: Island perspectives on "Global" change. *American Anthropologist, 99*, 30–42.

Kirch, P. V. (2004). Oceanic Islands: Microcosms of "Global Change". In C. L. Redman, S. R. James, P. R. Fish, & J. D. Rogers (Eds.), *The archaeology of global change: The impact of humans on their environment* (pp. 13–27). Washington, DC: Smithsonian Books.

Kirch, P. V., Steadman, D. W., Butler, V. L., Hather, J., & Weisler, M. I. (1995). Prehistory and human ecology at Tangatatau Rockshelter, Mangaia, Cook Islands. *Archaeology in Oceania, 30*, 47–65.

Klein, R. G. (1989). *The human career: Human biological and cultural origins*. Chicago: University of Chicago Press.

Klein, R. G. (1994). Southern Africa before the Iron Age. In R. S. Corruccini & R. L. Ciochon (Eds.), *Integrative paths to the past: Paleoanthropological advances in honor of F. Clark Howell* (pp. 471–519). Englewood Cliffs, NJ: Prentice-Hall.

Klein, R. G. (2000). Archaeology and the evolution of human behavior. *Evolutionary Anthropology, 9*, 17–36.

Koopman, K. F., & Steadman, D. W. (1995). *Extinction and Biogeography of Bats on 'Eua, Kingdom of Tonga*. American Museum Novitates No. 3125.

Krech, S., III. (1999). *The ecological Indian: Myth and history*. New York: W.W. Norton.

Krech, S., III. (2005). Reflections on conservation, sustainability, and environmentalism in indigenous North America. *American Anthropologist, 107*, 78–86.

Levy, S. (2010). Island fox paradox: Do species introduced by native people thousands of years ago deserve protection? *BioScience, 60*, 332–336.

Lyman, R. L., & Cannon, K. P. (2004). Applied zooarchaeology, because it matters. In R. L. Lyman & K. P. Cannon (Eds.), *Zooarchaeology and conservation biology* (pp. 1–24). Salt Lake City, UT: University of Utah Press.

Mannino, M. A., & Thomas, K. D. (2002). Depletion of a resource? The impact of prehistoric human foraging on intertidal mollusk communities and its significance for human settlement, mobility, and dispersal. *World Archaeology, 33*, 452–474.

Martin, P. S. (2005). *Twilight of the mammoths: Ice age extinctions and the rewilding of America*. Berkeley, CA: University of California Press.

Martin, P. S., & Klein, R. G. (1984). *Quaternary extinctions: A prehistoric revolution*. Tucson, AZ: University of Arizona Press.

Matisoo, S. E. (2009). The commensal model for human colonization of the pacific 10 years on—what can we say and where to now? *Journal of Island and Coastal Archaeology, 4*, 151–163.

Mcbrearty, S., & Brooks, A. S. (2000). The revolution that wasn't: A new interpretation of the origin of modern human behavior. *Journal of Human Evolution, 39*, 453–563.

McGovern, T. H., Vésteinsson, O., Fridriksson, A., Church, M., Lawson, I., Simpson, I. A., et al. (2008). Landscapes of settlement in Northern Iceland: Historical ecology of human impact and climate fluctuation on the millennial scale. *American Anthropologist, 109*, 27–51.

Miller, G. H., Magee, J. W., Johnson, B. J., Fogel, M. L., Spooner, N. A., McCulloch, M. T., et al. (1999). Pleistocene extinction of *Genyornis newtoni*: Human impact on Australian megafauna. *Science, 283*, 205–208.

Minnis, P. E., Whalen, M. E., Kelley, J. H., & Stewart, J. D. (1993). Prehistoric macaw breeding in the North American Southwest. *American Antiquity, 58*, 270–276.

Morales, A., Rosello, E., & Canas, J. M. (1994). Cueva de Nerja (prov. Malaga): A close look at a twelve thousand year ichthyofaunal sequence from Southern Spain. In W. van Neer (Ed.), *Fish exploitation in the past* (pp. 253–262). Tervuren, Belgium: Annales du Musee Royale pour L'Afrique Centrale.

Morrison, A. E., & Hunt, T. L. (2007). Human impacts on the nearshore environment: An archaeological case study from Kaua'I, Hawaiian Islands. *Pacific Science, 61*, 325–345.

Nagaoka, L. (2005). Declining foraging efficiency and moa carcass exploitation in Southern New Zealand. *Journal of Anthropological Archaeology, 21*, 419–442.

Owen-Smith, R. N. (1988). *Megaherbivores: The influence of very large body size on ecology.* New York: Cambridge University Press.

Pregill, K. P., & Dye, T. (1989). Prehistoric extinction of giant iguanas in Tonga. *Copeia, 1989*, 505–508.

Redman, C. L. (1999). *Human impact on ancient environments.* Tucson, AZ: University of Arizona Press.

Redman, C. L., James, S. R., Fish, P. R., & Rogers, D. (Eds.). (2004). *The archaeology of global change: The impact of humans on their environment.* Washington, DC: Smithsonian Books.

Reese, D. S. (1996). *Pleistocene and Holocene Fauna of Crete and its First Settlers.* Monographs in World Archaeology No 28, Madison, WI, USA

Rick, T. C. (in press). Hunter-gatherers, endemic island mammals, and the historical ecology of California's channel islands. In V. Thompson & J. Waggoner (Eds.), *Hunter-gatherers and shell midden archaeology.*

Rick, T. C., DeLong, R. L., Erlandson, J. M., Braje, T. J., Jones, T. L., Kennett, D. J., et al. (2009). A trans-holocene archaeological record of guadalupe fur seals (*Arctocephalus townsendi*) on the California coast. *Marine Mammal Science, 25*, 487–502.

Rick, T. C., DeLong, R. L., Erlandson, J. M., Jones, T. L., Braje, T. J., Arnold, J. E., et al. (in press). Where were the northern elephant seals? Archaeology and holocene biogeography of *Mirounga angustirostris. The Holocene.*

Rick, T. C., & Erlandson, J. M. (Eds.). (2008). *Human impacts on ancient marine environments: A global perspective.* Berkeley, CA: University of California Press.

Rick, T. C., & Erlandson, J. M. (2009). Coastal exploitation. *Science, 325*, 952–953.

Rick, T. C., Erlandson, J. M., Vellanoweth, R. L., Braje, T. J., Collins, P. W., Guthrie, D. A., et al. (2009). The origins and antiquity of the island fox (*Urocyon littoralis*): AMS [14]C Dates from California's channel islands. *Quaternary Research, 71*, 93–98.

Roberts, R. G., Flannery, T. F., Ayliffe, L. K., Yoshida, H., Olley, J. M., Prideaux, G. J., et al. (2001). New Ages for the late Australian megafauna: Continent-wide extinction of prey populations. *Nature, 412*, 183–186.

Simenstad, C. A., Estes, J. A., & Kenyon, K. W. (1978). Aleuts, sea otters, and alternate stable-state communities. *Science, 200*, 403–411.

Sluyter, A. (2001). Colonialism and landscape in the Americas: Material/conceptual transformation and continuing consequences. *Annuals of the Association of American Geographers, 91*, 410–428.

Smith, E. A., & Wishnie, M. (2000). Conservation and subsistence in small-scale societies. *Annual Review of Anthropology, 29*, 493–524.

Sonddar, P. Y. (2000). Early human exploration and exploitation of islands. *Tropics, 10*, 203–229.

Springer, A. M., Estes, J. A., van Vliet, G. B., Williams, T. M., Doak, D. F., Danner, E. M., et al. (2003). Sequential megafaunal collapse in the North Pacific Ocean: An ongoing legacy of industrial whaling? *Proceedings of the National Academy of Sciences, 100*, 12223–12228.

Starkey, D. J., Holm, P., Barnard, M. (Eds.). (2008). *Oceans past: Management insights from the history of marine animal populations*. London: Earthscan.

Steadman, D. W. (1989). New species and records of birds (Aves: Megapodiidae, Columbidae) from an archaeological site on Lifuka, Tonga. *Proceedings of the Biological Society of Washington, 102*, 537–552.

Steadman, D. W., & Kirch, P. V. (1990). Prehistoric extinction of birds on Mangaia, Cook Island, Polynesia. *Proceedings of the National Academy of Sciences, 87*, 9605–9609.

Steadman, D. W., Martin, P. S., MacPhee, R. D. E., Jull, A. J. T., McDonald, H. G., Woods, C. A., et al. (2005). Asynchronous extinction of late quaternary sloths on continents and islands. *Proceedings of the National Academy of Sciences, 102*, 11763–11768.

Steadman, D. W., Pregill, G. K., & Burley, D. V. (2002). Rapid prehistoric extinction of iguanas and birds in Polynesia. *Proceedings of the National Academy of Sciences, 99*, 3673–3677.

Steele, T. E., & Klein, R. G. (2008). Intertidal shellfish use during the middle and later stone age of South Africa. *Archaeofauna: International Journal of Archaeozoology, 17*, 63–76.

Stiner, M. C. (2001). Thirty years on the "Broad Spectrum Revolution" and paleolithic demography. *Proceedings of the National Academy of Sciences, 98*, 6993–6996.

Surovell, T., Waguespack, N., & Brantingham, P. J. (2005). Global archaeological evidence for proboscidean overkill. *Proceedings of the National Academy of Sciences, 102*, 6231–6236.

Vanhaeren, M., d'Errico, F., Stringer, C., James, S. L., Todd, J. A., & Mienis, H. K. (2006). Middle paleolithic shell beads in Israel and Algeria. *Science, 312*, 1785–1788.

Vigne, J. D., & Valladas, H. (1996). Small mammal fossil assemblages as indicators of environmental change in Northern Corsica during the last 2500 years. *Journal of Archaeological Science, 23*, 199–215.

White, J. P. (2004). Where the wild things are: Prehistoric animal translocations in the circum New Guinea archipelago. In S. M. Fitzpatrick (Ed.), *Voyages of discovery: The archaeology of islands* (pp. 147–164). Westport: Prager.

Williams, J. (2006). *Clam gardens: Aboriginal mariculture on Canada's West Coast*. Vancouver, BC: Transmontanus.

Wing, E. S. (1993). The realm between wild and domestic. In A. Clason, S. Payne, & H. P. Uerpmann (Eds.), *Skeletons in her cupboard: Festschrift for Juliet Clutton-Brock* (Oxbow Monograph No. 34, pp. 243–250). Oxford: Oxbow Books.

Wing, E. S. (1994). Patterns of prehistoric fishing in the West Indies. *Archaeofauna, 3*, 99–107.

Wroe, S., Field, J., Fullagar, R., & Jermin, L. S. (2004). Megafaunal extinction in the late quaternary and the global overkill hypothesis. *Alcheringa: An Australasian Journal of Palaeontology, 28*, 291–331.

Wroe, S., Field, J., & Grayson, D. K. (2006). Megafaunal extinction: Climate, humans, and assumptions. *Trends in Ecology and Evolution, 21*, 61–62.

Yellen, J. E., Brooks, A. S., Cornelissen, E., Mehlman, M. J., & Stewart, K. (1995). A middle stone-age worked bone industry from Katanda, Upper Semliki, Zaire. *Science, 268*, 553–556.

Zeder, M. A. (2008). Domestication and early agriculture in the Mediterranean basin: Origins, diffusion, and impact. *Proceedings of the National Academy of Sciences, 105*, 11597–11604.

Chapter 5
Predator–Prey Relationships: What Humans Can Learn from Horses about Being Whole

Judy Skeen

Overview

While the debate about the role of religion in environmental movements continues, the movement to care for creation is fueled by convictions shared by the nonreligious and the devout, the Judeo-Christian Westerner and the Tibetan monk. As life in industrialized culture becomes more insulated from the rhythms of seasons, climate, and wild creatures, those humans who are drawn to a kinship with all things resist ✓ this insulated living and work to restore the natural environment. Reconnection with human dependency upon, and participation in, nature's rhythms becomes a spiritual task, even when unrelated to religious practice. At the heart of this paradox is a foundational question about the value of nature and the role of humans. When the concept of human dominion over nature is questioned, the door opens for a multiplicity of relational bonds with fellow creatures and the world. If the role of nonhuman animals is greater than simply function or resource for humans, they may be able not only to teach about life and the world, but also about the interconnectedness of all life. When a hierarchy that places humans as more valuable is no longer assumed, measuring intelligent life by other than human intelligence standards is possible. This openness will challenge familiar ways of being—mentally, emotionally, and spiritually.

With the traditions within major world religions as a gathering place, this essay explores a possible way through the spiritual lens into a life of learning and growth alongside all living beings. If, beyond master or steward, humans can be partners with other living beings, the possibilities for a shared natural future expand, rather than narrow. Finally, through the example of one educator's experience of learning to communicate with horses, this chapter will illustrate stepping beyond the question of who is in charge, to the possibility of what can be learned when humans enter into relationship with other creatures with the goal of wholeness for all. With the seed of pondering predatory and prey behavior and communication, this experience of learning "natural horsemanship" has brought into view issues of identity, intuitive

J. Skeen (✉)
School of Religion, Belmont University, Nashville, TN, USA
e-mail: judy.skeen@belmont.edu

C. Blazina et al. (eds.), *The Psychology of the Human–Animal Bond*,
DOI 10.1007/978-1-4419-9761-6_5, © Springer Science+Business Media, LLC 2011

focus, intellectual gamesmanship, and development of meaningful work, spiritual depth, and the integrity of living with mindfulness.

The clearing rests in song and shade
It is a creature made
By old light held in soil and leaf,
By human joy and grief,
By human work,
Fidelity of sight and stroke,
By rain, by water on
The parent stone.
We join our work to Heaven's gift,
Our hope to what is left,
That field and woods at last agree
In an economy
Of widest worth.
High Heaven's Kingdom come on earth.
Imagine Paradise.
O dust, arise!
Wendell Berry (1998)

Introduction

While the field of religion and animals is relatively young as an academic discipline, the question of the human relationship to animals has existed as long as humans have. The connection between what humans believe about themselves and their world and how the "other" living beings fit into that view is reflected in the oldest of human artifacts, and in the images drawn in the walls of caves, telling the story of human life, full of animals who walked and worked alongside the humans. Embedded within these ancient images is the central question of the relationship from the human perspective: what are animals for? Within the question is the assumption that the human is more central and the "other animal" is here for the human; the human determines the value of the other. These ideas are given shape within the social and religious understandings of the human culture. To reflect as humans upon the presence of animals in the world is to call into question many assumptions: Is function central to the relationship? Is the human at the center of the question? Does what humans believe about hierarchy determine the worth and the "use" of the animal? As scientific discoveries continue to demonstrate how remarkably alike nonhuman brain physiology is to human brain physiology might it be worth asking: Are animals kin to humans in ways beyond physiology? Might humans and nonhumans animals be kin spiritually? Is it possible that to look from a religious or spiritual standpoint at the presence of creatures in the world offers alternative relational frameworks? And might the current crisis of degrading and declining natural resources in the face of increased population and multiplying industrial demands upon these same resources be an opportunity for revisiting these questions and perspectives with a new lens for finding the human place in the global setting?

By examining multiple traditional religious lenses which have given, and are giving, shape to humans relating to animals, some common threads develop. These common threads can then be used for exploring the potential of linking human spiritual development, shared global environmental sustainability, and partnership with animals.

Ecology and Religion as a Context for Animals and Religion

Using the academy as a marker, the organized theological conversation about animals and religion has existed since 1998 when the Animals and Religion group convened for the first time at the American Academy of Religion in San Francisco. Of course, the question has existed within the larger conversation about religion and ecology longer and before that existed within classic theological arguments about the nature of creation and the human responsibility toward other creatures. To narrow the conversation too quickly or perhaps at all is to lose the context of the interconnectedness of all life. This specialization is itself a symptom of the divided thinking being done by humans when they create a unique category for themselves from other creatures. Setting this particularity in the context of religious understandings of the human–animal relationship gives shape to the broader possibility as well as points to the complexity of defining by differentiation rather than discerning through the discovery of commonality.

Humans Relating to Animals in Religious Traditions

Each of the five major world religions (Hinduism, Buddhism, Judaism, Christianity, and Islam) contains within its traditions material which addresses ideal human behavior and also how to manage or deal with less-than-ideal human situations. Each has sacred texts and teaching which can be interpreted as valuing nonhuman animal life alongside humans; as well as material which can be interpreted to place nonhuman animal life below the life of humans. All of the major world religions have in their histories what would be considered cruelty toward animals by minimum standards today. Likewise, still existing in most wide-ranging traditions are practices and teachings which give support to the subjugation of nonhuman animals. Many sources are available which offer greater detail on the religious traditions and their teaching about animals. By looking selectively at classic texts, traditions, current practices, and new expressions, a broad, although not exhaustive, image of religious perspectives can be gleaned. Many other religious traditions exist and are worthy of investigation and discussion in this conversation about religion and the natural world.

The resources available from the world's religious groups addressing the environmental crisis are growing exponentially (e.g., Cummings, 1991; Foltz, 2003; Gottlieb, 2004; Maguire, 2000). Within these resources, the issue of human–animal relationship can be found both implicit and explicit. Waldau (2005) shows that trends of all the world religions toward nonhuman animals tend to deflate the importance of the animal's role, yet observes that in every tradition of record there are also voices calling these conclusions into question using the core values within the tradition. Often it is the common practice of the tradition which triggers the questioning. Embedded in these responses are insights into the particular question of human–animal relationships as taught and practiced in various traditions. While each religious tradition discussed will receive individual coverage, the traditions will be grouped into three patterned categories: Abrahamic/Monotheistic, Ancient Eastern, and, finally, Native/Indigenous.

Abrahamic/Monotheistic Traditions

From its earliest point, the Judeo-Christian scriptures demonstrate a complexity of the relationship between the Creator and creation that eludes one-dimensional doctrine. The foundational nature of these texts for Judaism, Christianity, and Islam bears consideration. It must be noted, however, that no summary of beliefs or practices can capture the diversity within each of these religious traditions either in the past or the present. Smith (2009) has identified three models of creation which can be evidenced in Genesis 1 and seen throughout the Hebrew scriptures:

(1) God as Divine Power in which God as creator is a warrior-king defeating cosmic enemies. It is believed that this was the prevailing view of creation in the Ancient Near Eastern cultures around ancient Israel, and that its presence in the Old Testament is fragmentary. (Psalm 89:11–13 and Psalm 74:12–17);
(2) God as Divine wisdom in which God is a craftsperson carefully building a world that operates in precise ways. (Psalm 104, Job 38, Isaiah 40:12–14, and Proverbs 8:22–31);
(3) God as Divine Presence in which the world is depicted as God's temple, a divine palace where God presides over the world. (Psalm 8, Psalm 150:1, Isaiah 40:22, and Ezekiel 1).

These models address the primal questions people may ask about a creator God or require of a creation narrative: does God have the power to help humans?; does the world make sense?; and is God here with humanity? In each of these models, humans and nonhuman animals have a purpose, although the model would indicate a variety of purposes within the overall work of the creator. In Judaism, Christianity, and Islam these questions appear to take on an ethic of anthropocentrism which is driven by the belief that the Creator intended humans to be the height of creation and therefore to rule over the other creatures. A closer look at these models allows for a broader understanding of the Creator's ways of relating to all that is created. And within Hebrew scripture, soon after these earliest narratives, come instructions to deal compassionately with the other creatures. The first narrative (Genesis 1:1–2:4a) tells of the creation of all other living forms as well by the same creator. The second narrative (Genesis 2:4b-25) which addresses different details shows the creatures as meant for companionship with the first human created. From that point the sheer number and variety of animals mentioned in Judeo-Christian scriptures demonstrates a creativity of the force of origin. In addition, the characteristics of many nonhuman animals are attributed also to God, as well as narratives showing that nonhuman animals are attuned to the voice of God when humans appear unable to hear or perceive it. In the Book of Job, a long monologue by God repeatedly makes the point (among others) that God created and holds the mysteries of a great many species of animals and that this ongoing creative force and participation in nature is cause for human humility.

Within Abrahamic traditions there is a current debate over the intent in their sacred scriptures toward the natural environment. One can find many examples of both the "wise use" mentality of nature as resource for humans, and the "shared stewardship/creation care" mentality that claims to rediscover in sacred texts the role of nature in human experience; both of these put into human hands the responsibility for caring for creation so that natural resources will be available for human use. The stewardship feature of these theories calls for responsible behavior by humans as a way of demonstrating devotion to God, the giver of the resources. Stewardship implied that God is the "owner" and that humans are the caretakers of God's possession. Patton (2000) argues that it sells these three traditions short to claim anthropocentrism as their primary foundational interpretation. Rather, she points toward theocentrism as the common root from which she asks "what light is shed on God and animals from the relationship with animals" (p. 408)? Putting human knowledge of God at the center creates a role for nonhuman creatures to point humans toward God, even clarifying what God is like by putting awareness of God, or characteristics of God in the qualities of animals for human observation and experience. Pointing out that monotheism in all its forms contains three aspects of this relationship—divine compassion for animals, communication and mutual awareness between God and animals, and animal veneration of God—she directs the conversation to the character of God. Central to her conclusions is the divine *ipseity*, the inexhaustible and reflexive creativity of God (p. 409). This view sees God as ongoing creative force rather than solely creator at the origin of human existence. For persons of faith, at the center of this conversation about what is possible in human–animal connection is the diverse evidence found within sacred texts to the intention of the creator. This question of the "use" of the human–animal relationship in relating to God will be considered in more detail below.

Judaism

In scholarly debates about the Hebrew scriptures, the question is raised as to whether the biblical narrative is primarily about God or primarily about the people of Israel. At the center of this question is the understanding that the Hebrew scriptures are a product of the priestly tradition and the questions it addresses are the questions of liturgy and morality. While these questions arise out of the source-critical work of scholars, they also open the conversation on how the scriptures were used by humans through history to understand their role in the world. The discussion then moves to the role of law or covenant in the beliefs and practices of Judaism. Central to both practice and interpretation is the narrative of Hebrew scripture. The law, which is central, rests within the narrative of God's reaching toward humans in covenant relationship (Shoemaker, 1998, p. xv). In other words, to reduce the stories found within the Hebrew scriptures to a backdrop for linear law codes is to misunderstand the intent of the text and to elevate the law above the community which shaped and received it. The text does not begin with law; it begins with the narrative of the world's creation, including all living beings, with God as life giver and humans and nonhumans as life receivers. The human response called for is first companionship and tending, delight in existence and enjoyment and instruction in the natural world, or original blessing (e.g. Fox, 1983; Shoemaker, 1998). The pattern of obedience and worshipful fellowship with the creator begins early but is only codified after much narrative ground is covered. According to Bernstein (2008), within Judaism creation is an ongoing process; creation is renewed daily and God is sustaining the world. While critics claim this is a form of reinterpreting classic texts, she would argue she is mining the gold of the text that has always been there but is overlooked in traditional interpretations embedded in paternalistic doctrine. She offers 10 Commandments of Creation Theology which she then shows to be deeply present in the text of Hebrew Scriptures. As presented above, these newly listed commandments point toward creation as God's first revelation, with the Law of Moses then coming as a succeeding revelation in the context of what has been revealed about the creating God.

1. God as creator: Rather than the warrior God, the God of Genesis 1 is the wind who pulses the energy of life into the world, who speaks the world into being. God is revealed as an artist who fashions clothing, plans gardens, trims trees, provides food, and, then beyond Eden, is encountered in harvesting and pruning, in cloud, mountain, and bush.
2. Goodness: In these same creation narratives all that has been created is valued and called good. Being itself is blessed.
3. Beauty: For Bernstein, beauty is the natural extension of everything being called good. The diversity of texture, sight, smell, and sound engages all creatures and opens the spirit to the fullness of creation—it draws humans beyond themselves.
4. Habitat: A Sense of Place: In both creation narratives found in Genesis 1 and 2 the habitat (air, water, earth) matters. The place is made or divided and then the creatures find their place in it. "Place and habitat are words from two different domains-culture and biology-that refer to the same thing: the physical environment in which a creature makes its home" (p. I-53).
5. Fruitfulness and Sustainability: The language of seed, generativity or fruitfulness, and the diversity "of every kind" permeates the narrative, giving intent and blessing to creatures sustaining their lives and the life of their habitat.
6. Interdependence, Relationship, and Community: The language of the creation narratives gives direction to the shared nature of creation. The earth "puts

forth vegetation" (Gen. 1:11). A voice of co creation is encountered in 1:26 as humans are created in the image of "us" and God's blessing follows the seeing that "everything that was made was very good" (Gen. 1:31). The connection to the earth is evident in the "matter" from which humans were created and when God searches for a partner for the first human creature he makes animals and shares the naming of these animals with the human (Gen. 2:18–20).

7. Language: Rabbis teach that there are no wasted words in Hebrew scripture. The language of creation is full of color and poetry. This language continues through the text in reference to natural resources and the sense of place carried throughout is " simultaneously an environmental principle, a literary principle, and a religious principle" (p. I-55).

8. Boundaries: The natural world from its creation has included limits and interconnectedness. The absence of attending to these limits by humans has contributed to the environmental crisis faced today. The practice of limits is a healthy part of human existence as designed by the Creator.

9. Humanity's Place: Dominion and Service: Still attending to the language of the creation narrative, Bernstein emphasizes that it is human privilege to "ensure the continuity and unfolding of creation on God's behalf" (p. I-55). Tilling, keeping, guarding, working, and serving are all words translated and used. The service of earth care can be seen as religious observance.

10. Shabbat: Time Out: Sabbath practice of ceasing the normal patterns of human behavior for one day a week draws together commandments 1–9. The "being" depicted in the blessing of creation is what is practiced on Sabbath and human creatureliness recognized becomes a restorative practice. The world held and moved by forces other than humans holds this practice of being and not doing and restores a balance of perception and anthropomorphic hubris.

Bernstein demonstrates that embedded in the ancient creation narratives of Judaism are principles that offer benefit not only for the planet in crisis, but also for the spiritual nurturance of humans who are caught in the grasping for more, the "obsession with progress and the future, the belief that more is better, and the conflating of wealth and status" (p. I-57). In addition, these principles offer clear and broad evidence that the Hebrew scripture contains plentiful evidence of the mandate to live as fellow creatures with all of life. Davis (2008) finds guidance which is both material and spiritual in these same writings. Drawing on the prophets she places the human responsibility for caring for the earth, literally the soil, in the context of God's covenant commitments, noting that the perspective here is both practical and visionary. The prophets called the people to faithfulness providing for now and the future and allowing no choice between the two. Faithfulness included acting on behalf of the created order.

Throughout the Hebrew text, themes arise which support a complex understanding of the interrelatedness of created life. A master theme developed by Zoloth (Maguire, 2000) is exile—an image which captures both the promise and the struggle of living on the earth. She points to the setting of Eden in Genesis as the image of the future, not the past. The Garden is intended as "a vision of the world that could be, where people would live in harmony with one another, with all of nature, and with God" (p. 105). Demonstrating that in Judaism, truth is located in paradox, Zoloth says "It is foolish to waste or ruin the land, to poison or to strip it, but in Jewish thought, it is not morally incorrect to manipulate it" (p. 108). Early Judaism struggled to distinguish the practices of following Yahweh from the practices of what some might call nature paganism. As they lived, moved, and resettled on land through their migration toward Israel, their connection to the land changed and broadened. Throughout Hebrew scripture are examples of nature having a voice to speak to and for God illustrating not only the character of God, but also the intimate connection between nonhuman animals and the creator. Later in their history as a people and a nation, conquering forces from other lands removed them from what had become home and they were not only removed from their place of worship, but also distanced from their sense of connection to the land.

The practices of Judaism today are closely tied, but creatively shaped, by ancient wisdom embedded in new ideas. One example is what Waskow (2000) calls "eco-kosher" observance of the sacredness of humans relating to the earth. He notes that the earliest connection of people with God as recorded in Hebrew scripture was through the earth. Humans—*adam*—were created from the earth—*adamah*, and relied upon the gifts of the earth to survive. So to observe Sabbath in the modern world is to restore this connection through actions and awareness.

Christianity

As with each of the modern world religions, the question is raised—does the Christian tradition hold within it the resources for environmental initiative or does it hold within it the teachings which continue to curtail helpful practice and progress? And, as with each tradition, it is difficult to reduce the practice and teachings of Christianity to any one strand of thought. Likewise it would be difficult to remove from the Christian tradition in the West a primary responsibility for the way humans have misused natural resources. While the debate rages about how the present environmental crisis was reached (and even that there is a crisis) there is little debate that Christian doctrine developed since the first century has been in partnership with societal practice, and more recently industrial greed, to provide philosophical and theological foundation for the abuse of natural resources. From earliest Christian understandings that Christ's return to earth was imminent to more recent apocalyptic teaching which encourages destruction of an earth that will be consumed in fire at Christ's day of victory (Moyers, 2006), the understanding from European to American traditions is that salvation through Christian teachings is for humans only. White (1967) wrote in what became a cornerstone of the modern argument that "Christianity is the most anthropocentric religion the world has seen" (p. 197). She tracked how in the early centuries of Christian teachings a well-developed doctrine of salvation included linking the uniqueness of humans in creation with the image of Jesus as second Adam. If the first Adam of Genesis is understood as the one who fouled creation, creating the need for humans and the earth to be "cleaned up" then Jesus, understood as the second Adam, is seen as the one sent to do the cleaning. This view reduces the extraordinary teaching of incarnation, God come in human form to live on the earth, and places it in the context of human dominion and human salvation. Built upon this through the voices of Tertullian and Irenaeus was "not only a dualism of [hu]man and nature but also that it is God's will that [hu]man[s] exploit nature for his proper ends" (p. 197). Peterson (2000) examines the tensions that have arisen in what she calls "theological anthropology." As humans within the traditions of Christianity have grown restless and asked what their role in the world might be, the answers have shaped not only Christian practices of worship and devotion, but also the view of nature which gives shape to lifestyle and industrial practice in predominantly Christian nations. Peterson traces the relationship of Christians to nature by beginning with the words in Romans, "do not be conformed to this world" (Romans 12:2) and accurately declares that even when biblical scholars inform the translation of this verse, the teaching itself has served to create a distance between all the elements of this finite life from the spiritual reality of the human. As Waldau (2005) points out, from this first generation of Christian teaching grew the conclusions of Augustine which served to shut down any discussion of the role of nonhuman animals. Augustine taught that the separation between the things of the earth and the things of God was necessary for a life of devotion. From this came the teaching that animals had no intellectual participation in the community of humans. Stunningly, Augustine's systematic and solid denial of any connection between humans and other creatures (other than that animals could be used for human benefit) held in practice until the inquiry into the place of animals in creation was revisited in the late twentieth century. With few exceptions Christian teaching simply ignored the presence of other creatures for centuries. During this time, layer upon layer of thought built conceptual walls to avoid seeing the relationship of animals to humans or to God. During the Reformation of the seventeenth century, which paralleled investigations into the distinct species of animals, the teaching developed that these specie designations were static, as determined by the literal understanding of the creation narrative in Genesis.

This layering of thought continued as the interest of Christian theologians in the questions concerning animals stayed in decline. This decline accompanied the growth of literalism and the development of scientific categories. Descartes is noted to have observed that animals are viewed as more like clocks than humans—their behavior instinctive only and completely predictable. Hence, this separation of humans from other animals developed theologically and scientifically. North American theological development over the past two centuries has included this separation as it further refined salvation as an individual human salvation. Waldau (2005) traces the resulting shift into a split awareness of animals in human life. The category of animals as domestic pets grew as humans distanced themselves from animals as tools in laboratory discovery, animals as resource for industrialization, and wild animals as pests or targets. Alongside these divisions was also the recognition of nature as powerful and majestic, primarily observed from a distance. This split awareness was relatively unchallenged in industrial societies until more recent crises of shared habitat forced new inquiries. This developed dichotomy of how humans think about relating to animals allows for detaching the spiritual wholeness of humans from their existence on earth and their relationship to any material reality which has been declared tainted. This detachment from a creation declared good in Genesis 1 and a coexistence with other creatures participated in by God in Genesis 2, has also supported unsustainable development in industrialized society. McKay (1995) summarizes this interplay of theology with economics:

> "The Industrial Revolution and recent technological development have brought us into a mindset which fits our theology. Economic gain is more important than caring for the creation. The pursuit of short-term gain renders the created order disposable. Materialism and militarism are served by science and technology. There is a critical imbalance in the circle of life when our life-style does not reflect a holistic and inclusive vision of the creation" (p. 217).

When looking for new and creative approaches to Christian theology in reference to animals, it becomes necessary to seek voices on the margin. One example requires a return to White's (2001) classic critique which also offers some fuel for hope. While some accuse White of being overly judgmental about the inherited Christian stance, it can be said that she is also optimistic about the role of "true religion" in responding to the environmental crisis. Unlike others who find religious devotion bankrupt in the ecological conversation, White is clear in saying that more technology and science will not in themselves bring resolution. She points to the potential of finding a meaningful connection between humans and nature and in that finds the possibility of turning around the present path of environmental destruction. Like most other sources investigating the relationship of Christian traditions to the environment and specifically animals, she points to St. Francis and his reform of impoverished theological assumptions about other creatures as a possible source for wisdom and change. Throughout the history of Christianity, dominant traditions have sought to denigrate, disregard, or even silence other voices. St. Francis is one rare example of a "marginal perspective" which survived and is remembered in mainstream teachings. One clear example of a marginal voice which was not preserved in a central way is the work of John Scotus Eriugena. Kowalski (1991) records that Martin Buber, a significant contributor in the twentieth-century theological development, found in Eriugena the deep traditions of delighting in creatures as fellow illustrations of God's own self. Philip Newell (2008) who is recapturing Celtic traditions for a modern audience, which is looking for insight into learning from creation, represents Eriugena as on who invited humans to listen to the book of creation "in stereo" with the book of scripture, teaching that to listen to either separately was to lose the harmony. To listen to either without the company of Christ is to risk losing the vastness or the intimacy of the song of the creator. Eriugena also offers an antidote to the dualistic view which dominated early Christianity within the Roman culture and offers a repair of the split and rigid teachings linking the purpose of the life of Jesus with the Greco-Roman interpretation of fallen creation mentioned above. For Eriugena, Christ's call was to the true nature of humanity, not separate from nature but a part of nature, a setting in which grace is not seen as opposed to the essential nature of humans but rather as grace and nature flowing together to offer a more complete view of God. As Teilhard de Chardin carries this teaching forward into the twentieth century, he reiterates that the work of grace in the human soul is not to make the person other than they are, but rather to restore them to their true nature. This is quite foreign to much of the Christian teaching of original sin and yet it is the very foundation of the idea that humans and nonhuman animals are kin in crucial ways and in fellow creatureliness. Newell steps further into the illustration by pointing to Alexander Scott, a nineteenth-century teacher, who illustrated that when a plant is blighted it is not named by its blight. Why then if humans are infected with evil are they named by this infection? Newell is quick to point out that Eriugena did not ignore the power of sin within humans. But crucial to the core of the argument is the acknowledgement that humans and nonhuman animals are rooted in God, created from God, rather than opposed to God. One final example of more recent reframing comes from Brian McLaren (2004), a primary voice in the conversation about how the Christian Church is undergoing significant transition in the twenty-first century. From the context of McLaren's volunteer work surveying species for the Department of Natural Resources comes his awareness that human behavior is interfering with the environmental provision for many other species with whom humans share the planet. As a Christian pastor he notes that many environmentalists are surprised to find him doing this work. The common view seems to be that Christians are part of the problem, not the solution. McLaren identifies six primary elements of theological succession related to environmental sustainability, which can serve as a summary of the above discussion of Christian theological history and contemporary shifts. He sees the former stagnant theology which gives emphasis to human evil (usually grounded in a much later doctrine of "original sin") as giving way to an understanding of the ongoing nature of the creative work of God. McLaren combines this with shifts occurring from a belief that this earth will be destroyed to an engaged teaching of the kingdom of God as present here and now as well as in the future. This flows into a greater concern for the poor and oppressed as well as the condition of the created world. This new understanding calls for a reconsideration of a rigid understanding of private ownership and a shift from rugged or selfish individualism to a new understanding of neighborliness. Finally the changing nature of technology combined with the worldwide nature of the environmental crises brings a shift toward a global/local way of thinking (p. 234–242).

Islam

The strict monotheism of Islam as well as the belief in the prophets of the Hebrew Bible place Islam well within Abrahamic traditions. The one Almighty God is the Creator of all that is and the aim of Islamic life is to live in accordance with these beliefs. Through its emphasis on human centrality in creation, Islam also has elements of teaching that humans will be judged by their treatment of animals. But it is unnecessarily limiting to Islamic thinking to try to encapsulate it within a Western, linear approach. Knowledge within Islam is for the sake of service to Allah and for the practice of righteous living. While vast diversity of thought and belief exist within Islam, the framework for devout practice is found almost universally in the five pillars, which are daily declarations of faith in one God, daily practice of prayer, fasting of Ramadan, the giving of alms to the poor, and pilgrimage to Mecca. Dempsey and Butkus (1999) offer an insightful and more thorough exploration of how the Islamic system builds knowledge incorporating science, philosophy, and religion so as to create a knowledge base for devout practice. The teachings of Islam concerning the treatment and relationship to animals then is based in this complex and concentric way of understanding the universe. Mohammed teaches that kindness to creatures of Allah is of the same importance as kindness to self. Like Judaism, Islam not only carried the ritualistic slaughter of animals, for food and for worship, but also carried the rules for taking care about how the killing is done so as to lessen the suffering of the animal. The practice of slaughtering an animal during the pilgrimage is to show their submission and willingness to give up something valuable to them for God. The Qur'an is clear that humans carry a particular responsibility for caring for the created order as the only creatures that can protect or destroy. When the slaughter of animals is practiced it is to celebrate the faithfulness of the prophet Abraham and the meat is used to feed the poor. The Qur'an teaches that neither the meat nor the blood reach to God, only the faithful practice of the people.

Ammar (2000) is a voice for Islam and the morality of environmental justice. Attention is directed to the focal text of the religious tradition, working for a new understanding of classic texts, pointing out that moral rules were a primary contribution of Mohammed. The rules of Islam for environmental stewardship and the honoring of community are: use nature and its resources in a balanced, not excessive manner; treat nature and its resources with kindness; do not damage, abuse, or distort nature in any way; share natural resources with others living in the habitat; and conserve (p. 297). To read this in the context of progressive Islam is to find what could also be called stewardship in other traditions. Islam's emphasis upon individual practice within community values gives new energy to shared resources and a view of a broader human community; the Islamic understanding of community includes nonhuman creatures.

Summary

Examination of Abrahamic traditions finds both diversity and similarity in practice, tradition, and theory. In addition, each tradition in modern forms is seeking to join ancient traditional understandings of creation with scientific and societal understandings of the nature of human existence now and the interdependence of life on the planet. Specifically, " the diverse streams of Judaism, Christianity, and Islam all indicate that once established by creation, God's relationship with animals does not stop then, but rather continues in an ongoing, vital way" (Patton, 2000, p. 409). All sacred texts describe the participation of God in the beginning and ongoing life of creation. This ongoing participation included relatedness to the well-being of animals as well as the demonstration by the behavior of animals concerning the character of God. Honoring God is central to devout practice in these three tradi-tions. Imitating the behavior of God is a bit more complex to discuss but it would certainly be fair to say that to imitate the valuing of all creatures and relating to all creatures by God is both a considerable and worthy goal for human behavior. What is apparent in the scriptures of all three traditions discussed is the acknowledgement of the life of animals as valuable to God, not primarily for food but for delight, for instruction and for companionship. While the stated laws in each tradition concern the use of animals and appear to give direction to a level of possession of animals by humans, the narrative sections of each scripture include a richer and broader treatment of the presence of animals in the world. Animals are cared for by God, animals are company for God and for humans, and animals can teach humans about their world and their God. Contemporary scholars in all three Abrahamic traditions are asking questions about more whole and healthy relations between humans and the created world. These questions all lead to new ways of encountering fellow creatures as well as the earth shared by all creatures.

Ancient Eastern Religious Traditions

As with the monotheistic religions already discussed, the traditions of Hinduism and Buddhism carry within them a variety of perspectives, both ancient and mod-ern. While each tradition presents unique perspectives, their similarities in cultural influence and geographical implications provide for considering their practices as related to each other.

Hinduism

Hinduism is marked by a central belief that all of life is lived according to one's beliefs, that religion is not a segregated part of life, but a way of life. Hinduism teaches that the divine is in everything. There is a supreme being but it is present in unlimited forms. While Hinduism evades any linear framework, its beliefs and practices can be gathered around the concepts of karma—all actions produce effects—and dharma—one's station in life or duty. These are discussed and interre-lated in the Bhagavad Gita. The goal is for the soul to be released from the cycle of being reincarnated, the cycle of suffering.

In early Hindu practice, animal sacrifice was common but by 500 B.C.E the practice was criticized and reformed. In the modern world, both in developed and underdeveloped countries, humans have been given a place of superiority to other nonhuman animals in theory and in practice. Within the Hindu teaching of reincar-nation lies the paradox of valuing animals and believing in a hierarchy of karmic reward. Being reincarnated as a human is karmic reward for living well as an ani-mal. Being reincarnated as an animal is the result of living a less moral life placing human existence higher than nonhuman at least in belief. Within this same paradox resides the awareness of the continuum of life and the human as model of life. One's ancestors and one's future human companions may currently be the animals living alongside. While this karmic hierarchy exists in theory and practice, so also does the teaching that all of life is sacred and to be carefully tended. Animals are believed to be creatures with souls who deserve care and protection from harm. It should be noted that while to be reincarnated as a nonhuman animal is seen as the outcome for living less than a moral existence, it is not taught that animals are worthless, rather that their lives are more full of suffering than the human existence; in other words, it isn't punishment to be an animal, it is simply more difficult.

This paradox continues in the teaching that animals are to be treated as one treats one's children, while many of the lower castes of humans are treated with less dignity or care. This alone would deter one from concluding that there is a line between humans and animals taught by Hinduism. The disparity between village life and city life in Hindu culture also brings into focus the practices which arise from the teachings and textual traditions. The treatment of animals which are believed to have particular divine worth is often in stark contrast to the mistreatment or neglect of other animals and humans.

Chapple (2001) writes in depth and with insight into the ancient and modern challenges and promise of Hindu contemplative practice as well as the inherent deep ecology present in living a devout Hindu life, even within modern challenges. New ideas, or ancient ideas revisited in response to modern environmental crises and tragedies, are developed in Hinduism as they are in other religions. A deep connection to place and to the sacredness of daily life in one's place is central to Hindu worship.

Buddhism

Similarities between Hinduism and Buddhism are found in language, practice, and teachings. Buddhism can be considered one of the sources which brought reform to Hinduism, particularly in relation to the treatment of animals.

The foundation of Buddhist wisdom, according to Moffitt (2008), is found in Four Noble Truths, an Eightfold Path to freedom from *dukkha*, and Twelve Insights. Dukkha can be described as a cycle of suffering found in life, an inevitable sorrow, pain, and frustration, and while the word "suffering" is insufficient in some ways for understanding the fullness of this philosophy, it will be used here. When the Buddha found freedom from his own suffering, he began teaching the Four Noble Truths. These Four Noble Truths are understood to be grounded in practice and are not a guideline or philosophy so much as an "actual practice of insight and realization: a teaching how to live wisely" (p. xxii). The Twelve Insights, three for each Truth, are patterned as first reflecting, then directly experiencing, and finally knowing (p. 2). Briefly, using Moffitt's language, they are: First Noble Truth: Your life is inseparable from suffering (the Buddha identified three kinds of suffering: the suffering of physical and mental pain, the suffering of constant change, and the suffering of life's compositional nature). Second Noble Truth: The cause of suffering is the craving for, clinging to, and identifying with one's desire.

Third Noble Truth: It is possible to be free of the clinging, to experience direct knowing of pure awareness. Fourth Noble Truth: By practicing the Eightfold Path one can experience purification of the mind which leads to ethical behavior, mindfulness, and wisdom. The Eightfold Path is right view, right intention, right speech, right action, right livelihood, right effort, right mindfulness, and right concentration. Central to Buddhist teaching, and found in the practice of the eightfold path, is kindness toward all living beings.

Similar to Hinduism's teaching, Buddhism views all forms of life as fellow participants in the flux and flow of existence. Unlike Hindu teaching which ranks various life forms in karmic order, Buddhism has two categories in its teaching: human and nonhuman. That which lives but is not human is grouped and placed lower than human existence. In part, this then carries the earlier mentioned teaching that animal existence is more full of suffering than humans and is deserving of compassion for this greater suffering and lesser level of agency in the flow of life. In Buddhist writings, it is taught that to be born an animal is the result of moral failure in a previous life. Buddha spoke of humans as a tangle and animals as simple so to live as an animal is to live a more simple life. Buddhist teaching and tradition offer, again, the paradox of creating a hierarchy which not only places humans above other animals, but also calls for fair treatment of animals. The lives of all are valued within Buddhism and the first precept taught is the valuing of all life. And yet, animals do not have their own agency, or intelligence, or individuality. While welcomed and valued in the living community there is also in some cases a denigration of the presence of animal life in that very community.

Within the wisdom tradition of Buddhist thought rest three primary movements: interdependence, mindfulness, and compassion. These three movements or concepts provide a rich resource for new models for life with fellow creatures, perhaps even for learning from animals about being human and being partners in the lessening of suffering for all.

Summary

Buddhism and Hinduism share some similar belief structures and practices while existing as separate traditions. Within each tradition are many groupings, both geographical and delineated by different practices and schools of thought. Both share a view of animals as fellow creatures and vessels of the divine. And both live within cultures where a distinct practice of both caring for and disregarding creatures is visible. As with the monotheistic traditions discussed earlier, the distinction between teaching and practice is apparent as is the struggle to honor the deepest concepts of valuing life.

While distinctions cannot be over looked it is possible to group Hinduism, Buddhism, Jainism, Taoism, and Bahaism into a category of religions which address the attachment of humans as the cause of suffering and the call of humans to protect all life through compassion and ethical living.

Native and Indigenous Understanding of Animals

Throughout native, indigenous, and more recently discovered religious traditions, the spiritual kinship of animals with humans is more commonly discussed, valued, and accepted. As Neihardt (1932) opened one door into Oglala Sioux tradition and more generally into Native American sensibilities and practice, the kinship of animals with humans is foundationally understood. The two-legged tribe of humans is understood to have always existed in the company of four-legged tribes. These four-legged kin are understood to be highly social and intelligent.

In other indigenous traditions, such as Druidism, Australian aboriginal religion, Pacific Rim Faiths (Maoris of New Zealand, Polynesians), and African indigenous religions, the legends and teachings about animals and the recorded and valued interaction with animals are foundational to the understanding of life on earth. In a deeply paradoxical reflection, humans and animals are individualized but no one of them is at the center of understanding life. In an interesting intersection, Waldau (2005) observes that the work of primatologist Jane Goodall and cognitive ethnologist Marc Bekoff call humans back to understanding animal behavior and spirituality in pursuit of better understanding human behavior and spirituality. Within this call for taking observation seriously is also a new way to listen to the wisdom of traditions found in many indigenous cultures which long have valued the presence and company of animals as fellow creatures (Sikhism, Jainism, Daoism, p. 22).

McKay (1995) writes beautifully but with hesitation from a Native American perspective which shudders to put that which is sacred into written words. He describes how the current view within Native American traditions is that the danger to the world has become so great that the risk of writing must be taken. The connection between Hebraic world views and other aboriginal world views becomes quickly evident. The division of human existence from the life of the planet or the other creatures on the planet is simply not understood. How can one separate that which is dependent upon each other for existence? The Western practices of individuality and ownership do not fit the native understanding of life as gift. The native spirituality does not receive the ideas of separate existence. Rather wholeness for each is wholeness for all and cannot be obtained through compartmentalizing. One cannot choose to heal oneself at the cost to the earth or another creature. It would not be health at this price. Hence, recognizing limitations of private ownership and individuality would be a gift to the modern West from indigenous traditions.

Foltz (2003) generates and informs this conversation in his anthology by directing attention to the movement among scholars and activists to honor, cultivate, and learn from native knowledge, or TEK (traditional ecological knowledge). From developing medicines to creating sustainable practices the knowledge of people groups who have continued to survive in close relationship to land and animals can enlighten the knowledge and practice of those who have developed life insulated from fellow creatures and natural rhythms. To accept this premise may also require openness to the developing trends in established religions as well as fledgling religious traditions which have existed or begun in less centralized ways.

Summary of Religions

From even a cursory look through major world religions and less-known traditions, a common thread begins to develop. Newly voiced awareness from the margins of all traditions is calling for greater attention to the human need for connection to habitat and recognition of the interdependence of life. Humans living on the earth are subject to the rhythms of the natural world. The cost of separating from this rhythm is not always immediately evident but becomes so as humans begin to develop hierarchical approaches to valuing themselves above nonhuman animals. In the modern scientific world this separation has existed through the parallel developments of science and religious traditions. In each tradition examined there are voices from the margin pointing not only to the crisis of limited natural resources, but also to ancient voices who called for a more cooperative way to live among creation. In Judaism, the arrogance and anxiety of humans were countered with reminders from nature. In Christianity, the fear and greed of humans were calmed and challenged by pointing to the natural order and restoration of shared existence with all creation. In Islam, humans are taught to quiet their hunger for more by sharing with all of life. In Hinduism and Buddhism, all forms are life are evidence both of suffering and of the presence of the divine in daily life.

The thread of relatedness to all creatures can be seen clearly in the environmental crisis which brings into focus the interconnectedness of all life. The loss of any species has effect on all other species. The more that is learned about any particular biosphere, the more the interrelatedness at a micro and macro level is evident. Within all these aforementioned systems of religion, humans have understood themselves to be the ones taking action. As the primary movers in civilization, humans must then also reflect upon the effects of human behavior.

Bringing together various cultures, traditions, peoples, and nonhuman creatures around a common hope is to also bring spiritual awareness and spiritual hope into the conversation. While it may not be progress to eliminate the distinctions of various historical religious traditions, it could be gain to listen to the voices of those traditions which value wholeness for all of life above the defense of particular doctrine or specialized perspectives. As stated at the start of the overview of religious traditions, every tradition carries within it the promise of its devout population and the danger of its imbalanced fanaticism. Also within each tradition are those voices which are today calling for moderation in stridency for the gain of shared earth and sustainable life for all. Zoloth (Maguire, 2000) illustrates this in her attempt to show that the particularity of the narrative of Judaism, while remaining a sacred text for observant and faithful Jews, is also the story of all people. As she focuses on exile as a central theme, she sets it alongside exodus as the basis for Jewish spirituality. She understands the narrative of Genesis not as the telling of creation which happened in the past to one group of people, but rather a vision of the future, a garden that can be. The harmony of life with all creatures and with God is the poetic language of what is possible. And as Maguire records her words, this experience of exile and vision of future harmony is a "panhuman experience." "... Humanity... searches for home in a fragile modern world... both lost and at fault, at risk and accountable, bearers of the scent of Paradise and lovers of the pleasure in the desert, easily seduced by idols, losing track of the column of fire in the night" (p. 105). This has grown from a Jewish story to a human story.

Many of the religious scholars noted above are examples of persons who are devoted and knowledgeable about one particular religion, while respectfully open to the wisdom of other traditions. This is a first step to recognizing unitive themes and future partnership. Weiming (1994) encourages this through the mobilization of spiritual resources, calling all of the world's religious traditions to offer their wisdom and allow themselves to transcend the tribalism inherent in exclusive dichotomies. The resources identified call for participation of Western, Eastern, and indigenous religious persons and thought.

Unitive Thought as a Way Forward

If the common thread being heard from the margins of world religions involves a restoration of awareness concerning the interconnectedness of all created life, the common thread for all humans which can reach through the separation that exists culturally, religiously, and geographically is that of suffering. At the core of all human religious experience is suffering and reverence. It can be said that these are the experiences of being creatures. Maguire (2000) considers all religion as born of reverence and epics of wonder, driven by justice and compassion, all bringing wisdom and difficulties. Is it possible that religious devotion, once freed from the need to be distinctive, could be the path toward a unified human experience? Unitive thinking as a new awareness opens one to seeing something other than what is expected, challenging humans to see beyond their inherited perspectives. This unitive approach does not preclude the role of particularity in religious traditions but it questions the power of particularity to divide and create conflict. To accept religious teaching, or any given conceptual approach as the final word on how the world works can prevent humans from participating in careful engagement with each other and the animals.

As one example, by shifting the focus to animal consciousness it can be seen how powerful curiosity and observation can be. Recent scientific observations call into question the idea of the simplicity of animal consciousness. The resulting openness can serve as an important companion to the interfaith inquiry into the role of animals in the spiritual life of humans. To call this new is to ignore the observational insights of Francis of Assisi who experienced kinship with everything around him. And Teilhard de Chardin who was banished to China by Roman Catholic authorities for his unorthodox perspectives and found in his new eastern home the very confirmation of what his religious experience in his European home had pointed him toward. The eyes of faith, or as Bourgeault (2008) calls this perspective, the eyes of the heart, allow us to see more than we are taught to see.

Palmer (2009) describes this very seeing as the maturing of the religious or faithful soul. The hardwiring of the primitive brain shapes humans to respond to tension or threat with fight or flight. As he reports, this is helpful when one is being chased by a hungry tiger, but not so helpful when a human is seeking a new insight or pressed with a new idea. In order for humans to grow beyond fight or flight, grow beyond enemy or kin, and step outside of tribal understandings, culture has offered language, art, education, and religion. As noted above, religion has as often served the tribal threat motif as it has made a way for engaging with new ideas and the tensions that exist in complex reality. As an antidote to this tribalism and its path of violence and degradation Palmer points toward the reality of suffering in all human existence. The pressure to resolve suffering can lead to destructive choices for all living beings.

The earth and its systems are suffering greatly. Along with it the inhabitants, human and nonhuman, share a breaking and painful existence. Human history is full of the attempts of one group or another to wrestle the suffering to the ground with force and violence; to wrest successful living from one group so that another can prosper.

But suffering also offers another route for all. "The alchemy that can transform suffering into new life is at the heart of every religious tradition I know anything about, including my own Christian tradition" (Palmer, 2009, p. 10). Bourgeault (2008) addresses the potential for this alternate route to justice for all living beings. She points to the latent operating system in humans (and perhaps animals) that has been driven underground by the dominant duality of conquering parties. The human mind has been raised to a level of reverence in modern post-Enlightenment culture. And it has cost humans the deeper "operating system" of heart, *intuition*, that which in the wisdom traditions of all religions is considered the heart, the organ of spiritual perception. The heart doesn't perceive as subject/object but rather seeks harmony. Bourgeault emphasizes that this isn't simply the development of a higher level of thought, but rather the ability to see from the seat of wisdom. And what is seen is what Jesus called for, the absence of division between humans and God, or between humans and other humans. This "christology" of redemption and transformation comes by different names but is present in all religious traditions. And in each it results from suffering, struggle with suffering, recognition that self is not the center of the universe, and seeing with eyes of non-duality (Keating, 2008). In all advanced spiritual traditions of the world, this non-duality is addressed. Keating (2008) says this is the paradox of God beyond all categories of existence, called to live beyond the "not this, not that; not one, not two" (p. 4). And Rohr (2010) expresses this conclusion succinctly, "Our very suffering now, our condensed presence on this common nest that we have fouled, will soon be the one thing that we finally share in common. It might well be the one thing that will bring us together. The earth and its life systems on which we all entirely depend might soon become the very thing that will convert us to a simple gospel lifestyle, to necessary community, and to an inherent and universal sense of the holy" (p. 2).

How might living in the common "fouled nest" of the earth in environmental crisis bring an opening for unitive thinking? How might voices of spiritual renewal also become voices of sustainable existence and creation care? What would be required of humans to move from defensive living and scarcity thinking toward a hopeful walking of the earth, participating in its rhythms and joining the conversation of nature beyond human philosophizing? Might more full and open relationship with other creatures, nonhuman animals, bring insight into this hopeful walking?

Openness, Observation, Curiosity, Respect, Humility: Horse–Human Communication as One Window Toward a Unitive Perspective

From a theological perspective, as shown above, the notion of control of nature and relationship to animals can be grounded in religious teachings. There is a common refrain among reformers of culture and religion. It is that nature is an avenue of spiritual renewal for humans (Taylor, 2009). If nature is an avenue to spirit for human experience, then being in the company of another species and working to communicate for mutual learning could be an act of spiritual growth. The natural world is where animals are found in their settings. Perhaps animals can be the company humans need to find and reconnect with natural rhythms, guides to undivided living.

Animals as teachers would require a reform of the most common patterns of human perspective on animals. One proponent of this reform, Temple Grandin, autistic educator and animal activist, describes her education in biology and behaviorism (Grandin, 2005). She captures the curriculum as taught to generations of American schoolchildren in the middle and late twentieth century. Animals were understood to be less developed forms of life and a practical necessity was developed for dealing with animals. Their value was determined by their worth to humans, their intelligence was measured against what humans deemed "smart" behavior, often meaning whether the animal did what the human wanted them to do. Animal survival was based on their usefulness to humans and/or their ability to dominate their setting. Behaviorism offered insight for how to control animals for human use. Efficiency and expediency became the determinants of domesticated life for animals in the developed world. Asking why an animal behaved as it did was a waste of time. Controlling their behavior was possible through the use of proper rewards and negative reinforcement. The formal scientific curiosity about what might be in the brain of animals was curtailed with the acknowledgement that their behavior was the only subject of interest. The potential of a creature was limited to the observation of the human. Fortunately, for animals and for humans, behaviorism proved its limits in time. And also, fortunately, for animals, some humans retained their fascination and respect for animals of many species.

Why the Horse?

While many species could be considered for the role of teacher, few are more suited to restoring wholeness to fast-moving, modern, overly mechanized humans than horses. The path of learning to partner with horses can lead to the examination of foundational assumptions about self, other creatures, and how the world works. The central question becomes what is possible in relation between humans and other animals. The development of natural horsemanship as a school of thinking has arisen from the observations of persons who in the company of horses chose to stop coercing and forcing. These men and women responded to what was app[r]ent suffering on the part of horses and chose to see what the horse might have to convey. They chose to stop following a traditional mind-set which said force was necessary for horse/human work. They chose to recognize that contrary to common wisdom, horses are not stupid. These people believe a horse as willing partner far exceeds horse as compliant service animal. Those who propose natural horsemanship as a method for developing horses would see the horse's sensibilities as more than half the equation (Brannaman, 2004; Dorrance & Porter, 1987; Parelli, 1993). Approaching horses with the self-knowledge as predator, the human must perceive the horse's, or prey animal's, state of mind as read through body language and respond with non-predatory body language to begin the conversation. (It is understood that even these categories of prey and predator are human conceived, but they allow for a starting point of communication and arise from observation). At the heart of what is now considered a movement of natural horsemanship is this understanding that not only are horses intelligent and perceptive, but that humans as predators have been the center of the problem in traditional approaches to horse work. A predator is linear, goal oriented, quick to grab, and slow to release. According to those who portray the physical differences between prey and predator, a predator can be identified as eyes in front, walking boldly and directly, straight up to what they want. They smell like what they eat, focus hard when trying to capture something, are unable to run fast and rely on tactics of surprise and force. In contrast, horses as prey animals are focused on their need to survive. As analogy they are more like deer than dogs, finding their first response to threat as movement, protecting their ability to move away, basing their prioritizing on safety first, then food, comfort, and play as alternating needs. They read the body language of all other animals including humans. Prey animals fear for their lives and perceive any threat as a mortal threat. They have acute hearing, and hesitation can mean death. Their first resort is to run away fast; speed is their best partner in survival and therefore they resist being confined. They will fight using all their means but only as a distant or learned second resort. It may be surprising therefore to see that horses are very social and enjoy play. Human knowledge about the complexity of animal perception, language, and response is growing exponentially as long-held conclusions are being set aside. The most powerful insight offered early in natural horsemanship is the need to understand the prey nature of a horse and the predatory nature of humans. This simple concept, if allowed to work on the modern human mind-set, can call into question every layer of communication and interaction. To accept oneself as predator can be difficult. To accept a large, fast, and reportedly aggressive animal as prey might also be a stretch in thinking. Certainly, a study of the history of humans and horses challenges the notion that horses are defenseless. But it also clearly sounds the verdict that horses have suffered greatly at the hands of humans for centuries. The horse/human history is fraught with tragic chapters. Humans have been forcing horses for centuries, perhaps millennia, to do what they want them to do. And the antidote of anthropomorphizing or sentimentalizing the connection has been equally unfair for the horse. Neither approach allows one to see the horse on its own terms, as a creature significantly different from humans.

Becoming Whole in the School of Natural Horsemanship: One Educator's Experience

I stumbled into the work of learning from horses about being human. As a professor of religion, trained in biblical studies and pastoral care, my theological and psychological training had shaped my sense that human wholeness and reconciliation with all life was at the heart of living well and making a contribution to a greater good. My presuppositions and my way of understanding the world are grounded in religious circles and theological education. As an educator, my work revolves around teaching-thinking and working to develop skills of critical analysis in the context of conversation about sacred texts and religious traditions. I thought I was busy doing the work of helping others to be open to new learning and never ending renovation of perspective. I thought I had developed a broad repertoire of books, activities, and classroom practices which could cultivate a hospitable place to risk being wrong in order to discover something new. And then I discovered how little I knew. I now know, whatever our preconceived notions about how the world works and who we are in its systems, attempting to communicate with animals, specifically horses, is fertile ground for learning and for becoming more whole.

I had enjoyed the company of animals my whole life. And yet, as a child of the 1960s I grew up disconnected from nature and unaware of its absence. I didn't know either of these concepts and didn't have words for them until my own spiritual brokenness and physical exhaustion took me into the natural world looking for something beyond the ancient texts and the teachings of religious traditions. Even then, it took me years to move from being comforted by a setting such as the grandeur of the Rocky Mountains to being conscious of walking the earth as human in the company of other creatures. While horses had always been fascinating to me, when I accepted the invitation to work through a system of natural horse development, I had little notion of how my way of seeing myself, the world, and other creatures would be challenged. I'd been a good and willing student since early years but discovered that my willingness faltered when asked to move from words and books into experience. My formal educational experience allowed and even encouraged learning without experiencing—learning in my mind, not in my bones. Working with horses and being open to new ways of seeing invites, and perhaps even requires, learning in the bones.

The methods of Pat Parelli (1993) are grounded in traditions that have been shaped since humans first encountered horses. Parelli himself is clear that what he teaches he learned from watching master horsemen. But these were horsemen who dared ask whether a traditional approach to horse training was working for both the horse and the human. These were people who were willing to set aside what they'd been told was true about horses and actually observe horses interacting with other horses. What they saw caused them to question what they'd been told about horse intelligence, or the lack of it. And some of them questioned the entitlement of humans to shape a horse's existence with misery and demand. What I found in this material, and in the strides made by the Parelli organization to make these methods accessible to everyone, was the invitation I didn't know I'd been waiting for. And I found what I unknowingly had hoped was true: that a person who didn't have years of experience with horses could begin this work, allowing the horse to participate with dignity.

None of this had fully prepared me for the teaching of a four-legged American quarter horse. The most powerful early and ongoing challenge was to understand the horse as prey and myself as predator.

Much as most acculturated religious training offers humans an insulated view of themselves within their system pointing out toward those who are not in the system, when I first began studying the Parelli method I resisted the notion that I was a predator. I meant these horses no harm. In fact, I would stand between them and harm. But my deeply held convictions about this meant nothing to the horses I approached. I looked and behaved as a predator. I gripped the rope firmly and held on tightly. When pressed or stressed I held my breath. The rigidity of my body and my determination dissolved the trust and curiosity that had been cultivated. Lesson #1—The horse knows I'm a predator by the set of my eyes and the rope in my hands. Lesson #2—Not every horse responds like every other horse. Of course I knew that dogs had individual characteristics, but did I believe that each horse came with their own characteristics? And what might that mean for other creatures? Are they individuals? Does recognizing animal consciousness require a broadened awareness from humans? As beginning learners we try to universalize what we learn and apply it. It didn't take long before it was easily observable that not every horse responded the same and not every skill or concept taught would fit every situation. And my methods of setting other humans at ease didn't appear to be working with the horses.

The cultivation of questions and curiosity in the horse and the human is at the center of this method. If as the predator I change my manner and become more demanding, more frustrated, more rushed, the horse's curiosity changes to fear or at least wariness. And the open line of communication closes with both reverting to prey and predator. This is the first of many moments when slowing down, relaxing, refocusing, and becoming internally clear allow the horse to re-approach and the communication to be reestablished. At the heart of this method is patience, curiosity, the belief that as Parelli says "it takes less time to take the time it takes" in gaining the horse's trust or attention the first time. As many of us have learned is true with humans as well: we cannot force horses to like us, respect us, choose to work with us. To do this requires a completely different approach and it is that approach which requires humans to live less divided, more whole.

As a member of the religion faculty at a private university, part of my role is one who tends souls. I bring to this a fascination with human wholeness. What I didn't know I brought to it was the recognition that when religion attempts to tame that which is natural and wild in human awareness, it robs power and passion. When I attempt to use my power to persuade a horse, or my power of emotion to connect with a horse, I am mistakenly using human analogies in a situation where humanness is not the language. To step outside of my language, or to attempt to, has become a learning experience with many layers. At present, it appears the layers will not come to an end. Each time I think I have waited long enough, or created enough interest or challenged the horse's ability to resist often enough, I see a new response. And each time I wait a bit longer, or get a bit more clear and transparent in my self-understanding, the horse's response is more immediate and clear. My resistance to being a predator has become the central question "how am I behaving as a predator in this situation?" I am learning to challenge the familiar by letting go of the certainty of the familiar. The methods of natural horsemanship require stillness and inner focus. Once we open ourselves to something not being what we expect, we can learn more about what it is and what we are. Horses are wonderful teachers and a wonderful metaphor for learning communication and developing rapport. In order to take responsibility when things don't go right we must let go of ego, let go of what we believe should be and see what is in front of us. Working with horses requires one to come to terms with denial, blame, anger, chaos, fear, insecurity, divided focus, and inattention.

The biggest change for me in my work with horses over the past two years grows from the foundational understandings gained in working to communicate with a prey animal. It has changed the way I walk through a pasture, the way I watch a rabbit eating in my backyard, the way I understand what deer along the road are doing, the way I hold the leash when I walk my dog. It has also changed the way I enter a classroom, or welcome a student to my office. When others appear to be angry or in distress my response is shaped by my understanding of what it means to be both prey and predator. When I find myself with clenched hands on the steering wheel, or gripping a paint brush or garden hose with force, I lessen my grip and ask a few questions: what am I trying to control, what is pushing me to be controlling, is there another approach, and what is this drive to control costing me?

Conclusion and Possibility

With the seed of pondering predatory and prey behavior and communication, this experience of learning "natural horsemanship" has brought into view issues of identity, intuitive focus, intellectual gamesmanship, and development of meaningful work, spiritual depth, and the integrity of living with mindfulness. Human self- and group understanding paired with conceptualized belief in the nature of the divine creates the framework for all religious traditions. In other words, religious experience happens in the context of one's self- and God understanding. As discussed earlier, religious traditions can direct humans toward particularity and tribalism or invite more broad self- and other understanding by seeking common experience. The major religious traditions of the world present creatures as "other" from humans. They each contain practices which value nonhuman animals less than humans. Some have well-developed theologies of domination and histories of animal sacrifice. But these traditions also carry patterns and possibility for shared life with creatures, even companionship as part of the blessing of the interconnectedness of created life.

Are there possibilities for humans and animals to relate in mutually helpful and fulfilling ways? While many human–animal relationships have been cast into the realm of sentiment, this determination appears reasonable only from a purely behaviorist perspective. The myth of domestication holds that an animal can be broken, that a living creature can become a tool, and that what one animal is capable of can be limited by the methods of the human and the needs of civilization. Even this is a step above the vision of animals as material goods to be birthed, manipulated, controlled, transported, slaughtered, and sold.

Mahatma Gandhi said, "The greatness of a nation and its moral progress can be judged by the way its creatures are treated." Perhaps recognition of the distance between humans and nature is captured in the distance between the developed world's view of itself as a measure of civilization and the reality of its disregard for life. A bridge can be built between the understanding of civilization and the perceived need to tame wildness.

The human illusion of controlling nature is parallel to the delusion that a wild animal can be tamed. As Parelli reminds his students, "inside every wild horse is a gentle horse and inside every gentle and domesticated horse is a wild horse" (Parelli, 1993, p. 11). What if rather than attempting to tame or domesticate these animals, what humans need from them is a tutorial on wildness, or naturalness? What if the loss of the notion that a wild animal can have soul has caused the human to disconnect from human soul as well? Parker Palmer (2009) describes the soul in a way that a natural horsewoman can't help but hear as describing a spirited horse:

> In our culture, we tend to gather information in ways that do not work very well when the source is the human soul: the soul is not responsive to subpoenas or cross-examinations. At best it will stand in the dock only long enough to plead the Fifth Amendment. At worst it will jump bail and never be heard from again. The soul speaks its truth only under quiet, inviting, and trustworthy conditions.
>
> The soul is like a wild animal-tough, resilient, savvy, self-sufficient, and yet exceedingly shy. If we want to see a wild animal, the last thing we should do is to go crashing through the woods, shouting for the creature to come out. But if we are willing to walk quietly into the woods and sit silently for an hour or two at the base of the tree, the creature we are waiting for may well emerge, and out of the corner of an eye we will catch a glimpse of the precious wildness we seek (p. 7–8).

Perhaps what is possible, even needed, is openness to how all creatures, including humans, can learn from each other about life and the giver of life. Perhaps faithfulness to discovering meaningful life is less about certainty and dogma and more about curiosity and participation in mutual suffering and joy. The work of the soul of humanity is the work of shared and interconnected life.

References

Ammar, N. (2000). An Islamic response to the manifest ecological crisis: Issues of justice. In H. Coward & D. Maguire (Eds.), *Visions of a new earth: New vision on population, consumption and ecology (pp. 230–260)*. New York: SUNY Press.

Bernstein, E. (2008). Creation theology: A Jewish perspective. In M. Sleeth (Ed.), *The green Bible*. San Francisco: HarperOne.

Berry, W. (1998). *A timbered choir: The Sabbath poems 1979–1997*. Washington, DC: Counterpoint.

Bourgeault, C. (2008). Seeing with the eye of the heart. *Radical Grace, 21*, 6–8.

Brannaman, B. (2004). *Believe: A horseman's journey*. Guilford, CT: Lyons Press.

Chapple, C. (2001). Hinduism and deep ecology. In D. Barnhill & R. Gottlieb (Eds.), *In deep ecology and world religions: New essays on sacred ground*. New York: SUNY Press.

Cummings, C. (1991). *Eco spirituality: Toward a reverent life*. New York: Paulist.

Davis, E. (2008). Knowing our place on earth: learning environmental responsibility from the Old Testament. In *The Green Bible* (pp. I-58-64). San Francisco: HarperOne.

Dempsey, C., & Butkus, R. (1999). *All creation is groaning: An interdisciplinary vision for life in a sacred universe.* Collegeville, MN: Liturgical Press.

Dorrance, T., & Porter, M. H. (1987). *True unity: Willing communication between horse and human.* Tuscarora, NV: Give It A Go Enterprises.

Eriugena, J. S. (1987). *Periphyseon (The Division of Nature)* (J. O'Meara, Trans.). Montreal, QC: Bellarmin.

Foltz, R. (2003). *Worldviews, religion, and the environment: A global anthology.* Belmont, CA: Wadsworth.

Fox, M. (1983). *Original blessing.* New York: Putnam.

Gottlieb, R. S. (2004). *This sacred earth: Religion, nature, environment.* New York: Routledge.

Grandin, T. (2005). *Animals in translation: Using the mysteries of autism to decode animal behavior.* New York: Scribner.

Keating, T. (2008). The paradox of non-duality. *Radical Grace, 21,* 4–6.

Kowalski, G. (1991). Somebody, not something: Do animals have souls?. In R. Gottlieb (Ed.), *Sacred earth: Religion, nature, environment* (pp. 351–354). New York: Routledge.

Maguire, D. (2000). *Sacred energies: When the world's religions sit down to talk about the future of human life and the plight of this planet.* Minneapolis, MN: Augsburg Fortress.

McKay, S. (1995). An aboriginal perspective on the integrity of creation. In D. Hallman (Ed.), *Ecotheology: Voices from south and north* (pp. 213–217). Geneva, Switzerland: WCC Publications.

McLaren, B. (2004). *A generous orthodoxy.* Grand Rapids, MI: Zondervan.

Moffitt, P. (2008). *Dancing with life: Buddhist insights for finding meaning and joy in the face of suffering.* New York: Rodale.

Moyer, B. (2006). *Welcome to doomsday.* New York: Review Books.

Neihardt, J. (1932). *Black elk speaks: Being the life story of a holy man of the oglala sioux.* Lincoln, NE: University of Nebraska Press.

Newell, P. (2008). *Christ of the Celts: The healing of creation.* San Francisco: Jossey-Bass.

Palmer, P. (2009). The broken-open heart: Living with faith and hope in the tragic gap. *Weavings, 24,* 7–16.

Parelli, P. (1993). *Natural horsemanship: The six keys to a natural horse-human relationship: Attitude, knowledge, tools, techniques, time, imagination.* Colorado: Western Horseman.

Patton, K. (2000). He who sits in heaven laughs': Recovering animal theology in the Abrahamic traditions. *Harvard Theological Review, 93,* 401–434.

Peterson, A. (2000). In and of the world. In R. C. Foltz (2003) *Worldviews: Religion and the environment, a global anthology.* Belmont, CA: Wadsworth.

Rohr, R. (2010). Creation as the body of God. *Radical Grace, 23,* 22.

Shoemaker, H. S. (1998). *Godstories: New narratives from sacred texts.* Valley Forge: Judson.

Smith, M. (2009). *The priestly vision of genesis 1.* Minneapolis, MN: Fortress.

Taylor, B. B. (2009). *An altar in the world: A geography of faith.* New York: Harper.

Waldau, P. (2005). *"Animals" published in the Encyclopedia of religion* (2nd Ed.). New York: Macmillan.

Waskow, A.(Ed.). (2000). Originally published in *Torah of the earth: Exploring 4400 years of ecology in Jewish thought* (Vol. 2). Woodstock, VT: Jewish Light Publishing. (reprinted in Worldviews, Religion and the Environment, edited by Richard C. Foltz, Belmont, CA Wadsworth/Thomson, 2003).

Weiming, T. (1994). Beyond the enlightenment mentality. In M. Tucker & J. Grim (Eds.), *Worldviews and ecology.* Cranbury, NJ: Associated University Presses, Inc.

White, L. (1967). The historical roots of our ecological crisis. *Science, 155,* 1203–1207.

White, R. (2001). Moving from Biophobia to Biophilia. Accessed from http://www.whitehutchinson.com/children/articles/biophilia.html

Chapter 6
Lapdogs and Moral Shepherd's Dogs: Canine and Paid Female Companions in Nineteenth-Century English Literature

Lauren N. Hoffer

Skill'd in each gentle, each prevailing art,
That leads directly to the female heart;
A soft partaker of the quiet hour,
Friend of the parlour, partner of the bow'r:
In health, in sickness, ever faithful found
Yet, by no ties, but ties of kindness bound

These verses by Samuel Jackson Pratt, excerpted from his epitaph to a lapdog in *Liberal Opinions, Upon Animals, Man, and Providence* (1775), articulate the function and characteristics of the ideal lapdog in the eighteenth century (quoted in Tague, 2008). A "Skill'd" "Friend," the "faithful" lapdog offers company and amusement to its, specifically "female," owner. The strength of the attachment is emphasized through the reference to partnership and the suggestion of intimacy implied by the bower; this diction, coupled with the allusion to common marriage vows in the fifth line of this passage, aligns the lapdog–owner relationship with that of husband and wife, a bond culturally understood as among the strongest connection between human beings. Indeed, this touching ode to *"woman's* best friend" could just as easily have been written to describe a human. Not only does the poet anthropomorphize his subject, but the characterization of the lapdog is equally applicable to another common companionate figure in eighteenth- and nineteenth-century England: the paid female companion. Paid female companions were the hired friends of other women and, like the lapdog, they were expected to provide their mistresses with company and entertainment in addition to serving as a confidant and chaperone. About seventy-five years after Pratt penned his epitaph, William Makepeace Thackeray drew an explicit connection between canine and paid female companions in his novel *Vanity Fair* (1847). Becky Sharp states that she requires a *"moral* shepherd's dog" or, as she goes on to explain, "A dog to keep the wolves off me, [...] a companion" who will act as "guardian of her innocence and reputation" (Thackeray, 1847).

L.N. Hoffer (✉)
Assistant Professor of Victorian Literature, Department of English & Theatre, University of South Carolina Beaufort, Bluffton, SC, USA
e-mail: lauren.hoffer@gmail.com

C. Blazina et al. (eds.), *The Psychology of the Human–Animal Bond*,
DOI 10.1007/978-1-4419-9761-6_6, © Springer Science+Business Media, LLC 2011

The parallels between canine and human companionate figures suggested implicitly in Pratt's poem and more explicitly in Thackeray's novel signal significant discourses in Britain during the eighteenth and nineteenth centuries regarding bonds between humans and animals and among humans with one another. In the wake of the Enlightenment, pervasive cultural concerns addressing natural and social hierarchies, interspecies distinctions and relations, ownership, and dominance all circulated around these two analogous figures. The various ways each figure was represented in literature provides valuable insight into contemporary perceptions of lapdogs and paid female companions as well as offers a contextual framework for our understanding of similar relational dynamics today. Writing in the early decades of the nineteenth century, Jane Austen falls between Pratt's and Thackeray's two literary representations of canine and human companions. Austen's novel *Mansfield Park* (1814) features both a lapdog and a human companion and engages with the cultural perceptions and anxieties surrounding these twin figures.

As Jodi Wyett writes, "The idea that dogs were reflections of their owners was common in the eighteenth century" (Wyett, 2000). This tendency to equate pets with their owners has dominated literary scholarship on fictional lapdogs and owners as well. For example, Ayres-Ricker argues that "dogs are often projections of their masters. [...] the reader is able to learn more about the characters and their actions because of the narrator's extension of character to the dogs" (Ayers-Ricker, 1991). However, my concern here is not with the resemblance between owner and lapdog in Austen's novel, but with the narrative alignment of the two companionate figures in *Mansfield Park* and what this reveals about contemporary tensions surrounding domestic hierarchies and intra- and interspecies relationships. Austen's novel addresses the parallelism, dynamic interplay, and confusion that can arise in relationships among humans as a result of relationships with animals. *Mansfield Park* depicts a triangulated relationship between Lady Bertram, her lapdog Pug, and her niece Fanny Price, who becomes, over the course of the novel, a companion to her aunt by fulfilling all the duties that prescribed that role in the time period. The complex position of Pug in the household, and Lady Bertram's privileging of her lapdog's service and well-being over that of her niece/companion, serve as both exemplar and indictment. Although the companion figures in *Mansfield Park* are "trained" to perform their respective, corresponding roles within the text, ultimately the novel seeks to train their mistress, Lady Bertram, and readers themselves, in the proper valuation of individuals, both canine and human, in the domestic space.

"Skill'd in Each Gentle, Each Prevailing Art": Lapdogs and Companions in the Nineteenth Century

There is some debate over when the modern practice of pet keeping began; while Harriet Ritvo argues pet ownership as we know it commenced in the nineteenth century, Tague claims that "it was during the eighteenth century that pet keeping first developed as a widespread phenomenon, and this period also saw the rapid growth of literary works dealing with pets" (Tague, 2008). The creation of pets:

Required the demarcation of space that was a characteristic of the early modern period, when those who could afford it separated living from working quarters, moved livestock into separate outbuildings, and designated certain spaces as more private or public. [...] Once most animals were moved away from intimate human contact, it became possible for some to be marked out as special by virtue of their sharing the same domestic space as their human owners (Tague, 2008).

This "demarcation of space" altered hierarchies, both within the animal kingdom, as those species granted access to the domestic realm rose to a greater level of human concern and intimacy, and within human hierarchies as pets became new members in the family circle, taking their place there. Pet keeping also required significant disposable income: "Thanks to the financial and commercial revolutions, eighteenth-century English people could indulge in an ever-growing number and range of consumer goods. In this context, when consumption was no longer simply a matter of necessities, it became possible to consider keeping an animal for the purposes of pleasure alone" (Tague, 2008). The concept of keeping an animal for "pleasure alone" defines the phenomenon of the lapdog in particular. A creature whose primary purpose was to act as a status symbol with no measurable socioeconomic utility, the lapdog's function is solely to sit with its mistress and accompany her idle hours with the pleasures of comfort and diversion.

Laura Brown specifies the timeline of modern pet keeping to canine pets, writing, "The foundations for the canine obsession were laid before [the eighteenth century]: toy spaniels were kept by upper class women in the sixteenth century, and pugs in the seventeenth. But it was in the eighteenth century that the canine house pet rose to the status of companion and acquired recognition for intelligence, affection, and loyalty" (Brown, 2001). As pets were increasingly anthropomorphized and came to be seen as "companions," their status in the household often came to equal that of human family member. Markman Ellis argues that "the variety of dog known as the lapdog was primarily a social construction, not a product of natural history or zoology. [...] The lapdog trope is a concise bundle of received ideas and commonplace associations" (Ellis, 2007). As Jodi Wyett makes clear, this "bundle" included a vast array of meaning and contention: "During the long eighteenth century, the specific figure of the lapdog appears within a wide range of cultural discourses where it seems to represent a number of social and sexual anxieties [...] especially when conflated with their aristocratic, female owners, lapdogs often reified social anxieties surrounding class, gender, sexuality, trade, nation, and empire" (Wyett, 2000). Lapdogs' physical closeness with their mistresses—their access to their owners' private quarters and bodies (sitting in laps, licking, petting, cuddling, and so on)— as well as their tendency to bark and bite male strangers who came to the home as suitors, often led lapdogs to be viewed, satirically or literally, as sexual rivals. Similar satire regarding wives who were more intimate with their lapdogs than their husbands also pervaded the cultural discourse surrounding lapdogs (Wyett, 2000).

Notably, foreign breeds, such as Lady Bertram's Pug in *Mansfield Park*, signified international relations and trade and acted as subtle markers of imperialism within the English estate: "The ancestry of the lapdog, in all its varieties, is an important issue precisely because such dogs were not indigenous to England. [...]

many seventeenth- and eighteenth-century lapdogs were imported from Holland, Italy, France, most breeds of lapdog originated in the East" (Wyett, 2000).[1] Beyond their associations with the world beyond the borders of Great Britain, the most widespread cultural understanding of lapdogs pertained to their function as status symbols: markers of wealth, social standing, and refinement. As Wyett writes, the lapdog's "long association with the aristocracy, and the royal family in particular, is clear enough. The restoration of the kind in 1660, one possible demarcation of the beginning of the 'long' eighteenth century, entrenched the lapdog as a symbol of English royalty. [. . .] Second only to Charles II for dog-owning fame amongst royals were William and Mary" (Wyett, 2000). Thus, the lapdog became a way for the aristocracy and upper middle class to align themselves with the highest representatives of their own social hierarchy: the monarchy.

Ideally, lapdogs functioned to provide their mistresses with all the best a pet could offer: "Pets, they say, provide pleasure, companionship, and protection, or the feeling of being secure" (Shell, 1986). However, this job description could be filled by another popular figure, one that was equally embroiled in questions of social and domestic hierarchy. Paid female companions in the nineteenth century were generally genteel or middle-class "redundant" women, either single or widowed. The role was one of the few available employment options for women of this social status and was the only respectable choice that did not involve teaching. A companion's duties ranged from keeping her mistress company at home and abroad, amusing her and tending to her whims, to serving as chaperone whenever the mistress entertained men. The companion read to her mistress, played music for her, ran errands; she acted as both lackey and confidant—a "friend" who was always at her employer's disposal as a sympathetic receptacle for blame and frustration, light-hearted gossip, or intimate conversation. To fulfill the diverse and often contradictory requirements of her position, a companion's qualifications included good breeding, an array of feminine accomplishments with which to entertain her mistress, and, like the lapdog, a capacity for loyalty, obedience, and humility. A companion's compensation for her work varied as widely as the catalog of her duties often did. While some companions were paid a salary, others simply received room and board in exchange for their services.

Companions blurred the lines between family, friend, employee, and object. Definitively a member of the "upstairs" region of the home, the companion was the constant, genteel attendant to her mistress, and there was rarely, if ever, any question of where the companion should take her meals, where she would sit in a coach, or how she was to be treated by her mistress's domestic servants. She

---

[1] Both Wyett and Precious McKenzie Stearns have interpreted the pug in Austen's novel along these lines. Wyett contends that Austen's "characterization of a favored lapdog on English soil not only serves to indict its mistress, but also emphasizes the indignity of a lapdog living in luxury made possible by the unspoken sufferings of human slaves on West Indian soil" (292), while Stearns reads Pug as an "imperial presence in the mistress's lap" and argues "the lapdog's symbolism is less about femininity, gender roles, and confinement than the silent presence of imperialism in British family life" (451).

was superior to the servants, but her status as neither equal nor servant to her mistress left her in an indistinct position within the household. Although usually of the same or only slightly lower class position than their mistresses, companions were often expected to act with servility and endure disrespect and disdain from their employers. Forced to work for their self-preservation despite their social status, and victimized by their personal situations as well as the stigma associated with being single, these women often suffered from the coarsening and demeaning effects of their sycophantic, dependent occupation.[2]

Thus, the most significant points of comparison between lapdog and paid female companion lay not only in their function, but also in their status in the household and, consequently, in the ways they were treated. As Ingrid Tague writes, "One of the issues that became increasingly important during the eighteenth century was the question of the morality of pet keeping itself. Thinking about pets inevitably raised difficult questions about the unequal power relationship inherent in pet ownership and about pets' liminal status as both chattel and individuals" (Tague, 2008). For this reason, lapdogs and other animals were often depicted in literature and other discourses as comparable to slaves. Likewise, Harriet Ritvo claims that in the nineteenth century "animals became significant primarily as the objects of human manipulation [...] Animals were uniquely suitable subjects for a rhetoric that both celebrated human power and extended its sway" (Ritvo, 1987). In keeping with a Judeo-Christian worldview that animals were set upon the earth for man's use (as God tells Adam, the first man, in the Bible's book of Genesis), animals—including domestic pets—were viewed in terms of what they could offer humanity and simultaneously provided an outlet for the exercise of human authority. Focusing on human–animal relations in the Romantic Period in which Austen wrote, David Perkins asserts, "Even in this sentimental age, it was possible to analyze the motive for keeping pets as love of power."

Like the lapdog, which relies solely on its owner for shelter, sustenance, and human interaction, the paid female companion was utterly dependent upon her mistress. To hire and compensate another human being for the services expected of her places the individuals involved in a formal hierarchy of master, or "owner," and servant- a dynamic in which the companion figure exists, like the lapdog or other pet, only to serve the master's needs. The mistress–companion dynamic was fundamentally different from other contemporary employment relationships, which were generally located in the public realm outside the home. Because the mistress–companion relationship was situated within the domestic space and was defined as a dynamic between two women, traditional codes of paternalism and even increasing government regulation often did not apply or could not reach within the private sphere to protect the companion from mistreatment at the hands of her employer.

---

[2]There has been almost no scholarship on the companion in literary or historical studies. My work on the figure thus draws heavily upon fictional representations of the companion in nineteenth-century literature and has also benefited from valuable studies by scholars such as Kathryn Hughes and Bronwyn Rivers, whose work on the analogous but distinct figure of the governess provides some insight into the daily conditions of actual companions.

If "the best animals were those that displayed the qualities of an industrious, docile, and willing human servant," this set of expectations also applied to paid female companions (Ritvo, 1987). Both companionate figures existed to serve and served as a site for the exertion of others' power. In what ways, then, might the paid female companion—even one who is an extended family member—also be viewed and treated "as both chattel and individual" due to her role in the household? How did those in the early nineteenth century understand the place of lapdogs and companions in society and in the home? What ethical dilemmas arose from the existence of these figures within the family circle, and how can these two parallel figures help to illuminate one another? Austen's *Mansfield Park* explores the effects when one of these figures is an animal and the other is a human being.

"A Soft Partaker of the Quiet Hour": Pug and Fanny as Companionate Figures in *Mansfield Park*

Jane Austen's third published novel, *Mansfield Park,* is the story of the aristocratic Bertram family and their lives on the eponymous estate. At the beginning of the novel, the Bertrams decide to take in Fanny Price, the daughter of Lady Bertram's sister, who married beneath her caste and now lives in poverty with more children than she can care for. Fanny Price and Lady Bertram's lapdog, Pug, are introduced almost simultaneously and, in this way, Austen sets up a parallel between the two companionate figures from the beginning of the novel. As Sir Thomas Bertram and Mrs. Norris discuss their plans to take Fanny in, Lady Bertram interjects her only personal concern in the matter: "'I hope she will not tease my poor pug'" (Austen, 1814; 9). Unlike her interlocutors, Lady Bertram is not concerned with the well-being of Fanny, or even that of her own children; instead, her concern lies with Pug—that he might not suffer any adverse effects from the addition of a new member to the Bertram household. Austen makes Lady Bertram's privileging of Pug over her own children even more explicit in a famous passage that delineates Lady Bertram's character:

> To the education of her daughters Lady Bertram paid not the smallest attention. She had not time for such cares. She was a woman who spent her days in sitting, nicely dressed, on a sofa, doing some long piece of needlework, of little use and no beauty, thinking more of her pug than her children, but very indulgent to the latter when it did not put herself to inconvenience [. . .] Had she possessed greater leisure for the service of her girls, she would probably have supposed it unnecessary, for they were under the care of a governess, with proper masters, and could want nothing more (16).

As this description of Lady Bertram's day-to-day activity (or lack thereof) makes clear, the lady of the manor has nothing *but* "time" and "leisure"; yet, she turns the care of her children over to hired hands while she sees to the care of the dog herself. According to Wyett, this was a common trope in eighteenth-century literature: "Servants, children, and husbands were often thought to suffer at the preferred treatment of a lapdog. [. . .] Throughout the century, literary representations of women who nurture relationships with their lapdogs while shunning or neglecting more conventional heterosexual or familial ties suggests a fragile foundation for such domestic hierarchies" (Wyett, 2000). Evidently aware of these contemporary criticisms, Austen depicts a lapdog that has achieved an inappropriately high ranking in the domestic hierarchy and is causing issues among the household's human members.[3]

A better pet owner than mother, Lady Bertram's endlessly idle, sedentary pondering of her own and her lapdog's comfort epitomizes cultural indictments against aristocratic women as well as their lapdogs. As Tague writes, there is a "long tradition of using animals to satirize women. [. . .] Pets—especially lapdogs, monkeys, and parrots—could be seen as useless luxuries, just as women themselves were useless; women's love of pets proved their misplaced values as well as their susceptibility to the whims of fashion" (Tague, 2008). Lady Bertram's preference for Pug seems to lie in the dog's own identical lack of energy. Pug's simplicity and stillness doesn't require her to exert herself physically or mentally. After all, in order for a lapdog to take its customary place in its mistress's *lap*, the pet owner must be sitting, stationary, inactive—just like her lapdog. Exemplifying the cohort of critics who have interpreted literary lapdogs as symbolic reflections of their owners, Sally Palmer asserts that "Austen readers are clearly to associate the Bertram pug with its mistress's caste and personality" (Palmer, 2004).[4]

However, an examination of the parallel between Pug and Fanny, rather than between the lapdog and his owner, offers us new insight into the role of both companionate figures in the novel and in the nineteenth century. In contrast to Lady Bertram's lack of concern for the potential repercussions of allowing her niece to move in with them, Sir Thomas worries about the class distinctions between his family and that of his wife's sister. His description of Fanny, before ever meeting her, shows his social biases and situates Fanny far beneath the pedigree of the Bertrams: "'We shall probably see much to wish altered in her, and must prepare ourselves for gross ignorance, some meanness of opinions, and very distressing vulgarity of manner'" (8–9). As if Fanny is almost subhuman in her "meanness" and "vulgarity," even less well-bred than the aristocrat's lapdog at Lady Bertram's side due to her poor, working-class upbringing in Portsmouth, Sir Bertram voices his concerns that her presence could have a debasing influence on his daughters. Therefore, he makes plans "'to preserve in the minds of my *daughters* the consciousness of what they are, without making them think too lowly of their cousin; and how, without depressing

---

[3] The only human being Lady Bertram seems willing to set Pug aside for is her husband, and this only after Sir Thomas has been away on an extended, dangerous trip to Antigua: "She had been *almost* fluttered for a few minutes, and still remained so sensibly animated as to put away her work, move Pug from her side, and give all her attention and all the rest of her sofa to her husband" (140).

[4] Regarding this particular scene, Palmer writes, "[Austen] points up the faults in Lady Bertram's character not so much by anthropomorphizing the pug, as by caninizing its owner. Yet she judges the dog's personality, along with Lady Bertram's, by using human standards of behavior. The pug is lazy, selfish, worthless; it sits and dozes on the couch all day rather than accomplishing some constructive purpose. This is the criticism Austen makes of Lady Bertram" (Palmer).

her spirits too far, to make [Fanny] remember that she is not a *Miss Bertram*'" (9). Established within a firm familial hierarchy before she ever sets foot in Mansfield Park, Fanny is viewed as separate—"not a Miss Bertram"—and "lowly," beneath those whose home she is to share. In lieu of Lady Bertram's own system of importance and privilege within the household, in which Pug takes precedence over her own flesh and blood, this familial hierarchy places Fanny beneath even the lapdog.

Upon Fanny's arrival at the age of ten, Austen quickly shows that Sir Thomas's fears regarding his daughters' sense of status versus that of their cousin are unnecessary; Maria and Julia Bertram interact with Fanny in a way strikingly akin to Lady Bertram's relationship with Pug. Austen writes, "To her cousins she became occasionally an acceptable companion. Though unworthy, from inferiority of age and strength, to be their constant associate, their pleasures and schemes were sometimes of a nature to make a third very useful, especially when that third was of an obliging, yielding temper" (14). For the Bertram sisters, Fanny's function, and thus their treatment of her, resembles the function and treatment of a pet. Her "obliging, yielding temper," a description equally suitable for an ideal lapdog and a characterization which seems just as appropriate to Pug, makes her a desirable plaything. Yet Fanny is also implicitly presented as inferior to Pug here: if her "inferiority" makes her only "occasionally an acceptable companion," then we must view her as less worthy than Pug, who is nothing if not Lady Bertram's "constant associate."

It is clear that as the years pass and the girls of Mansfield Park age into young adulthood, this dynamic of Fanny as a kind of pet to the Bertram sisters remains in place. When the family decides to put on a play in Sir Thomas's absence, Maria and Julia insist that Fanny assume an empty role in the dramatis personae, despite Fanny's resistance: "'We cannot excuse you. It need not frighten you; it is a nothing of a part, a mere nothing, not above half a dozen speeches altogether, and it will not much signify if nobody hears a word you say, so you may be as creepmouse as you like, but we must have you to look at'" (115). Not only is Fanny directly associated with an animal in this passage—and, notably, one that would not make a desirable pet—but her participation is required only as a kind of placeholder, much in the same way lapdogs were meant to function: an object to be seen and not heard. Lapdogs, because by definition small, vocal breeds, were often criticized for their loud, yappy nature. In this scene, Maria and Julia want Fanny to act as a well-behaved pet: simply something "to look at."

Yet, despite her eventual acquiescence to this and all her cousins' demands, Fanny is perpetually undervalued, ignored, and treated as if she were an object or animal with no feelings of her own. After she agrees to participate in the play, Austen reveals that although "Every body around her was gay and busy, prosperous and important [...] She alone was sad and insignificant; she had no share in any thing; she might go or stay, she might be in the midst of their noise, or retreat from it to the solitude of the East room, without being seen or missed" (125). In contrast, as Sally Palmer points out, Austen "include[es] Lady Bertram's pug in almost every Bertram family scene" (Palmer, 2004). Again, Austen implicitly contrasts Fanny's position in the family with Pug's. The lapdog, as Austen's descriptions of Lady Bertram's attachment to Pug make clear, is always "seen" as the center of (Lady

Bertram's) attention and would be immediately and desperately "missed." Fanny serves as an exemplary literary example of the contemporary historical situation Wyett describes: "Lapdogs, though indeed members of a lower species, were also certainly members of the upper classes, and thus enjoyed better treatment than many humans" (Wyett, 2000).

Nevertheless, as the novel progresses, the Bertram girls are not the only characters who begin to see Fanny as a potential pet-like companionate figure. Eventually, Fanny begins to serve her Aunt Bertram as a companion.[5] Austen foreshadows this later development in Fanny's position in the family at the beginning of the novel in her description of Fanny's first day at the estate. In describing Fanny's fear and awe in the presence of the refined, wealthy Bertrams, Austen notes how each of the adults attempts to welcome their niece: "In vain were the well-meant condescensions of Sir Thomas, and all the officious prognostications of Mrs. Norris that she would be a good girl; in vain did Lady Bertram smile and make her sit on the sofa with herself and pug" (11). Austen aligns Fanny with Pug as Lady Bertram invites her young niece to assume a place at her side, joining her in her perennial residence on the sofa, opposite Pug, as a kind of pet. The tableaux created here depicts a stereotypical aristocratic lady flanked in her indolent repose by her two companions—one canine, one human. What Austen suggests here is that Lady Bertram sees little, if any, distinction between the two species of companionate figures. In fact, Lady Bertram seems to signify an attitude toward Fanny that is mediated through the lapdog.

In these early chapters of the novel, before Fanny assumes the mantle of actual companion, Austen further establishes Lady Bertram's opinion that Fanny possesses the qualities that make her a suitable companionate, lapdog-type figure. In response to reports that Fanny is ignorant and has difficulty learning her lessons, Lady Bertram "could only say it was very unlucky, but some people *were* stupid, and Fanny must take more pains: she did not know what else was to be done; and, except her being so dull, she must add she saw no harm in the poor little thing, and always found her very handy and quick in carrying messages, and fetching, what she wanted" (16). First, the language in this passage is rife with allusions to animals. That Fanny should be "dull," inferior in intellect to the other *people* in the household, transforms her into a kind of object: she is a "poor little *thing*." Lady Bertram's remark that Fanny is adept at "carrying" messages not only suggests she has begun to employ Fanny in companion-like errands but also recalls older British conceptions, predating the practice of pet keeping, of the usefulness of animals as beasts of burden, serviceable for their ability to bear people, crops, and other materials from place to place. Austen's most explicit diction here, the idea that Fanny is

---

[5]Like governesses, companions usually found employment by posting or answering advertisements or through familial connections; in fact, many ladies served as companion to extended family members when their financial situations required that they find some form of genteel labor. As the daughter of her "mistress's" sister, Fanny falls into this category. Companions who are also relations or close family friends, at least as they are represented in the literature of the eighteenth and nineteenth centuries, rarely received an actual salary but were instead compensated with room and board, as Fanny is in *Mansfield Park*.

capable of "fetching" whatever her aunt desires, is a direct reference to a common activity of dogs.[6] Thus, Fanny's aunt begins to view her as a potential companion, even while Fanny is still a child, and one that can fulfill many of the same functions that a lapdog or other animal might.

Executing sundry errands and chores were among the least of a companion's duties in the nineteenth century. While "pets have two defining characteristics: they live in the domestic space, and their primary purpose for humans is entertainment and emotional companionship" (Tague, 2008), Edmund Bertram addresses the similar attributes Fanny possesses to make her an ideal companion: "'You have good sense, and a sweet temper, and I am sure you have a grateful heart, that could never receive kindness without wishing to return it. I do not know any better qualifications for a friend and companion'" (21). Fanny exhibits the temperament, gratitude, and capacity for loyalty one could wish for in a companion—human or canine. Tague points out that "dogs were widely recognized in natural histories as well as in traditional lore as the best of animals because they combined intelligence with loyalty" (Tague, 2008). What sets Fanny apart and distinguishes her from her lapdog counterpart, however, is her degree of intelligence, her "good sense," and Edmund privileges this quality by listing it first in his catalog of a proper companion's qualifications. This capacity is one that allows the *human* companion to exceed the talents of a lapdog, and one that enables Fanny to fulfill needs that Pug cannot. The human companion can speak, can listen and comprehend, can engage in conversation. As a young adult, Fanny begins to perform these functions for her aunt:

> Fanny had no share in the festivities of the season; but she enjoyed being avowedly useful as her aunt's companion, when they called away the rest of the family [. . .] she naturally became everything to Lady Bertram during the night of a ball or party. She talked to her, listened to her, read to her; and the tranquility of such evenings, her perfect security in such a *tête-à-tête* from any sound of unkindness, was unspeakably welcome to a mind which had seldom known a pause in its alarms or embarrassments. (28)

Fanny seems "naturally" fitted for this role as an attendant to her aunt. Fulfilling the traditional duties of a hired companion by providing company and amusement through conversation and reading, Fanny herself finds "tranquility" and "security." As for Lady Bertram, she benefits from, if not a more active companion, then at least a more interactive and entertaining one. Austen represents the mistress–companion dynamic as one that is mutually beneficial: useful and comforting to each party.

Like any good dog, it appears that Fanny eventually becomes trained to perform her companion duties, whether through force of habit, through the positive reinforcement she receives, or through the contentment and sense of purpose she gains from her duties. It is interesting that when Fanny leaves the Bertrams to visit

---

[6]The etymology of the word "fetch" as a reference to the actions of a dog dates back to at least early modern England, according to Oxford English Dictionary. William Shakespeare's *Two Gentleman of Verona* (1591) contains the line "Her Masters-maid. . .hath more qualities then a Water-Spaniell. . .Imprimis, She can fetch and carry"; like Austen and her contemporaries, the bard draws a parallel between a female and canine figure here (III. i. 274; qtd. in *OED*).

her nuclear family at Portsmouth—where she is a full and equal member of the household—the companion longs for her subservient position at Mansfield Park:

> Could she have been at home, she might have been of service to every creature in the house. She felt that she must have been of use to all. To all, she must have saved some trouble of head or hand; and were it only in supporting the spirits of her aunt Bertram, keeping her from the evil of solitude, or the still greater evil of a restless, officious companion, too apt to be heightening danger in order to enhance her own importance, her being there would have been a general good. She loved to fancy how she could have read to her aunt, how she could have talked to her and how many walks up and down stairs she might have saved her, and how many messages she might have carried (339).

Despite the fact that her understanding of her position there seems to be one of "service" in which her role in the family is to be "of use to all," Fanny refers to Mansfield Park as her "home." Furthermore, Fanny has come to view herself not only as a companion, but also as the epitome of what a companion should be: one who will *not* attempt to "enhance her own importance" but, instead, one who knows her place as a "supporting" figure. No doubt due to her own unassuming disposition, but also through the "training" she has received at Mansfield Park in always being treated and referred to as "inferior" and put to "use," Fanny actually craves her companion duties to the point where she "love[s] to fancy" fulfilling her function in the household and experiences discontentment at her inability to be useful in her own proper home.

Fanny's drive to be actively useful, and the companion's status as a figure hired and compensated to fulfill a variety of useful functions for her mistress, places the companion in direct opposition to Pug and to larger cultural discourses about the uselessness of lapdogs. Palmer explains that "Much current discussion of animals in fiction mentions the anthropocentrism with which past authors viewed animals. Certainly in Jane Austen's world in 1814, dogs both real and literary were valued not objectively, but according to their usefulness to humankind. By this yardstick, pet lapdogs tended to be disparaged as useless in British fiction, by Austen as well as other writers" (Palmer, 2004). According to Ellis, "Most clearly associated with the domestic and the private, the lapdog was far removed from the scene of work and utility" (Ellis, 2007). In the long tradition of Britain's history with stalwart, hearty working dogs—the tireless shepherd dogs tending flocks and the vigorous hounds leading the hunt—the lapdog was the odd dog out in its lack of definable, productive utility.

Oblivious to Fanny's true value as the superior, because more useful, companionate figure, for a time Lady Bertram continues to privilege Pug in both her affections and her consideration. When Fanny falls ill after being compelled by her aunts to work outdoors all day in the hot sun, picking roses in the garden and running errands between houses on the estate, Lady Bertram admits, "'I am very much afraid she caught the headache there, for the heat was enough to kill anybody. It was as much as I could bear myself. Sitting and calling to Pug, and trying to keep him from the flower-beds, was almost too much for me'" (59). Lady Bertram betrays her awareness of the heat, but, as the reader has come to expect by this point in the narrative, her concern over whether "anybody" might be killed by the sweltering weather is reserved for herself and for Pug. It is clear that, at the time, Fanny's well-being—her "body" or her status as "anybody"—never crosses Lady Bertram's mind. Ellis calls this phenomenon, in which a canine is pampered while a fellow human being suffers nearby, "counter-sensibility": lapdogs "emblematize the malevolent, spiteful, and hypocritical quality of their female owners, who demonstrate an 'unfeeling' nature. Their canine bodies are luxurious in themselves (expensive commodities consuming expensive commodities), and in their snappy, biting ways they literalize the cruel violence of their owners, even as they are shown to be the recipients of misdirected sentimental feeling, inordinate caresses, excessive affection and grief" (Ellis, 2007). However, a distinct turning point occurs mid-way through the novel when, first, the Bertram children leave the family home (due to marriage, school, or travel), and more substantially when Tom Bertram, the eldest son and heir falls dangerously ill.

As the Bertram children make their way in the world, their parents begin to suffer something akin to empty nest syndrome. As a result, "Fanny's consequence increased on the departure of her cousins. Becoming, as she then did, the only young woman in the drawing-room, the only occupier of that interesting division of a family in which she had hitherto held so humble a third, it was impossible for her not to be more looked at, more thought of and attended to, than she had ever been before; and 'Where is Fanny?' became no uncommon question, *even without her being wanted for any one's convenience*" (160; emphasis added). Although Lady Bertram has been more interested in Pug than her children throughout their upbringing, Austen suggests that she and her husband feel their absence deeply. Ironically, it isn't until all of her children are away that Lady Bertram seems to become more interested in her human family members than in Pug. Consequently, Fanny's position in the household shifts; where she was ignored and neglected before, she becomes "more thought of" and is even "attended to" for the first time in her life at Mansfield Park. Rather than being noticed solely for the attendance she can provide for everyone else, Fanny begins to be valued as a *person*, even when she is not required to perform some kind of companionate service.

While the Bertram elders finally begin to realize Fanny's personhood and value, at this point there is still a lingering degree of objectification and a sense of ownership in their views of, and interactions with, their niece. In their longing for their own children, Sir and Lady Bertram not only appreciate Fanny's presence, but also take it for granted. Lady Bertram states, "'Sir Thomas, I have been thinking—and I am very glad we took Fanny as we did, for now the others are away we feel the good of it,'" to which Sir Thomas responds, "'Very true. We shew [sic] Fanny what a good girl we think her by praising her to her face, she is now a very valuable companion. If we have been kind to *her*, she is now quite as necessary to *us*.' 'Yes,' said Lady Bertram presently; 'and it is a comfort to think that we shall always have *her*'" (223). Like a pet who remains forever in its owner's care onto its death, loyal and obsequious—like Lady Bertram's ever-present Pug—the Bertrams fail to take into account any desires or prospects Fanny might have in her future, believing that she will always be present to serve their needs. Indeed, Lady Bertram can no better bear the thought of being without Fanny for a single evening than she would let Pug wander from her side. When Fanny is invited to dinner at a neighboring home,

Lady Bertram repeatedly asks "'But how can I spare her?'" and "'But can I do without her?'" (169–171). It is not until Fanny herself departs from Mansfield Park, on her trip home to Portsmouth, that Lady Bertram truly recognizes not only her niece's inherent value as a person, but also the superiority of a human companion to a canine one.

During Fanny's sojourn at home, as Tom Bertram falls ill and both Maria and Julia fall into social scandal, the narrative focuses on Fanny's experiences with her mother and siblings, but upon her return to her aunt's estate, it is clear how Lady Bertram has suffered without her companion. As Fanny enters the estate, Lady Bertram, "falling on her neck," exclaims, "'Dear Fanny! now I shall be comfortable'" (351). Lady Bertram's exclamation indicates that she had not been, and could not be, "comfortable" in Fanny's absence. Austen subtly implies here that, in the face of true distress and familial tragedy, Pug has become insufficient. Despite his intimacy and constant attachment with Lady Bertram, the lapdog fails to offer its mistress any true, lasting comfort. After all, "the lapdog cannot reciprocate the act of sympathy: there is not mutual understanding to the sympathetic scene. The dog's sympathetic look or extended paw simulates but does not manifest sympathy. The lapdog trope depicts an extreme example of this sympathetic failure by instancing an animal lavished with benevolent care and sympathy but neither interested nor capable of reciprocation" (Ellis, 2007). Fanny, on the other hand, is able to provide all her mistress could hope for or expect in such times of trial: "Fanny devoted to her aunt Bertram, returning to every former office with more than former zeal, and thinking she could never do enough for one who seemed so much to want her. To talk over the dreadful business with Fanny, talk and lament, was all Lady Bertram's consolation. To be listened to and borne with, and hear the voice of kindness and *sympathy* in return, was everything that could be done for her" (352; emphasis added). By the end of the novel, Fanny emerges as the ultimate *compassionate*, companionate figure in the text—she is "all" to Lady Bertram. Again, it is notable that it is exactly what distinguishes Fanny from Pug that makes her so crucial, so *useful* to her "mistress" and the household; she can "talk," "listen," and offer the demonstrable "kindness and sympathy" the family requires in their hardship, all activities beyond the lapdog's capacity. In fact, Pug is never mentioned in these final chapters of the narrative, once Fanny's character seems to reach the apex of the familial hierarchy in which she was once at the bottom.

At the end of the novel, the Bertram family, and perhaps Austen's reader, have learned an important lesson about the dynamics of human–animal and human–human bonds and the proper place of each in a relational hierarchy. Fanny ascends from animal/object to valued human companion to, ultimately, the wife of Edmund Bertram and full-fledged member of the Bertram household. Only Lady Bertram expresses some qualms about her niece's new position: "Selfishly dear as [Fanny] had long been to Lady Bertram, she could not be parted with willingly by *her*. No happiness of son or niece could make her wish the marriage. But it was possible to part with her, because Susan remained to supply her place" (371). Having clearly realized Fanny's value, and no longer viewing her as a pet that she owns, Lady Bertram still would have her niece forever in her attendant role. However, Lady Bertram is pacified and eventually accepting of the marriage not because of the companionship Pug can still provide, but because she has acquired a new human companion in Fanny's younger sister, Susan. Austen *could* have written, "but at least she still had her darling Pug," but instead she presents a, at least somewhat, reformed Lady Bertram who seeks companionship in another human being rather than in the listless lapdog at her side. The reader can expect that—having learned through her relationship with Fanny—Lady Bertram will treat her new attendant with more of the respect and consideration due to a true companion.

"Yet, by No Ties, But Ties of Kindness Bound": What Austen Can Tell Us About Canine and Human Companions Today

The myth created by the final line in the excerpt from Pratt's poem, with which this chapter began, is a telling glimpse into the way eighteenth- and nineteenth-century Britons wished to view their relationships with family pets. The lapdog, however, is of course bound not by "kindness" but by its status as an object owned and mastered by its human mistress; similarly, the paid female companion was tied to her mistress in an employment relationship in which she too was dependent upon her employer for her well-being. While the poem romanticizes the lapdog's "ties" to its owner, effacing the realities of domination and dependence, Jane Austen turns a probing, critical eye on canine and human companionship in *Mansfield Park*. Although one rarely hears the term "lapdog" used to describe a pet in the twenty-first century, and the hiring of paid female companions is no longer in practice today, Austen's novel—and the discourses it engages with regarding bonds between humans and animals and humans with one another—remains relevant for us, both as a representation of our past relational dynamics and as a touchstone upon which we might examine our own interpersonal bonds with pets and people alike.

Almost two centuries after Austen wrote her novel, pets are still considered companionate figures. As David Perkins writes of modern-day pets, "Pets amuse by their play, valuably distract us by their demands, and offer companionship" (Perkins, 2003). However, the same ambiguities and tensions Austen portrays regarding pets' place in the home remain and are perhaps even more pronounced in the twenty-first century. Mark Shell notes that, today, "For pet lovers, [the] interspecies transformation of a particular animal into a kind of human being is the familiar rule" (Shell, 1986). Many pet owners consider their pets to be companions, full-fledged members of the family who enjoy human-like luxuries such as gourmet food, plush bedding, "spa days," and even a wardrobe of clothing fit for all occasions and climates. Perhaps more than ever before, people talk to their pets, sharing with them the ins and outs of their day at work, or the pain of a broken relationship; they take their pets on family vacations, throw them birthday parties, buy gifts for them to unwrap during the holidays, and mourn them intensely when they pass. In this sense, Lady Bertram's treatment of Pug as one of her children is an apt forecast of the direction pet keeping was heading in the future.

Yet, the potential dangers of this heightened relationship with pets linger as well. Shell points out that "The ordinary definition of the family pet as an *animal* tends to obscure the essential demarcation between human beings and other animals since it implies that any animal, including a human being, can be a pet," suggesting that our fellow human beings may, in some cases, still be treated as pets or experience treatment inferior to that a family pet receives (Shell, 1986). An individual may refuse a homeless person a dollar on her way to buy the latest new accessory for her dog's closet of outfits; a small business owner might treat his employees with far less consideration and compassion than that which he shows to the cat waiting for him at home. Now that the keeping of paid female companions, domestic servants, and the like has fallen out of practice, however, the threat of privileging pets over people within the household circle itself has faded. In fact, of particular pertinence to my argument here, Shell asserts that one of the reasons pets have achieved such heightened status within the home is as a result of the decline in hiring domestic help: "Pets are especially useful to us here in America, in the age of the small, 'nuclear' family, because this age puts unique pressures on the kinship structure of the family. In the past, there were family slaves, nursemaids, servants, mistresses, and domestic working animals [. . .] The general disappearance of such metakinship institutions as domestic servants has left a lacuna that pets often fill" (Shell, 1986). In this formulation, pets are considered to be, and treated like, people because they have *literally* taken the place of people—the extended network of unrelated, but often intimate, domestic workers who populated the private space of the home in days gone by.

But, if pets bear the role of extra-familial family member today, in effect serving as both pet *and* companion—if pets, say, enact the roles of Austen's Pug and Fanny both—then they are not only invested with all the more affection, but also bear the brunt of all humankind's craving for mastery. Yi-Fu Tuan has explored the dynamic interplay of love and dominance that exists in our current relationships with our pets: "numerous reports, stories, and anecdotes attest to the personal devotion of owners to their charges. On the other hand, pets exist for human pleasure and convenience" (Tuan, 1984). Tuan points out that "Domestication means domination" and claims that the dog, in particular, "exhibits uniquely a set of relationships we wish to explore: dominance and affection, love and abuse, cruelty and kindness. The dog calls forth, on the one hand, the best that a human person is capable of— self-sacrificing devotion to a weaker and dependent being, and, on the other hand, the temptation to exercise power in a willful and arbitrary, even perverse, manner. Both traits can exist in the same person" (Tuan, 1984). Without fellow humans on whom to exert our cravings for authority and mastery, pets are left to fulfill this role. Consequently, it is up to us to remember Austen's lesson to Lady Bertram and her readers, to be mindful of our valuation and treatment of one another, both pet and otherwise.

References

Austen, J. (1814). *Mansfield Park*. Oxford: Oxford University Press. 2003.
Ayers-Ricker, B.. (1991). Dogs in George Eliot's Adam Bede. *The George Eliot, George Henry Lewes Newsletter, 18–19,* 22–30.

Brown, L. (2001). *Fables of modernity: Literature and culture in the English eighteenth century.* Ithaca, NY: Cornell University Press.

Ellis, M. (2007). Suffering things: Lapdogs, slaves, and counter-sensibility. In M. Blackwell (Ed.), *The secret life of things: Animals, objects, and it-narratives in eighteenth-century England* (pp. 92–113). Lewisburg, PA: Bucknell University Press.

Palmer, S. (2004). Slipping the Leash: Lady Bertram's Lapdog. *Persuasions, 25.*

Perkins, D. (2003). *Romanticism and animal rights.* Cambridge: Cambridge University Press.

Ritvo, H. (1987). *The animal estate.* Cambridge, MA: Harvard University Press.

Shell, M. (1986). The family pet. *Representations, 15,* 121–153.

Tague, I. (2008). Dead pets: Satire and sentiment in British elegies and epitaphs for animals. *Eighteenth-Century Studies, 41,* 289–306.

Thackeray, W. M. (1847). *Vanity fair.* New York: The Modern Library. 2001.

Tuan, Y. -F. (1984). *Dominance and affection: The making of pets.* New Haven, MA: Tale University Press.

Wyett, J. (2000). The lap of luxury: Lapdogs, literature, and social meaning in the 'Long' eighteenth century. *Literature, Interpretation, Theory, 10,* 275–301.

Part II
Psychological Issues of Attachment and Well-being

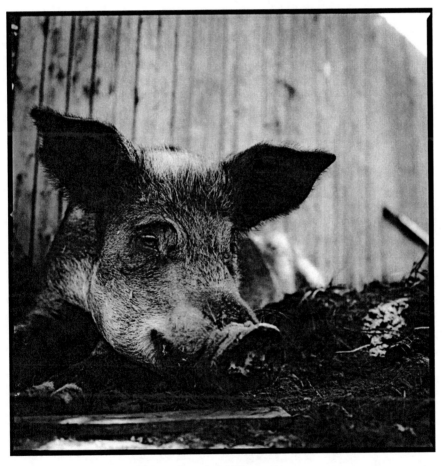

Maryjane, Resident of Grateful Acres Farm Animal Sanctuary
She was found abandoned on a farm. Rescued and since nursed back to health.

Chapter 7
Understanding the AAT Rx:
Applications of AAI in Clinical Practice

Aubrey H. Fine

The Status of Animal-Assisted Therapy

> *Mary Hessler-Kay once stated that, 'When we open our hearts and accept what our companion animals have to teach us, we gain not only the secrets to a more fulfilled life, but also a greater sense of peace and compassion.'*
> *A companion animal's love for life and for its human companions can inspire us to live each day to the fullest, learn to treat others with kindness, and become sensitive to the challenges others face (*Fine & Eisen, 2008*).*

As many chapters in this book will attest, the unique bond between humans and animals has been documented for hundreds of years. Over the decades, we have watched our relationships with domestic animals flourish and our appreciation of their significance in our lives increase. More than ever, we are realizing the sentience within animals and their contributions to our lives in general. Although, many believe that an animal-assisted intervention (AAI) is a new phenomenon, the history of animals used therapeutically dates back to the ninth century. Reports indicate taking care of an animal as part of rehabilitation was utilized in Belgium to help persons with disabilities (Fine, 2008a). One of the earliest documented trials of investigating the benefits of incorporating animals into the therapeutic lives of the mentally ill occurred at the York Retreat in England (Fine, 2008a). The staff believed that having animals on the grounds enhanced patients' morale and behavior. However, it wasn't until the early 1960s that child psychologist Boris Levinson became the leading disciple for utilizing animals in therapeutic settings. He made this discovery serendipitously when his dog, Jingles, was left with a particularly noncommunicative child client. Levinson was very impressed that the child began engaging in a deep conversation and interacting with the friendly pup (Gonski, 1985; Mason & Hagan, 1999; Reichert, 1998). Consequently, Levinson began to utilize Jingles more often in his therapy with his clients. Although not a panacea, Levinson began to argue that animals could begin to make a major difference in the overall therapy of children with various psychiatric disorders. However, its early

A.H. Fine (✉)
College of Education and Integrative Studies, CA State Polytechnic University, 3801 W. Temple Ave. Pomona, CA 91768, USA
e-mail: ahfine@csupomona.edu

C. Blazina et al. (eds.), *The Psychology of the Human–Animal Bond*,
DOI 10.1007/978-1-4419-9761-6_7, © Springer Science+Business Media, LLC 2011

reception by fellow psychotherapists was received with great skepticism. Coren (in press) in his Foreword to the third edition of *The Handbook on AAT* noted he attended Levinson's first formal presentation on animal-assisted therapy (AAT) at an American Psychological Association conference in New York. At the lecture, Levinson incorporated several findings from his case studies applying animals in therapy and provided the audience with a rationale of the value of animals in therapy. Unfortunately, Coren reports the session was not well received by the delegates. Many treated his session as trivial and with little credibility. This continued for several other years wherein the scientific community has reacted indifferently to the field. Many believe that it wasn't until National Institutes of Health (NIH) convened a workshop on the health benefits of pets in 1987, that the scientific community began to appreciate and became more willing to consider the therapeutic power of the human–animal bond.

Animal-Assisted Interventions: Definition of Terms

Before going into the major purposes and applications of AAI, it seems logical that a definition of terms be given. Although AAI is considered a relatively new field, there have been numerous terms used to describe the phenomena of incorporating animals in working with humans (Fine & Beiler, 2008). For example, LaJoie (2003) in her dissertation indicated that there were over twelve different terms in existence today to describe various animal-assisted interventions. Terms such as "pet therapy," "animal-facilitated counseling," "pet-mediated therapy," and "pet psychotherapy" have been commonly used interchangeably as descriptive terms. Nevertheless, the two most widely utilized terms are "animal-assisted therapy" and "animal-assisted activities." Both of these alternatives could be classified under the rubric of animal-assisted interventions.

The Delta Society's *Standards of Practice for Animal Assisted Therapy* (1996) defines *animal-assisted therapy* as an intervention with specified goals and objectives delivered by a health or human service professional with specialized expertise in using an animal as an integral part of treatment. For example, to help a client deal with issues of touch, a therapist may use the holding of a rabbit as a strategy to open a discussion with the child. Whether provided in a group or individual setting, Delta Society reports that AAT promotes improvement in physical, social, emotional, and/or cognitive functioning. However, these findings are primarily based on anecdotal evidence rather than empirical findings (which is one of the major weaknesses presently confronting AAI). The need for more research and empirical evidence will be discussed later in this chapter.

In contrast, *animal-assisted activities* (AAA) occur when specially trained professionals, paraprofessionals, or volunteers accompanied by animals interact with people in a variety of environments (Delta Society, 1996). In AAA, the same activity can be repeated for many different people or groups of people, the interventions are not part of a specific treatment plan and are not designed to address a specific emotional or medical condition, and detailed documentation does not occur. The familiar sight of volunteers taking their pets to visit patients at an assisted living facility meets the criteria for AAA. It is important to point out that there needs to be a clarification on what constitutes AAT, and how the recreational use of animals, although possibly therapeutic, shouldn't be viewed as therapy. For example, Beck and Katcher (1984) agree with this position and suggest that not all activities that apply to animals and are enjoyed by patients are kind of a therapy.

Present Evidence Demonstrating Efficacy

One of the greatest challenges that AAI continues to be plagued with is the lack of empirical support. Although the field continues to get an enormous amount of attention, the evidence to support AAT primarily comes from anecdotal comments and poorly designed research. (Fine, 2002, 2003, 2008b; McCulloch, 1984; Serpell, 1983). In fact, in an early paper written by Voelker (1995), he emphasized that the biggest challenge facing AAT was the lack of empirical evidence. This lack of scientific research seems to plague the acceptance of AAI, especially as many become more concerned about evidence-based forms of psychotherapy.

Before we actually address some solutions to a research agenda, which could help elevate the status of AAT, it may be helpful to highlight some of the current findings supporting the application of AAI with various special populations.

Nimer and Lundahl (2007) conducted a thorough search of all existing literature investigating the efficacy of AAT. They reviewed over 250 studies, with only 49 that met inclusion criteria into their meta-analytic procedures. Their findings suggested that AAT had moderate effects in the treatment of persons with autistic spectrum symptoms, medical difficulties, and persons with behavioral problems. Attention will now be given to a few studies (not necessarily those highlighted in the Nimer and Lundhaul study).

There have been several studies that have been conducted that have demonstrated the efficacy of AAI with persons with autistic spectrum disorders (ASD). For example, Martin and Farnum (2002) noted several improvements in children with ASD when they interacted with therapy dogs. The researchers observed improvements in children's playful moods, and they also appeared more attentive as a direct consequence of being around the dogs. It was also observed that participants laughed more and had an increase in energy during the sessions. They were more likely to talk to the dogs, and engage the therapist in discussions regarding the dogs. Finally, the subjects also focused more on related tasks when the dogs were present. These improvements were not noticed in the control condition of playing with a ball, or in the second experimental condition of playing with a stuffed dog.

Grandin, Fine and Bowers (in press) provided a rationale of why AAI may be valuable therapeutic alternative for persons with ASD. Within their paper they also pointed out specific concerns for applying AAI with this population and provided various suggestions that should be considered. For example, maybe one of the advantages that may have an impact on these relationships is perhaps that both populations (persons with ASD and various species of animals) seem to use sensory-based thinking. The authors also note that special attention needs to be given to the sensory oversensitivity within the person with ASD. It is evident that ASD impacts the manner in which persons relate to their environment. These issues (although variable with all people) may also have a tremendous impact on the person's inter-action with an animal. Some individuals may not be able to tolerate smells, others may have more difficulties with sudden sounds from an animal, while still others will have no difficulties at all. An individual needs to be evaluated to assess if any of these variables will have an impact on the outcome.

On the other hand, there have been several studies that have stressed the value of AAI in enhancing health. For example, Friedmann, Son and Tsai (in press) point out that dog owners reported that their dog was a strong source of motivation, compan-ionship, and social support. Many noted that it was the dog that encouraged them to walk more often. Friedmann et al. (in press) also reported several studies that incor-porated dog walking as an AAI and many of them demonstrated health benefits including healthier cardiovascular outcomes (Cutt, Giles-Corti, Wood, Knuiman, & Burke, 2008; Motooka, Koike, Yokoyama, & Kennedy, 2006).

Baun and Johnson (2006) have argued that animals play an important role in the lives of persons with chronic illnesses. They report that in health care set-tings, companion animals have been found to be extremely beneficial. For example, they noted that animal-assisted therapy in an oncology day hospital, with elderly patients receiving chemotherapy, resulted in decreased depression. Furthermore, Jessen, Cardiello, and Baun, (1996) reported that elderly persons hospitalized for short-term rehabilitation experienced less depression when a caged bird was placed in their rooms for seven days (Jessen et al., 1996).

Many studies have been conducted looking at the role of animals in the residential setting for the elderly. In a study by Banks and Banks (2002) residents in long-term care facilities reported feeling less loneliness when receiving animal-assisted therapy (AAT) than those not receiving AAT.

It is apparent that relationships with animals may have an impact on quality of life, especially with those who are suffering from terminal illnesses. Phear (1996) prepared a report that surveyed the attitudes to companion animals in a day hospice in the United Kingdom. The report suggested that all hospice patients enjoyed the companionship and interaction from visiting animals. Phear (1996) concluded that one of the strongest benefits derived from the animals was the fact that the animal was an attentive audience to individual patients and provided the needed affection. Additionally, Chinner and Dalziel (1991) pointed out that the use of a therapy dog in a hospice setting appeared to enhance the patient–staff relationship and enhanced the morale of the living environment. They also observed that the dog had a relaxing and comforting effect on the patients.

Nevertheless, as previously noted, although the results of these studies show promise, there are limits to the designs presently in place to evaluate their effi-cacy. Fine and Mio (2006) suggest that those interested in advancing AAT into more accepted evidence-based intervention must consider the steps that need to be taken to document its efficacy. According to Kazdin (in press), there are several methodological standards now in place for establishing evidence-based psychotherapies. Most researchers would agree that RCTs (randomized controlled trials) are a beginning point and regarded as the "gold standard." He emphasized that key questions need to be answered by the researchers to support the application of AAI. Basically, the questions are as follows: Does the presence of an animal improve the effectiveness of therapy and if so, what is it about the animal contact that makes a difference? Additional questions, such as what clients and with what types problems are most likely to respond to AAI, would be excellent focus questions to be addressed. Kazdin (in press) concludes by arguing that the future research in AAT must match the other designs put into place by other disciplines in psychotherapy for its status to be more elevated and respected.

The Foundation of AAT: Understanding the Basic Tenets

Fine (2009) has suggested that there are several basic tenets to consider when incorporating animals into therapeutic practice. For the AAI to be effective, the procedures need to be integrated into the therapeutic goals of the therapy. Fine (2006) developed a simple problem-solving template that therapists could use as they plan on applying AAT interventions with their various patients. The following three questions should be considered:

A: What benefits can AAT/AAI provide this client?
   The clinician needs to consider the benefits animals will have in the therapy. What benefits will the animals provide in the clinical intervention?
B: How can AAT strategies be incorporated within the planned intervention?
   A clinician must begin to conceptualize the vast array of opportunities that the therapy animals can provide. A plan must be formulated so the outcome will not be purely serendipitous.
C: How will the therapist need to adapt his/her clinical approach to incorporate AAT?

Chandler (2005) also agrees that the therapist needs to integrate the goals of the therapy into the animal-assisted intervention. She points out the therapist should design interventions to involve a therapy animal in ways that will move a client toward treatment goals. The decisions regarding if, when, and how a therapy animal can or should be incorporated into therapy depends on (1) the client's desire for AAI along with the appropriateness of the client for AAI (which may be prohibited by such things as animal allergies, animal phobias, or client's aggressive tendency); (2) the therapist's creative methods to design AAI consistent with a client's treatment plan; and (3) the therapy animal's ability to perform activities that assist in moving a client in a direction consistent with treatment goals (Chandler, 2005).

Animals as Social Lubricants

Many believe that one of the most natural aspects of integrating animals into therapy is their role in enhancing therapeutic alliance. O'Callaghan (2008) investigated the various animal-assisted interventions incorporated by mental health professionals as part of their therapeutic regime and their intended purposes. Results from her study found that the vast majority of mental health counselors reported using AAT to *build rapport in the therapeutic relationship*. They often did this by reflecting on the client's relationship with the therapy animal, encouraging the client to interact with the therapy animal, and sharing information about the therapy animal. Arkow (1982), in an earlier publication, suggested that the animal might act as a link in the conversation between the therapist and the client. He called this process a rippling effect. Others, such as Corson and Corson (1980), describe this process as a social lubricant. It appears that the presence of the animal allows the client a sense of comfort, which then promotes rapport in the therapeutic relationship.

Mallon (1992) emphasizes in his paper that the animals must be considered as adjuncts in the establishment of a therapeutic relationship and bond. Fine (2006) suggests that when relating to a therapist with an animal, people with difficulties sometimes find the animals the catalyst for discussion, which previously may have been blocked.

Parish-Plass (2008) suggests that AAT is based on the very strong emotional connection and evolving relationship between the therapist, client, and animal. She points out that animal's presence in the environment contributes to the perception of a safe environment. She also believes that the client's perceptions that the therapist makes the therapy animal feel safe contributes to the client's impression that s/he will feel safe as well. This perception agrees with the work of Kruger, Trachtenberg, and Serpell (2004) who also suggested that a therapist who conducts therapy with an animal being present might appear less threatening. A gentle animal helps a client view the therapist in a more endearing manner.

Fine and Eisen (2008) in their book, *Afternoons with Puppy,* highlight many case studies which demonstrate the value of having a therapy animal to act as a social catalyst. The following is one case study. Meet Sarah and Hart (a black Labrador).

Sarah was thirteen when she first attended therapy. Her school counselor referred her because of apparent depression and anxiety. She entered her first session wearing a baseball cap pulled low on her head. She seemed to use the brim of the cap to cover her eyes. Sarah was overweight and trembled most of the first session. Her mother reported that Sarah had significant difficulties with various family members. To complicate matters, her parents had recently divorced and her mom had taken a job outside the home. This left Sarah and her sister alone much of the time.

At her first visit, Hart simply went to her side, ready to be petted if and when Sarah felt like it. Initially, Sarah didn't look at Hart or mention the dog's presence, but after a few seconds, she reached out and stroked Hart's head. She petted the dog without much show of emotion. It seems that she primarily used the action of petting Hart to avoid looking at me. Yet her trembling decreased. The physical contact with Hart eased her tension and anxiety.

Early in our relationship Sarah revealed, *"I have no real friends and feel like an outcast. They ignore me because I'm different. They can't see my fear, that I'm just afraid all the time. "* Adding to her fear was the high incidence of violence and crime in her neighborhood; because of this, she felt her two primary environments, home and school, held no comfort or safety. To help deal with her fear, she wore clothes that she could hide in: an oversized army jacket, matching army green pants, sneakers, and always a baseball cap pulled low over her eyes.

Sarah was hospitalized after a few sessions because of cutting. After Sarah was released from the facility, the turning point in our relationship was the day she showed me the healing scars. When she lifted her sleeve after a few moments, Hart looked at the scars and slowly walked over to her and began to lick them. This action connected the two and Sarah began to weep. She found her soul mate, but in this case she was wrapped in fur. Hart then became a large part of her treatment. Sarah loved having the chance to walk Hart, and her special affection for Hart helped initiate a new openness in our discussions.

Over the course of our treatment, Sarah made great progress. I placed her on independent study, and also I integrated volunteering at a preschool and an animal shelter into her treatment. Her outside experiences seemed to provide her with more comfort and security and she began to blossom.

After we reached our therapeutic goals, Sarah was dismissed from therapy. It had been over two years since I had heard from or seen Sarah, when one day, I received a wonderful e-mail from her. She wrote:

Hello Dr. Fine:
You may not remember me, but I was "seeing" you for a while when I was younger. I was doing research about animals in psychology and I read about a book you were writing about your animals. It reminded me of how when I had "seen" you, I was so scared and nervous about saying the wrong thing, that I usually didn't talk about much. I remember how whenever I was nervous, Hart and Shrimp would be right there, as if telling me that your not a "bad" guy and the such. Hart especially seemed to be the one being the psychologist, always sitting near me, comforting me from everything that I would worry about. She is what I remember most about my visits. She also gave me an excuse to talk to my Mom about what was going on at the time.
In the end, I don't remember talking to you about much, but all that I did tell you was for those two...and some of the fish, (though one isn't able to pet a fish) and the bearded dragon. My Mom and I still talk about one of the fish in the waiting room that would swim in a repetitive motion, and looked like it was the happiest fish in the world, and I still tell my friends about how I went on a walk with a bird. (they still don't believe me.)
I hope all is well with you and the animals. Good luck on the book.

Six months after her e-mail, we had a reunion. She looked so different. Her hair was longer and there is a positive air in the way she carried herself. There was a simple but beautiful glow in her eyes. She now spoke clearly and her voice was strong. Sarah was excited to tell me all about her accomplishments, but even more she delighted in telling me about her new life. She was a full-time student at a local high school, earning A's and B's. Additionally, since going back to school she had become more outgoing, joining a hiking club and an animal advocacy and support group. She told me that she became a member of a service group that raises money to send livestock to underdeveloped countries. For a short while, she explained her love of all these new opportunities, but then she focused more on her relationships with people: "I like the volunteer work with the animals, but I like hanging out with friends more."

After talking for a short while, I knew it was not really me that she came to visit. I looked at her and said, "Do you want to see your friend?" She smiled and said yes. A moment later out pranced Hart from the backroom.

Hart wandered over to Sarah, just the way she used to. Her tail was wagging and her body swayed back and forth. Sarah looked into Hart's eyes and said, "You are the one who got me through the tough time. You got me to talk." It was a touching moment. They embraced, as though no time has passed and Hart was still the blanket of fur that comforted her. It is evident when reading this case study that Hart fulfilled numerous roles for this client. She initially acted as the social catalyst that engaged Sarah to become more comfortable and involved in therapy. As time proceeded, with the support and attention from Hart, Sarah was able to reveal more in therapy and progress was made.

The Benefits of Animals as an Extension to a Therapist: A Method for Rapport Building

Animals are known for the zealous greetings they provide to visiting clients they encounter. Levinson (1965), in a seminal article on the use of pets (in the treatment of children with behavior disorders), implies that bringing in the animal at the beginning of therapy assisted frequently in helping a reserved client overcome his/her anxiety about therapy. Many therapy dogs are more than willing to receive a client in a warm and affectionate manner. Imber-Black (2009) points out that animals in therapy provide healthy support for spouses being yelled at by their partners and shy children who are anxious to attend therapy.

A Therapeutic Benefit of Animals in Therapy: A Catalyst for Emotion

Fine and Beiler (2008) point out that for many clients, the mere presence of an animal in a therapeutic setting can stir emotions. Simply interacting with an animal in a therapeutic setting can lighten the mood and lead to smiling and laughter. Animals may also display emotions or actions that may not be professionally appropriate for therapists to display. For example, the animal might climb into a client's lap or sit calmly while the client pets him. Holding or petting an animal may sooth clients and help them feel calm when exploring difficult emotions in treatment that might be overwhelming without this valuable therapeutic touch. Animals within therapeutic settings can also elicit a range of emotions from laughter to sorrow.

Animals as Teachers

Teaching animals and supporting their growth can also have therapeutic benefits for the clients. There have been many therapists that have used animals as part of therapy in a teaching manner. Arluke (2007) investigated five settings utilizing AAI while treating teens at risk. The major goal of all the programs was to give the youths an opportunity to act as mentors and teachers for animals that needed their support. Although there has been limited empirical evidence supporting these programs, anecdotal comments and qualitative feedback seemed to suggest they helped the youth develop more appropriate pro-social skills. The paper also gives some good insight on how one should apply these practices so that there will be more generalization of the behaviors.

There have been numerous other researchers and clinicians who have studied and written on how animals can be used in different teaching capacities with other diverse group of children. For example, Katcher and Wilkins (2000) have written on the role of therapeutic farms and children with Attention Deficit/Hyperactivity Disorder (ADHD) and the tremendous impact thy have made. Baról (2007) and Gee, Sherlock, Bennett, and Harris (2009) have used animals as a catalyst for teaching children (preschoolers and children with autism) developmental skills such as counting, cutting, expressing oneself, and problem solving.

Considerations for Applying AAI

Training and Liability

Therapists considering incorporating animals within their practice must seriously consider the factors of liability, training, as well as the safety and welfare of both the animal and the client. The Delta Society's Pet Partner Program strongly advocates that health care professionals must have training in AAT techniques. Clinicians also need to be aware of best practice procedures ensuring quality, as well as safety, for all parties.

There are numerous references that therapists should consider reading to help them understand dog behavior and possible training techniques. The *Other End of The Leash* by Patricia McConnell (2002) and *The Power of Positive Dog Training* by Pat Miller (2001) are two excellent guides. Fine's (2006) third edition (2010) of the *Handbook on Animal Assisted Therapy* is also a tremendous guide that could be used to answer numerous questions. Attention is not only given in the chapters to discuss how one builds and designs an effective intervention, but is also given to helping clinicians recognize their ethical responsibility to safeguard and preserve the therapy animal's welfare.

Conclusions and Directions for the Future

The field of animal-assisted interventions continues to evolve. More attention continues to be given to these interventions as a plausible adjunct to treatment. Although glorified and sometimes misrepresented, it is apparent that animals can make a significant difference to the well-being of many persons, especially those in need. Nevertheless, process mustn't be misrepresented and appear too simple. Quality

✓ AAT occurs only when a tandem relationship between a trained therapist and a therapy animal is applied and works well. It is a process that utilizes clinical problem solving, just like any other form of psychotherapy.

Fine and Eisen (2008) point out that the relationships between animals and people shouldn't be viewed for only the extraordinary outcomes, but rather the impact of an evolving relationship. If people focus only on the outcomes, they will miss the brilliance of the process. The magic within these interventions is found in the daily actions that are at the heart of animal-assisted interventions.

The author fully supports the need for a stronger research agenda to document the efficacy of this intervention. Positive findings should help elevate the status of the field and hopefully provide those who are skeptical with stronger evidence to follow. However, some information that seems simple to understand may be more difficult to measure. One may marvel, if this is one of the apparent roadblocks in measuring the effect of the human–animal bond. As Albert Einstein once insinuated, *"everything that can be counted does not necessarily count; everything that counts cannot necessarily be counted."* Maybe our quest to document and study this impact may lead us to new roads of understanding and maybe even more unclear answers. Only the future will know for sure.

References

Arkow, P. (1982). *Pet therapy: A study of the use of companion animals in selected therapies.* Colorado Springs, CO: Humane Society of Pikes Peak Region.

Arluke, A. (2007). *Animal assisted activities for at-risk and incarcerated children and young adults: An introductory ethnography of five programs.* Unpublished paper presented at the National Technology Assessment Workshop on Animal Assisted Programs for Youth at Risk, Baltimore.

Banks, M. R., & Banks, W. A. (2002). The effects of animal-assisted therapy on loneliness in an elderly population in long-term care facilities. *Journal of Gerontology, 57*(7), 428–432.

Baról, J. (2007). *The effects of animal assisted therapy on a child with autism.* Unpublished doctoral dissertation. New Mexico Highlands University, Las Vegas, NM.

Baun, M., & Johnson, B. (2006). Human-animal interactions and successful aging. In A. Fine (Ed.), *The handbook on animal assisted therapy* (3rd Ed.). San Diego, CA: Elsevier Press.

Beck, A., & Katcher, A. H. (1984). *Between pets and people: The importance of animal companionship.* New York: G. P. Putnam's Sons.

Chandler, C. K. (2005). *Animal assisted therapy in counseling.* New York: Routledge.

Chinner, T., & Dalziel, F. (1991). An exploratory study on the viability and efficacy of a pet-facilitated therapy project within a hospice. *Journal of Palliative Care, 7*(4), 13–20.

Coren, S. (2010). Forword. In A. H. Fine (Ed.), *Handbook on animal assisted therapy: Theoretical foundations and guidelines for practice* (3rd Ed.) (pp. 247–264). San Diego, CA: Academic Press.

Corson, S., & Corson, E. (1980). Pet animals as nonverbal communication mediators in psychotherapy in institutional settings. In S. Corson & E. Corson (Eds.), *Ethology and nonverbal communication in mental health* (pp. 83–110). Oxford: Pergamon Press.

Cutt, H. E., Giles-Corti, B., Wood, L. J., Knuiman, M. W., & Burke, V. (2008). Barriers and motivators for owners walking their dog: Results from qualitative research. *Health Promotion Journal of Australia, 19*, 118–124.

Delta Society. (1996). *Standards of practice in animal assisted activities and therapy*. Renton, WA: Delta Society.

Fine, A. H. (2002). Animal assisted therapy. In M. Hersen & W. Sledge (Eds.), *Encyclopedia of psychotherapy* (pp. 49–55). New York: Elsevier Science.

Fine, A. H. (2003, November 1). *Animal assisted therapy and clinical practice*. Psycho-Legal Associates CEU meeting, Seattle, WA.

Fine, A. H. (2006). Animals and therapists: Incorporating animals in outpatient psychotherapy. In A. Fine (Ed.), *Handbook on animal assisted therapy* (2nd Ed., pp. 179–211). San Diego, CA: Academic Press.

Fine, A. H. (2008a). Building a bond: Three principles lead the way to a close human-canine relationship. *Dog Fancy, 39*(10), 51.

Fine, A. H. (2008b, September 30–October 2). *Understanding the application of animal assisted interventions*. National Institute of Child and Human Development meeting on the Impact of Animals in Human Health, Bethesda, MD.

Fine, A. H. (2009, October 20–25). Animal assisted interventions from a researcher/practitioner point of view: Bridging the gap and strengthening efficacy. *2008 ISAZ Conference*. Kansas City, MO.

Fine, A. H., & Beiler, P. (2008). Demystifying animal assisted intervention: Understanding the roles of animals in therapeutic settings. In A. Stozier (Ed.), *Handbook of alternative therapies*. Binghamton, NY: The Hayworth Press.

Fine, A. H., & Eisen, C. (2008). *Afternoons with puppy: Inspirations from a therapist and his animals*. West Lafayette, IN: Purdue University Press.

Fine, A. H., & Mio, J. (2006). The future of research, education, and clinical practice in the animal-human bond and animal-assisted therapy. Part C: The role of animal-assisted therapy in clinical practice: The importance of demonstrating empirically oriented psychotherapies. In A. H. Fine (Ed.), *Handbook on animal-assisted therapy: Theoretical foundations and guidelines for practice* (2nd Ed., pp. 167–206). San Diego, CA: Academic Press.

Friedmann, E., Son, H., & Tsai, C. (2010). The animal/human bond: Health and wellness. In A. H. Fine (Ed.), *Handbook on animal assisted therapy: Theoretical foundations and guidelines for practice* (3rd Ed.) (pp. 85–110). San Diego, CA: Academic Press.

Gee, N. R., Sherlock, T. R., Bennett, E. A., & Harris, S. L. (2009). Preschoolers' adherence to instructions as a function of presence of a dog and motor skills task. *Anthrozoos, 22*(3), 267–276.

Gonski, Y. (1985). The therapeutic utilization of canines in a child welfare setting. *Child & Adolescent Social Work Journal, 2*(2), 93–105.

Grandin, T., Fine, A. H., & Bowers, C. (2010). The use of therapy animals with individuals with autism spectrum disorders. In A. H. Fine (Ed.), *Handbook on animal assisted therapy: Theoretical foundations and guidelines for practice* (3rd Ed.) (pp. 247–264). San Diego, CA: Academic Press.

Imber-Black, E. (2009). Snuggles, my cotherapist, and other animal tales in life and therapy. *Family Process, 48*, 459–461.

Jessen, J., Cardiello, F., & Baun, M. M. (1996). Avian companionship in alleviation of depression, loneliness, and low morale of older adults in skilled rehabilitation units. *Psychological Reports, 78*, 339–348.

Katcher, A. H., & Wilkins, G. (2000). The centaur's lessons: Therapeutic education through care of animals and nature study. In A. Fine (Ed.), *Handbook on animal assisted therapy* (1st Ed., pp. 153–178). San Diego, CA: Academic Press.

Kazdin, A. (2010). Methodological standards and strategies for establishing the evidence base of animal-assisted therapies. In A. H. Fine (Ed.), *Handbook on animal assisted therapy: Theoretical foundations and guidelines for practice* (3rd Ed.) (pp. 519–546). San Diego, CA: Academic Press.

Kruger, K., Trachtenberg, S., & Serpell, J. A. (2004). *Can animals help humans heal? Animal-assisted interventions in adolescent mental health*. Retrieved from http://www2.vet.upenn.edu/research/centers/cias/pdf/CIAS_AAI_white_paper.pdf

LaJoie, K. R. (2003). *An evaluation of the effectiveness of using animals in therapy.* Unpublished doctoral dissertation, Spalding University, Louisville, KY.

Levinson, B. M. (1965). Pet psychotherapy: use of household pets in the treatment of behavior disorder in childhood. *Psychological Reports, 17,* 695–698.

Mallon, G. P. (1992). Utilization of animals as therapeutic adjuncts with children and youth: A review of the literature. *Child and Youth Care Forum, 21*(1), 53–67.

Martin, F., & Farnum, J. (2002). Animal assisted therapy for children with pervasive developmental disorders. *Western Journal of Nursing Research, 24,* 657–670.

Mason, M., & Hagan, C. (1999). Pet-assisted psychotherapy. *Psychological Reports, 84*(3), 1235–1245.

McConnell, P. (2002). *At the other end of the leash.* New York: Ballantine Books.

McCulloch, M. J. (1984). Pets in therapeutic programs for the aged. In R. K. Anderson, B. L. Hart, & L. A. Hart (Eds.), *The pet connection* (pp. 387–398). Minneapolis, MN: Center to Study Human-Animal Relationships and Environment.

Miller, P. (2001). *The power of positive dog training.* New York: Hungry Minds.

Motooka, M., Koike, H., Yokoyama, T., & Kennedy, N. L. (2006). Effect of dog-walking on autonomic nervous activity in senior citizens. *Medical Journal of Australia, 184,* 60–63.

National Institute of Health Workshop (1987, September 10–11). *The health benefits of pets. Workshop summary.* Bethesda, MD: National Institute of Health, Office of Medical Applications of Research.

Nimer, J., & Lundahl, B. (2007). Animal-assisted therapy: A meta-analysis. *Anthrozoos, 20,* 225–238.

O'Callaghan, D. (2008). *Exploratory study of animal assisted therapy interventions used by mental health professionals.* Unpublished doctoral dissertation, University of North Texas, Denton.

Parish-Plass, N. (2008). Animal assisted therapy and children suffering from insecure attachment due to abuse and neglect: A method to lower the risk of intergenerational transmission of abuse? *Clinical Child Psychology and Psychiatry, 13,* 7–30.

Phear, D. (1996). A study of animal companionship in a day hospice. *Palliative Medicine, 10,* 336–339.

Reichert, E. (1998). Individual counseling for sexually abused children: A role for animals in storytelling. *Child and Adolescent Social Work Journal, 15*(3), 177–185.

Serpell, J. A. (1983). Pet psychotherapy. *People – Animal – Environment, 1,* 7–8.

Voelker, R. (1995). Puppy love can be therapeutic, too. *The Journal of the American Medical Association, 274,* 1897–1899.

Chapter 8
Self Psychology and the Human–Animal Bond: An Overview

Sue-Ellen Brown

Self Psychology and the Human–Animal Bond: An Overview

Why is it that some people will stop short at paying for an injury to their animal and elect for euthanasia, while others will go into financial ruin to pay for their animal's radiation and chemotherapy to prolong their animal's life for just one year? Why is it that some people are extremely bonded to one of their animals and not the others? And what makes some people become desperate at even a hint that their animal may be sick? Finally, how can family members or significant others convey their understanding of the loved one's extraordinary bond in an empathetic way?

The answer to these questions lies in an application of a psychological theory called self psychology developed by a prominent psychoanalyst named Heinz Kohut (1971, 1984). Self psychology is a psychoanalytic theory that is primarily used in applied clinical situations between a therapist and a patient. The theory is used by psychotherapists both as a developmental model and as a method of conducting psychotherapy (Banai, Mikulincer, & Shaver, 2005). Self psychology helps psychotherapists gain an in-depth understanding of the patient's needs and relationships and to guide the therapist's empathic responses. But self psychology can also be applied to the human–animal bond. Self psychology can help define the kind of relationship a person has with his/her animal and also explain why some animals are so crucial to a person's sense of self and well-being.

This work was funded in part by the Department of Health and Human Services' Health and Services Administration, Bureau of Health Professions under Tuskegee University's Center of Excellence Grant.

S.E. Brown (✉)
Paoletta Counseling Services Inc., Mercer, PA 16137, USA
e-mail: sebi2i@aol.com

Previous Research

Although many theoretical articles and case studies appear in the literature of self psychology, there are very few quantitative or qualitative research studies that utilize self psychology. One reason for the lack of research is that selfobject needs are thought to be primarily unconscious, only occasionally reaching consciousness (Kohut, 1971). Therefore, it would be difficult for people to consciously assess their own selfobject needs and rate them on a questionnaire.

Silverstein (1999) applied self psychology concepts to a person's time-limited sample of discourse in *Self Psychology and Diagnostic Assessment: Identifying Selfobject Functions through Psychological Testing*. In this book, he describes how he identifies the mirroring, idealizing, and twinship selfobject needs in the psychological testing protocols of various patients. He describes in detail each of the selfobject types and gives many examples of each. Silverstein's examples consist of humans using other humans or objects and ideas as selfobjects, but not animals.

Self psychology as a field lacks quantitative and qualitative research to define and examine Kohut's concepts empirically (Banai et al., 2005). Banai et al. point out that there are scales measuring narcissism, but those are mostly based on a psychiatric definition of narcissism and not specifically on Kohut's ideas. Also, some researchers have created scales to measure other concepts that Kohut used, such as grandiosity and idealization, but they did not measure specific selfobject needs (Banai et al., 2005). Obviously, more research is necessary on Kohut's selfobject concepts before they will be as well accepted and useful for quantitative research studies.

Banai et al. (2005) created a self-report measure that was based on self psychology concepts, such as the selfobject needs for mirroring, idealization, and twinship. Following a series of survey studies, they concluded that their 38-item questionnaire called "Selfobject Needs Inventory" (SONI) was able to measure a person's hunger for selfobject needs for mirroring, idealization, and twinship as well as the avoidance of these needs. However, the SONI is designed to measure selfobject needs with people, not companion animals.

Brown (2007) used the theory of self psychology to design a semi-structured, 16-question interview to explore the types of selfobjects a companion animal fulfilled for 24 participants, many of whom rescued animals. The interviews were intended to identify whether the horse/dog/cat/rabbit was a selfobject—that is, a provider of self-cohesion, self-esteem, calmness, soothing, and acceptance—for the participant and, if so, whether the primary type(s) of selfobject was mirroring, idealizing, or twinship. She found that companion animals provided strong selfobject functions to the participants and that the type of selfobject relationship could be determined to be of a mirroring, idealized, or twinship nature from the interview data. In this sample, animals rivaled and even surpassed humans in their ability to provide important selfobject needs for the participants.

Alper (1993) applied self psychology concepts to her case studies of children seen in psychotherapy. Alper did not collect data in any systematic way other than using case studies as examples of self psychological concepts.

Hartmann, M. and Walter, H. (2009) also attempted to quantify the human–animal bond through using self psychological concepts in a questionnaire; however, their work is published in German only.

Basics of Self Psychology

In self psychology, two of the main concepts are "self" and "selfobject." The self is a psychological structure that is the core of the personality and gives a person a sense of well-being, self-esteem, and general cohesion (Wolf, 1988). A selfobject need is provided by an animal, person, thing, idea, or experience in the environment which gives a sense of cohesion, support, or sustenance to a person's sense of self (Kohut, 1984). To be considered as fulfilling a selfobject function, the person, animal, thing, idea, or experience must play a crucial role in sustaining the self of the person. If the selfobject is taken away, the person will feel a sense of fragmentation or falling apart. Does this mean that a person may be held together psychologically by an animal? The answer to this question is, "yes."

Is the Animal a Selfobject?

Technically, the animal is not the selfobject, but the supportive function the dog provides to the person is the selfobject function. Some important aspect of the particular external "object" stirs an inner experience (feeling validated and connected) inside the person. The objective, external aspects of a selfobject (whether a person or animal) would make little difference for the self or person (Kohut, 1984). The important aspect for the person is the inner experience stirred by the selfobject. For example, a snake kept as a companion animal may not appear to most people as a creature that would fulfill a selfobject function. However, for someone, that snake could be providing a vital selfobject function, perhaps making a person feel calm and powerful in the snake's presence.

Most people are held together or sustained by other important people in their lives, such as spouses, parents, friends, or other loved ones. The most important of those people are probably serving a selfobject function to the person. The true test of whether or not someone is serving a selfobject function is to find out what the person's reaction would be if the selfobject were to be lost. If the person would feel devastated and have trouble functioning, then the person or animal would probably be fulfilling a selfobject need.

The reliance or dependency on an animal selfobject can also be quite intense and crucial to a person's sense of well-being. Kohut (1971) believed that sometimes the selfobject may even be experienced as not separate but as part of the self. Therefore, if separated from an animal selfobject, the person may feel a sense of emptiness, depression, or disintegration until reunited with the animal (Brown, 2007).

Given the internal turmoil that is possible when losing an important animal as a selfobject, it is easy to understand why people can become desperate to save their animal's lives at any cost. In such cases, the people may be (consciously or unconsciously) striving desperately to maintain the core of their whole personality by keeping their companion animals alive (Brown, 2007).

If the relationship with an animal is not that crucial to the person's sense of self, then it is not a selfobject experience (Wolf, 1988). It is possible to feel protected by, enjoy the company of, be amused by, or even love a companion animal, but these functions may not necessarily be crucial for the integrity of the person's self structure. An example of this might be a dog that is kept strictly for the protection of the home and family. The owner may appreciate the protective function the dog serves but will not experience a sense of falling apart if the dog dies. In this case, the dog was not functioning as a selfobject (Brown, 2007).

In self psychology, the objective reality of the animal selfobject is not important to determine for the animal to be a selfobject (Kohut, 1971). Therefore, how the animal really feels or the true meaning of their behavior is not really relevant to what they give to the person. The animal may make a person feel special and loved even if they are not objectively demonstrating behavior that would lead most people to conclude that is what the animal is in fact indicating. This explains how an animal hoarder can state that the animals make them feel loved even if the animals may be sick or dead. It is the internal experience of the person receiving the selfobject function that is important.

Three Types of Selfobject Experiences

According to Kohut (1984), there are three types of selfobjects: (1) mirroring, (2) idealizing, and (3) twinship. Wolf (1988), a psychiatrist, and Silverstein (1999), a psychologist, further defined these three types of selfobjects. Finally, Brown (2007), a psychologist, added animal examples to these selfobject types.

Mirroring selfobjects sustain the self by providing the experience of affirmation, confirmation, and recognition of the self in its grandness, goodness, and wholeness (Wolf, 1988). These feelings promote positive self-esteem, healthy pride, buoyancy, and energy. A mirroring selfobject animal would make one feel loved in spite of any flaws, imperfections, or "warts" (Wolf, 1988). In the study by Brown (2007), there was a woman who owned an Australian Shepherd–Border Collie mixed breed dog. That dog was extremely devoted to the woman and stayed by her side whenever possible. This behavior made the woman feel special, loved more than anyone in the world, and accepted unconditionally.

Idealized selfobjects sustain the self by allowing the person to have the experience of being part of an admired and respected selfobject. Idealized animals provide the opportunity to be accepted and be part of a stable, non-anxious, wise, powerful, protective, or calm selfobject (Wolf, 1988). For example, in the study by Brown (2007), an elderly woman relied on her Rottweiler to keep her safe. He protected her from unwanted intruders as well as aggressive stray dogs. Her dog made her feel strong, protected, and powerful. Horses also often serve as idealized selfobjects, making people feel strong, protected, and calm when around their horses (Brown, 2007).

√ Finally, twinship selfobjects sustain the self by providing the experience of essential likeness of another's self (Wolf, 1988). According to Silverstein (1999), the core characteristics of the twinship selfobject relationship shows the experience of intimacy and shared understanding in depth or a sort of communion with each other, like a "soulmate." There may be the wish for a feeling of oneness or a deep and close bond. There may also be a shared worldview, thinking the same thoughts, having the same feelings or mutuality of needs (Silverstein, 1999). An example of this from the study by Brown (2007) is a woman who felt like she was sharing her spine with her horse when doing dressage and they communicated by breathing alone. She felt as though she was one with her horse, physically, psychologically, and spiritually.

Additional Self Psychology Concepts

Self psychology emphasizes that what happens during infancy is critical to the development of a secure, cohesive self (Banai et al., 2005). The availability and responsiveness of parents or other caregivers is essential for healthy self-development as well as secure attachment. Kohut (1971) stated that during infancy, the self is immature and totally dependent on caregivers for soothing, distress regulation, and self-cohesion. But through a process of empathic interactions with the mothering figure (or selfobject) he or she develops the internal capacity for self-regulation of emotional states and becomes less dependent on others. Kohut felt that empathy from a caregiver is as important to human development as is oxygen.

Self psychology emphasizes that when a mothering figure is inconsistent, absent, or abusive the stage is set for lifelong issues in relating to others and/or psychopathology (Banai et al., 2005). Kohut (1971) described the resulting pathologies in terms of unmet selfobject needs and the development of disorders of the self, such as pathological narcissism. According to Kohut, people with a disordered self become extremely vulnerable to criticism and failure, focused on their deficiencies, overwhelmed by negative emotions, pessimistic thoughts, and feelings of alienation and loneliness. They may also remain heavily dependent on selfobjects throughout their lives to maintain emotional stability, unable to regulate internal states on their own.

Another important concept in self psychology is that the ability to self-regulate emotions and to maintain self-esteem and self-cohesion are obtained through a developmental process involving interactions with significant others in the environment (Banai et al., 2005). The process begins in infancy with parents and eventually the person becomes able to self-regulate internal states. Kohut (1971) called this process "transmuting internalization." √

According to self psychology, the support from others in the environment is necessary throughout the life span (Banai et al., 2005). According to Kohut, people will always need external support to maintain a healthy sense of self (or narcissism) throughout life, especially during times of crisis, life transitions, or traumatic experiences.

According to Schore (2003), Kohut worked to deepen the understanding of four basic areas: (1) how is the self developed in early relations within the self–selfobject (or infant–mother) dyad, (2) how the early interactions with the social environment become internalized as the structuralization of the self, (3) how the early deficits in self-structure lead to self-pathologies, and, finally (4) how can a therapeutic relationship lead to a restoration of the self. Also, Kohut developed the three kinds of selfobject needs: mirroring, idealizing, and twinship. Kohut not only created a model of development, but he also created a systematic way of doing psychotherapy to heal disorders of the self.

Self psychology has been used primarily by psychotherapy clinicians as a theoretical model to understand the development of psychopathology, as the structure of a person's self (both healthy and pathological aspects), and also as a method to treat people with disorders of the self. Because of the fact that there is a current emphasis on using evidence-based treatment (EBT) in psychotherapy techniques, self psychology may become less evident as a psychotherapeutic technique unless more empirical evidence is forthcoming.

Companion Animal Selfobject Questionnaire

One selfobject, self-report assessment tool already exists. Banai et al. (2005) developed a 38-item Self-Oobject Needs Inventory (SONI). Through a series of several survey studies, the authors found that the selfobject needs for mirroring, idealization, and twinship could be operationalized by a reliable and valid self-report measure, the SONI. The SONI also measures the level of hunger for, or avoidance of, the three selfobject needs. However, the SONI is designed to measure selfobject relationships with people, not companion animals. Also, Europeans have proposed an instrument to measure selfobject functions of companion animals; however, that research and the resulting scale are published only in German at this time (Hartmann & Walter, 2009).

The purpose of the Companion Animal Selfobject Questionnaire is to allow people to get a general idea of what kind of selfobject role a companion animal may have in their lives. To find out which type of selfobject your animal may be for you, take the Companion Animal Selfobject Questionnaire below. Keep just one animal in mind as you fill it out. If you have more than one animal, fill it out separately for each animal. It is important to remember that the questionnaire is only meant to give a general idea about the selfobject type—that is, mirroring, idealized, or twinship—and your animal may fulfill more than one selfobject function. Also, these selfobject functions can change over time, depending on what the person needs at various times in his life. For example, it is possible to have a strong mirroring need at one point in life and then have that change to an idealizing need at a later point. Furthermore, selfobject needs can vary depending on life circumstances. During times of crisis or stress, selfobject needs may be intensified but become less crucial during times of peace and contentment. Therefore, the questionnaire results are only meant to be an approximation of what role your animal companion plays in your life at this time.✓

This Companion Animal Selfobject Questionnaire has been designed by taking the interview questions used in the Brown (2007) study as well as some additional questions. All questions were created by using the selfobject descriptions given by Silverstein (1999) and Wolf (1988). Silverstein's (1999) descriptions of selfobject functions were developed to measure selfobject needs in projective testing. No psychometric data exist on this preliminary selfobject questionnaire. Therefore, the questionnaire was devised from only face validity derived from the theory, so some ✓ caution may be warranted when using this. This questionnaire would not necessarily be expected to be reliable, as selfobject needs can change over time. Hopefully, future research could address the validity of the questionnaire. (See appendix for the Companion Animal Selfobject Questionnaire.)

Mature vs Archaic Selfobjects

Kohut discussed archaic and mature selfobject relating but never completely defined the terms (Tonnesvang, 2002). As described in Brown (2011), the main differentiation between the two types of relating is the ability to empathize with the selfobjects and see them as independent others, with needs and lives separate and different from their own. Hagman (1997) referred to this as "self-centeredness" versus "other-centeredness." Hagman says the sense of differentiation of the object from the self is fundamental to mature selfobject experiences and is the main concept for distinguishing between mature and archaic ways of selfobject relating.

If people are relating to their companion animals as archaic selfobjects who are, more or less, extensions of themselves, they may be able to relate only in an anthropomorphic way (Brown, 2011). They would see animals as part of themselves and be unable to empathize with how the animals really feel or to understand what the animals really need. People with archaic selfobject relationships can only imagine what they feel themselves and therefore what the animal feels is only a projection of how they feel or how they expect the animal to feel (Brown, 2011).

As described by Brown (2011), the extreme example of archaic selfobject relationships with animals would be the animal hoarder. The definition of animal hoarding includes (1) failure to provide minimal standards of care for the animals, (2) lack of insight about that failure, (3) denial of the consequences of that failure, and (4) obsessive attempts to maintain and even increase the number of animals in the face of these failures and deteriorating conditions (Patronek, 1999). The consequences of animal hoarding include starvation, illness, and death of animals; neglect of self and others; and household destruction (Patronek & Nathanson, 2009).

Animal hoarding is not classified as a sign of any specific psychological disorder and is not recognized as a clinical entity or psychiatric diagnosis (Hoarding of Animals Research Consortium or HARC, 2002). According to Arluke and Killeen (2009), the inability to come up with one diagnosis is due to possible factors such as animal hoarders suffer from multiple pathologies, a novel pathology may under-lie their behavior, or that too few animal hoarders have been studied to define their actual pathology (Brown, 2011). Another problem with trying to find a psycho-logical model for animal hoarding is that animal hoarding appears to be a very heterogeneous behavior. Patronek, Loar, and Nathanson (2006) have proposed that three types of animal hoarders may exist: the overwhelmed caregivers, the rescuer hoarders, and the exploiter hoarders. It is possible that the psychology, etiology, and treatment for the three types could be different.

One frequent finding with animal hoarders is that they often believe they are rescuing the animals from horrible fates (such as euthanasia), while seeming to be completely oblivious to the fact that they themselves are inflicting tremendous pain, suffering, starvation, disease, or even death on the animals (Patronek & Nathanson, 2009). As Patronek and Nathanson point out, there is no theory of the human–animal bond that explains the animal hoarders' profound attachment to their animals while at the same time inflicting extreme animal suffering.

According to Patronek and Nathanson (2009), for some people, especially those who have suffered from a dysfunctional primary attachment experience in child-hood, animals can provide a comforting, protective relationship which forms strong and lasting imprint. In adulthood, when human relationships become chronically problematic, compulsive caregiving of animals can become the primary means of maintaining or building a sense of self.

As described by Brown (2011), Hagman (1997) outlined nine factors that define the differences between mature and archaic selfobjects: (1) The experience of rela-tionship, (2) Mature confidence, (3) Flexibility of function, (4) Personal agency, (5) Other recognition, (6) The experience of reciprocity, (7) The capacity to be empathic, (8) Self-transformation, and (9) Altruism. These factors, as defined by Hagman (1997), are outlined below. See Brown (2011) for specific examples of how these factors might be seen in an animal hoarder.

The Experience of Relationship. The mature selfobject way of relating would be to experience the other as a separate being. It would require the participation of the person in securing, using, and nurturing relationships with people or ani-mals to meet selfobject needs. A person with archaic selfobject functioning would just expect for the relationship with the selfobject to just happen with no effort on his part.

Mature Confidence. Mature confidence in the selfobject experience with another is something that is learned. People learn to trust that the other person or animal will continue to meet their needs in spite of some failures, shortcomings, or uncertainties. The archaic selfobject relationship is just assumed. There is a naïve confidence in the objects providing the selfobject experiences that they will always be there and never fail to meet the needs of the person.

Flexibility of Function. Mature selfobject relating is characterized by flexibil-ity in both level of need and ways to get the needs met. Times of stress, loss, or frustration may intensify the need for selfobject experiences with others or even the need for archaic selfobject needs. A person with mature selfobject relating can find the people or animals to meet those selfobject needs during those times and can be flexible in how they get the needs met—that is, they may get mirroring from one animal or strength from another idealized animal.

Personal Agency.   Obtaining mature selfobject experiences requires an active role for the person in seeking out, nurturing, and maintaining selfobject responses from others. The maturely functioning person acts, within a selfobject milieu, to "make it happen." By contrast, the person functioning on an archaic level just expects to be the passive recipient of love and care from the selfobject milieu.

Other Recognition.   Kohut (1984) stressed that in mature selfobject relating, the other is experienced as a separate and distinct center of initiative. Hagman (1997) argues that the concept of recognition of the subjectivity of the other is perhaps the key aspect of mature development. The other would be perceived as having a unique and differing perspective and center of experience. In the archaic selfobject experience, the subjectivity of the other is only dimly perceived and plays little, if any, part in the experience of its key functions. In other words, a person relying on an animal for archaic selfobject needs would not see the animal as a separate being with thoughts, feelings, and needs of its own. The animal would be seen as being there simply to fulfill the needs of the person, regardless of the animal's true state of being.

The Experience of Reciprocity.   In mature selfobject relating, the recognition of the other as a separate self is an integral part of the experience and the person or animal involved will reciprocate based on his assessment of the other's needs. There is a give-and-take process of mutual recognition and reciprocity. However, in archaic selfobject relating, the other person or animal is perceived as giving selflessly. The self of the other is not considered when the archaic needs are being met. There is no mutual engagement. The exchange would be one sided.

The Capacity to be Empathic.   Hagman (1997) explains that true empathy is an important characteristic of maturity. Mature empathy requires both the experience of the other from a subjective and an objective point of view. This allows one to experience both what might be inside the other's head and how that other might perceive or feel from outside his head. Hagman believes that mature selfobject experience involves a sense of empathic connection that involves a simultaneous recognition of self and other, characterized by cognitive and emotional sharing. True empathy is very limited or nonexistent in archaic selfobject relating.

Self-Transformation.   Mature selfobject experience is transformational. By engaging with others in creative and unpredictable way, we grow to include other-than-me experiences. Through our relationships with others who may be serving selfobject functions, our boundaries can expand and we can include new elements into our self. On the other hand, archaic selfobject relating only serves to meet the needs of the self and does not allow for change.

Altruism.   Self psychologists stress that the ability to offer to another the opportunity for a selfobject experience is the most developed capacity of mature selfobject relating. This would mean serving the needs of another because their emotional needs are perceived as having priority over your own. The most obvious example of this is the psychotherapist who offers himself to a patient as an opportunity for a healthy selfobject experience. Or it might be the parent who puts his/her own needs aside to be the mirroring selfobject that his/her child may need at that moment. Altruism characterizes the most advanced form of mature selfobject relating. Altruism is not possible for people functioning only at archaic levels of selfobject experience. To be altruistic requires the awareness of the other as well as empathy to perceive their needs.

The more mature the selfobject relationship with a companion animal is, the more likely the relationship will be beneficial to both the human and the companion animal. The ability to be mindful of the needs, feelings, anxieties, and desires of the companion animal requires empathy, sensitivity, and, at times, selflessness. The lack of mature empathy is one factor that can lead to animal abuse or neglect. The example of the animal hoarder is one example of a person whose own needs and lack of empathy have led to massive suffering on the part of animals.

Animals and Selfobject Merger Needs

Individuals who rely on relating in primitive ways (such as lack of recognition of the otherness of the animal or an inability to empathize with the animal) often want to merge with the selfobject to get their selfobject needs met. Wolf (1988) describes this as a person can only receive confirmation of their sense of self by seeing the mirroring or idealized selfobject as being an extension of them, with no boundaries between them. For example, Brown (2011) describes an animal hoarder who would lie in bed next to her large dog, back to back, and she imagine they shared a spine. Kohut (1984) states that the merger needs can appear as any of the three selfobject types: mirroring, idealized, or twinship. They all have in common the need to merge with or be one with the selfobject.

Animals as selfobjects lend themselves to being good merger selfobjects (Brown, 2011). Relationships with animals leave more room for projection of a human's emotions. Animals cannot disagree with a human's interpretation of how they feel or what they want. People can believe animals feel and think like them, whether they actually do or not. Humans are less likely to tolerate another person's inaccurate perception of themselves. This would make it easier to believe an animal (vs a human) is a soul mate, is one with the person or is able to read one's mind. Therefore, animals may create better merger selfobject experiences than humans do.

Special Qualities of Animals as Selfobjects

Sometimes, the animals in our lives become as important, or even more important, than the people in our lives. This is increasingly true as more people live alone and many people no longer live close to their extended families (Hart, 2000). However, animals are not just important to those who are isolated from other people. Many of the participants in a study by Brown (2007), who clearly had animals as selfobjects, also had spouses, children, or significant others.

It may be that some people have a special affinity for animals or that animals have unique qualities that make them better suited to provide selfobject functions. In the study by Brown (2007), animals were found to be especially adept at being silent, soothing selfobjects to people.

Part of the reason animals make good selfobjects is because they can be intensely focused on their humans and very adept at reading nonverbal cues (Brown, 2007). The nature of nonverbal relationships may lead to a deeper bond. Animals cannot verbally disagree, criticize, judge, or give advice. Animals are also capable of a single-minded focus on their humans that exceeds what most humans are capable of doing. Often, an animal's sole purpose in life is to be near to and devoted to their humans (Brown, 2007). It would be difficult for any human to match that level of devotion.

Self psychology also can explain why people in general may bond strongly to one animal and not others. Sometimes one particular animal may have the selfobject qualities someone is seeking, such as being protective. An example of this from the study by Brown (2007) is buckskin mare that was an idealized selfobject and was extremely protective of her owner. The owner said the horse's protective behavior reminded her of her recently deceased mother who was also very protective. This particular owner did not have the same strong bond with her other four horses. This person needed the idealized selfobject function and found it in this one particular horse, but not in the others.

Conclusion

Self psychology can help understand the depth and meaning of the extraordinary bond with animals. A companion animal may be providing an individual with perceived empathy, love, comfort, confidence, joy, protection, energy, and strength which all contribute to a sense of positive self-esteem. One, small, companion animal may be the powerful sustenance of a person's whole sense of self.

Appendix: Companion Animal Selfobject Questionnaire

Select one specific animal to answer the questions. You may select animals that are alive or deceased. If you have more than one animal, complete the quiz separately for each one.

Part I: Is your animal a selfobject?

(1) Would you feel devastated if you lost your animal?   True False
(2) Would you feel a sense of falling apart or have trouble functioning   True False
    if you lost your animal?

If your answers to both questions in Part I were true, then your animal is probably a selfobject to you. If so, continue to Part II. If you answered only one as true, continue on as they may still be a selfobject.

Part II: What type of selfobject is your animal?

Answer the following questions to find out what type of selfobject your animal may be. Circle T for True and F for False.

Mirroring Selfobject   True False

(1) Does your animal give you a feeling of being loved, special,   T   F
     treasured or important?
(2) Would you say your animal calms, soothes, comforts or reassures   T   F
     you?
(3) Does your animal make you feel loved and accepted in spite of   T   F
     any flaws or imperfections?
(4) Does your animal make you feel vibrant, invigorated or   T   F
     energized?
(5) Do you feel your animal sometimes shares in your emotional   T   F
     states, reflecting back to you your own happiness, sadness or other
     emotions?

                                            Mirroring Selfobject Sub-Total _____

Idealized Selfobject

(6) Do you feel stronger (psychologically or physically) when near   T   F
     your animal?
(7) Do you feel proud when out in public with your animal (or   T   F
     showing photos of your animal) or when other people admire
     them?
(8) Would you say your animal has abilities or qualities that you wish   T   F
     you had or you admire?
(9) Do you admire your animal's strength, power, confidence or   T   F
     assertiveness?
(10) Do you perceive your animal as having a stable, calm,   T   F
     non-anxious, powerful, wise, or protective presence?

                                            Idealized Selfobject Sub-Total _____

Twinship Selfobject

(11) Would you say that you consider your animal to be a soul-mate or   T   F
     that you have a special kinship with him/her?
(12) Do you sometimes feel a sense of being one with your animal?   T   F
(13) Does it seem to you that you are similar to your animal in some   T   F
     meaningful and deep way(s)?
(14) Do you feel an unspoken capacity to know and understand each   T   F
     other's inner states?
(15) Do you believe that you and your animal are often thinking the   T   F
     same thoughts or that you can read each other's minds?

                                            Twinship Selfobject Sub-Total _____

Add 1 point for each True item above. Add item points for each type of selfobject to obtain the 3 sub-totals. The highest sub-total number is an indication of which type of selfobject your animal is for you. It is also possible that your animal is more than one type of selfobject.

References

Alper, L. S. (1993). The child-pet bond. In A. Goldberg (Ed.), *The widening scope of self psychology: Progress in self psychology* (Vol. 9, pp. 257–270). Hillsdale, NJ: The Analytic Press.

Arluke, A., & Killeen, C. (2009). *Inside animal hoarding: The case of Barbara Erickson and her 552 dogs*. West Lafayette, IN: Purdue University Press.

Banai, E., Mikulincer, M., & Shaver, P. (2005). Self-object needs in Kohut's self psychology: Links with attachment, self-cohesion, affect regulation and adjustment. *Psychoanalytic Psychology, 22*(2), 224–260.

Brown, S. E. (2007). Companion animals as self-objects. *Anthrozoos, 20*(4), 329–343.

Brown, S. E. (2011). Theoretical concepts from self psychology applied to animal hoarding. *Society & Animals, 19*(2), 175–193.

Hagman, G. (1997). Mature self-object experience. In A. Goldberg (Ed.), *Progress in self psychology* (Vol. 13, pp. 85–107). Hillsdale, NJ: The Analytic Press.

Hart, L. A. (2000). Psychosocial benefits of animal companionship. In A. H. Aubrey Fine (Ed.), *Handbook on animal assisted therapy: Theoretical foundations and guidelines for practice* (pp. 39–78). New York: Academic Press.

Hartmann, M., & Walter, H. (2009). Konnen (Heim) Tiere die Funktion eines Selbstobjekts ubernehmen? *Self psychology: European journal for psychoanalytical therapy and research, 38*, 365–388.

Hoarding of Animals Research Consortium (2002). Health implications of animal hoarding. *Health & Social Work, 27*(2), 125–136.

Kohut, H. (1971). *The analysis of the self: A systematic approach to the psychoanalytic treatment of narcissistic personality disorders*. New York: International Universities Press.

Kohut, H. (1984). *How does analysis cure?* Chicago: University of Chicago Press.

Patronek, G. I. (1999). Hoarding of animals: An under-recognized public health problem in a difficult-to-study population. *Public Health Reports, 114*, 81–87.

Patronek, G. J., Loar, L., & Nathanson, J. N. (2006). Animal hoarding: Strategies for interdisciplinary interventions to help people, animals, and communities at risk. Boston: Hoarding of Animals Research Consortium. Available at: http://www.tufts.edu/vet/cfa/hoarding/pubs/AngellReport.pdf. Accessed Sept 16, 2009.

Patronek, G. I., & Nathanson, J. N. (2009). A theoretical perspective to inform assessment and treatment strategies for animal hoarders. *Clinical Psychology Review, 29*, 274–281.

Schore, A. N. (2003). Advances in neuropsychoanalysis, attachment theory, and trauma research: Implications for self psychology. In A. N. Schore (Ed.), *Affect regulation and the repair of the self* (pp. 108–148). New York: W. W. Norton & Company.

Silverstein, M. L. (1999). *Self psychology and diagnostic assessment: Identifying self-object functions through psychological testing*. Mahwah, NJ: Lawrence Erlbaum Associates Publishers.

Tonnesvang, J. (2002). Self-object and self-subject relationships. In A. Goldberg (Ed.), *Postmodern self psychology: Progress in self psychology* (Vol. 18, pp. 149–166). Hillsdale, NJ: The Analytic Press.

Wolf, E. S. (1988). *Treating the self: Elements of clinical self psychology*. New York: The Guilford Press.

Chapter 9
A Developmental Psychological Perspective on the Human–Animal Bond

Nancy A. Pachana, Bronwyn M. Massavelli, and Sofia Robleda-Gomez

Introduction

Companion animals have been part of our human experience for centuries. Archaeological evidence reveals that over 14,000 years ago, domesticated wolves—ancestors of our modern companionable canines—lived in settlements with humans (Serpell, 2008). By 9,000 years ago, both dogs and cats assumed crucial roles in developing agricultural communities and became increasingly valued by humans as companions as well as contributors to human society. During the early Greek and Roman empires, dogs were kept as hunters, herders, and guardians, and also cared for as loyal beloved pets (Coren, 2002). In Peru, archaeologists have discovered cemeteries where early Chiribaya people buried their dogs with blankets and food alongside human companions (Begley, Contreras & Hays, 2006).

In modern times, pets are a part of people's lives, sometimes for only a portion of their lives, and sometimes throughout their life. The term *pet* comes from the root of the French word 'petit' (Grier, 2006). However, most professionals prefer the term *companion animal* to connote a psychological attachment and a reciprocal relationship (Walsh, 2009). Some people experience companion animals as an integral part of their lives from birth (or nearly so). Others come to have animal companions later in life, perhaps acquiring a pet as part of marriage, or getting a pet for their children. The idea of acquiring a puppy or kitten for a child introduces the idea of companion animals being a part of lifespan development. Regarding children, animals are often given to a child not only to bring pleasure, but also to teach about the responsibilities of caring for a living being. This happy developmental milestone can be contrasted with the unfortunate situation of older adults having to part with a beloved animal companion when they are no longer able to look after it, or when they enter a nursing home which does not allow animals. These two examples illustrate the importance of considering the human–animal bond from a developmental perspective.

N.A. Pachana (✉)
School of Psychology, University of Queensland, Brisbane, Australia
e-mail: npachana@psy.uq.edu.au

C. Blazina et al. (eds.), *The Psychology of the Human–Animal Bond*,
DOI 10.1007/978-1-4419-9761-6_9, © Springer Science+Business Media, LLC 2011

The Human–Animal Bond

In Childhood and Adolescence

Growing up with a companion animal can prove one of the most satisfying experiences for a child or an adolescent, as this is the time of their lives where core emotional bonds with animals are established. Children learn how to relate to, care for, and love animals within a social learning theory framework, using classical and operant conditioning (Brickel, 1985; Cohen, 2002). In many cases, families teach their children how to relate to animals; exposure to a dog or cat, for example, can shape a child's attitudes and behaviours about the world. Bryant (1982) states that intimate chats with grandparents and pets were highly important factors related to increased socioemotional functioning for a group of seven- to ten-year-old children. Moreover, their pets were viewed as special friends with whom they could share happy moments and secrets comfortably, because they perceived their pets as displaying constancy, empathy, and warmth. Similarly, the children reported they also confided in their pets when they felt angry, upset, and scared. This suggests that pets play a role similar to that of another sibling. Moreover, pets are said to be reinforcing for children because they provide constant attention in addition to unconditional positive regard.

Pets promote positive psychosocial development of children (Melson, 2001, 2003), who demonstrate enhanced empathy, self-esteem, cognitive development, and increased participation in social and athletic activities. Most children see companion animals as peers and they can learn to read an animal's body language. In fact it is easier to teach children to be empathic with an animal than with a human, because an animal is straightforward in expressing feelings and behaviour. This bond contributes to higher confidence, improvements in mood, and greater empathy with humans (Melson, 2001, 2003; Serpell, 2008).

Adolescence can be a difficult time (Triebenbacher, 1998) for most families, and is a time when children are shaping their identities as well as their perceptions of the world. Further, although bonds with animals may have already been established by adolescence, the focus then turns to maintaining these bonds. Adolescents also perceive pets in ways that are similar to children. Davis and Juhasz (1985) reported that although adolescents ranked a pet below their parents, companion animals were ranked higher than other social choices on a list of things that helped them to feel good about themselves in times of low self-esteem. Animals can also be thought of as a friend and confidant by adolescents. In a time that is turbulent for a majority of adolescents, animals can serve as a buffer during this transition into adulthood. Having contact with an animal during the early years into adolescence enables a child to develop stable attributes of personality, such as warmth, empathy, and compassion, that can shape and assist them in their interactions with peers as well as prepare them to cope with various stressors later in life (Van Houtte & Jarvis, 1995).

As patterns of individual and family life continue to evolve and change, adults and children increasingly move in and out of a range of living situations and relationships over a lengthening life course (Walsh, 2003). Companion animals meet relational needs for consistent, reliable bonds and facilitate transitions through disruptive life changes. Beyond the family unit, a growing number of studies have found that pets increase neighbourhood interactions and a sense of community (e.g. Triebenbacher, 1998; Wood, Giles-Corti, Bulsara, & Bosch, 2007).

In Adulthood

For many persons, by the time they reach adulthood their human–animal bond(s) are flourishing. Various studies with adults have reported that pets continue to provide much of the same benefits as those reported by children and adolescents. These benefits include companionship, serving as an aid to health and relaxation, providing protection, love, and loyalty, and acting as an outlet for the adult to express their inner child, as well as offering continuing non-judgemental and unconditional acceptance (Cohen, 2002; McNicholas et al., 2005; Walsh, 2009). Indeed, in a 1996 survey by the American Animal Hospital Association, 75% of pet owners considered their animals akin to children, and nearly half the women surveyed reported that they often relied more on their dogs and cats than on their husbands and children for support (Serpell, 2002). In addition, relationships with pets are less subject to provider burnout or to fluctuations, and they do not impose a strain or cause concern about continuing stability. For example, companion animals seem to be of value in early stages of bereavement (Headley, 1998) and after treatment for breast cancer (Ownby, Johnson, & Peterson, 2002).

Pet ownership is becoming more common for adults, and this trend is international. At least half of the households in Western societies own pets (Podbercek, Paul, & Serpell, 2000). For example, the 2005–2006 US National Pet Owners Survey showed that 63% of all American households owned a pet of some sort, which equates to more than 69 million households (Walsh, 2009). Over three-quarters of US children live with pets—a number which exceeds that of children living with both parents (Walsh, 2009a). In Australia, 53% of families own a pet dog or cat (Australian Companion Animal Council, 2006). Six of every ten Spanish homes have at least one pet, meaning that the 20 million companion animals existing in that country are spread across approximately 8.5 million homes (Terra Noticias, 2008). Market research in Argentina shows that there are 22 million domestic pets in the country, with 44% of households owning any type of pet (Euromonitor International, 2009). In China, where the smaller Chinese family unit use pets as a replacement for more children or as a companion for an only child, the latest market research shows that the dog population has risen from 20.4 million in the year 2000, to just under 27 million in 2008 (Euromonitor International, 2008). Also, the increased trend for spending significant amounts of money on the care and, indeed, pampering of animals has also been noted in the popular press. For example, the amount of money spent on companion animals has doubled over the past decade, exceeding the gross national product of many developing countries (Walsh, 2009).

Melson (2003) extends attachment theory to better understand relationships with pets. Beck and Madresh (2008) applied attachment theory in a web-based survey of pet owners and found pets to be a consistent source of attachment security. Compared to relationships with romantic partners, attachments with pets were more secure on every measure. Brown (2007) found that companion animals rivalled and even surpassed humans in their ability to provide important self-object needs, such as self-cohesion, self-esteem, calmness, soothing, and acceptance.

In Later Life

The human–animal bond continues into later life. Older age is a time where there can be multiple losses for an older person, particularly in a short period of time. When an older person loses someone close to him or her, it is often the case that it is not a single loss. The person lost may have also been his or her best friend, confidant, or financial support. Similarly pets often live their full lives with their human companions, and profound bereavement at the loss of a cherished pet is normal and commonly as strong as for a significant human companion (Walsh, 2009a).

The power of the human–animal bond has been documented across numerous studies that have looked into the effects of companion animals with older adults. The evidence is that animals play a positive role for older persons living alone (Siegel, 1990, 1993). For example, animal owners appear to experience improvement in life satisfaction and levels of personal safety after retirement compared to non-owners (Norris, Shinew, Chick, & Beck, 1999).

For some older people, an animal *is* their family. One study that looked at attitudes in older people caring for pets compared to older adults caring for only plants reported that the older adults with animals experienced continued improvement in their attitudes towards other people (Mugford & M'Cominsky, 1975), while others have reported a positive relationship between happiness and the extent of the attachment in older people (Johnson & Meadows, 2002).

Various studies support the buffering effect that human–animal relationships can have on stress, illness, mood, and loneliness. In turn, the particular social support that animals can provide is increasingly recognized as an important modulator for stress. Animals can provide a special type of social support, one that is nonjudgemental and unconditional. Where individuals feel that they cannot talk to anybody for fear of being judged, ridiculed, or not taken seriously, animals are their safe option (Hafen, Rush, Reisbig, McDaniel, & White, 2007).

Developmental Issues with Respect to Therapeutic Effects of Companion Animals

Having a companion animal in the family can be beneficial on a number of levels. As noted earlier, many families acquire pets in order to teach children responsibilities and provide companionship. Pets can also enhance the quality of life of families, through promoting a positive attitude, giving and reciprocating affection, and increasing interaction and communication between family members. Some families may even use their pet as a means of redirecting and diffusing tension or conflict among family members (Cohen, 2002; Mueller, 2004).

Pets in the family can also shed light on how a family system may be functioning. For example, the manner in which the human–animal bond is introduced to the child can be significant (Brickel, 1985). From a classical conditioning perspective, the child may learn to associate having a pet with the family home. From an observational or modelling perspective, the child may gauge from the parents the way to interact with an animal, thus setting the foundation for future human–animal bonds. From an operant conditioning model, the child learns through consequence which behaviours will elicit a positive outcome from his/her pet. In fact, it is thought that by age five, having a pet within the family serves to shape a child's attitudes and behaviours towards a pet (Brickel, 1985).

The role of pets can also become important when the 'empty nest' syndrome is experienced. This can be a particularly lonely time for older people, especially if they live alone or do not report a satisfying relationship with their significant other. At this time, the family pet can fill the void, allowing family members to redirect their need to care and shower affection on another being (Cain, 1983).

Companion Animals and Physical and Emotional Wellness

Carefully designed studies which explore the benefits of pets for children in both classroom as well as therapeutic environments suggest this is an area worthy of attention (Jalongo, 2005; Jalongo, Astorino, & Bomboy, 2004). The research highlights physiological, emotional, and social impacts of companion animals. Nagengast and colleagues (1997) found the presence of a dog significantly lowered behavioural, emotional, and verbal distress in children when participating in a mildly stressful activity, such as a visit to the doctor's office. In another study, Friedmann and colleagues (1983) found that the presence of an animal lowered blood pressure and heart rate when a child read aloud. Students tend to be more attentive, responsive, and cooperative with an adult when a dog is present in a classroom (Limond, Bradshaw, & Cormack, 1997). Dogs have been found to contribute to elementary students' overall emotional stability, and more positive attitudes towards school in children diagnosed with severe emotional disorders (Anderson & Olson, 2006). Animals can enhance students' self-esteem by providing a 'friend' to bond with and love in the classroom setting (Zasloff & Hart, 1999). In therapeutic settings, children have experienced increased alertness and attention span, and an enhanced openness and desire for social contact, when involved in therapy sessions with dogs (Prothmann, Bienert, & Ettrich, 2006).

There are numerous studies offering evidence that interactions with companion animals contribute to good health, psychosocial well-being, and recovery from serious conditions in adults (Friedmann & Tsai, 2006; Wells, 2009). For example, one of the most solid areas of research links pet ownership with improved physiological measures, such as decreased blood pressure, serum triglycerides, and cholesterol levels (Allen, Blascovich, & Mendes, 2002; Anderson, Reid, & Jennings, 1992; Dembicki & Anderson, 1996; Serpell, 1991). In fact, merely stroking a dog notably reduces blood pressure in both the person and the animal (Charnetsky, Riggers, & Brennan, 2004). Companion animals have also been found to help improve depression in AIDS patients (Siegel, Angulo, Detels, Wesch, & Mullen, 1999) and increase the quality of life and motivation of those with schizophrenia (Barker & Dawson, 1998; Beck, 2005). Virues-Ortega and Buela-Casals (2006) found strong evidence that ongoing human–animal interactions moderated psychosocial and physiological reactions by providing relaxation and stress-buffering effects through stroking or holding, bolstering health by maintaining exercise, and catalysing social exchanges or conversations about pets, which helped to reduce isolation and loneliness.

Better physical and psychological well-being in community-dwelling older people who live with companion animals has also been found (Raina, Waltner-Toews, Bonnett, Woodward, & Abernathy, 1999). In their study, Raina and colleagues (1999) found that the ability to perform activities of daily living was relatively higher as well as better maintained by pet owners compared to non–pet owners over a one-year period. Furthermore, pet ownership cushioned the harmful impact of lack of social support on psychological well-being, and emerged as a possible factor that could facilitate successful ageing.

Evidence suggests that feeling closer to a pet than to others is not uncommon, and the vast majority of pet lovers are not socially inept or trying to replace their human companions (Hines, 2003). Most people who connect strongly to animals also have a large capacity for love, empathy, and compassion. In another study, the presence of a pet was found to be more effective than that of a spouse or friend in ameliorating the cardiovascular effects of stress (Allen et al., 2002). Moreover, although companion animals do not speak our language, they clearly understand and communicate with us in a myriad of ways. For example, dogs demonstrate an uncanny ability (better than our closer primate relatives) to read human cues and behaviour and accurately interpret even subtle hand gestures and glances (Katz, 2003).

There have been several studies linking cardiovascular health and companion animals. For example, following a heart attack, patients with pets had a significantly higher one-year survival than those without pets; those with dogs were 8.6 times more likely to still be living (Friedmann & Thomas, 1995; Friedmann, Katcher, Lynch, & Thomas, 1980).

Yet, the protective effects of companion animals have also not been supported, being confounded with other variables—for example, rural or urban place of reference (Pachana, Ford, Andrew, & Dobson, 2005). Gillum and Obisesan (2010) demonstrate in a nationwide cohort of American adults that living with companion animals was not associated with greater survival after controlling for key health confounders. However, people do not own pets specifically to enhance their health, rather they value the relationship and contribution their pet makes to their quality of life (Podberceck et al., 2000), which has its own value.

Larger studies, including longitudinal studies, are important in looking at long-term health and well-being trends associated with having companion animals. Longitudinal research over two decades in Germany (N = 9,723) and Australia

(N = 1,246) found that people who have continuously owned a pet were the healthiest group, whereas those who no longer had a pet or never had one were the least healthy (Headley & Grabka, 2007). The relationship remained significant after controlling for gender, age, marital status, income, and other variables associated with health.

Recovery from Illness: Role of Companion Animals

A great deal of stress surrounds a hospital visit for children undergoing treatment for cancer and other serious illnesses. These children have had to leave the relative safety of their homes and familiar home environment, and face often extremely unpleasant and extended treatment regimes. However, studies have shown improved mood and emotional well-being in hospitalized children following a visit from a pet (Kaminsky, Pellino, & Wish, 2002), thus providing support that companion animals and animal-assisted therapy (AAT) can facilitate the recovery process of hospitalized children.

Children from households with pets have stronger immune systems and take fewer days off sick from school (McNicholas, Collis, Gilbey, & Seghal, 2004). Pets have also been found to influence the course and optimal functioning of children with pervasive developmental disabilities (Martin & Farnum, 2002).

A well-replicated, intensive animal care intervention programme has had remarkable success with children and adolescents with severe conduct disorder in residential treatment (Katcher & Wilkins, 2000). The programme elicited a range of pro-social behaviours—nurturing, affection, play, lower aggression, peer cooperation, responsibility, teaching others, and responding to adult authority, and also produced greater calming and focused attention than comparison programmes (such as Outward Bound). Recently, the programme has been effective with children with attention deficit disorder and other learning disabilities in public school special education programmes (Katcher & Teumer, 2006).

Companion animals also have a role to play with older adults who are recovering from a period of illness or who may have been diagnosed with a chronic or terminal condition. Older adults who own a pet make 21% fewer visits to their family doctor (Siegel, 1990). Avian companionship was found to alleviate depression, loneliness, and low morale of older adults in skilled rehabilitation units (Jessen, Cardiello, & Baun, 1996). Companion animals ease suffering and anxiety at end of life for those in palliative care and hospice care (Geisler, 2004).

Special Populations and Companion Animals

Autism

A wide variety of animals, including horses, rabbits, service dogs, and even dolphins, are also implicated with special populations, such as those with intellectual or physical disabilities (Spence & Kaiser, 2002). The interactions of autistic and attention-deficit-hyperactivity-disordered (ADHD) children with dolphins has also been reported as a largely positive experience, with these children showing increased verbalizations, speech intelligibility, and motor co-ordination (Nathanson, Castro, Friend, & McMahon, 1997).

The effects of animal-assisted therapy on individuals with medically based speech and language disabilities are also documented. In one study involving a canine co-therapist, an older participant experienced significant improvement regarding one-word answers, object identification, and verbalization behaviours (Walter-Esteves & Stokes, 2008). Alzheimer's patients have also benefited from contact with animals; positive effects have been shown in terms of increased frequency of smiles, touch, laughter, and verbalizations (Filan & Llewellyn-Jones, 2006). AIBOS, commonly known as robotic pets, are also beneficial for children with intellectual or physical disabilities, and older adults who may have behavioural and psychological symptoms associated with dementia, as this eliminates the possibility of harm coming to the animal.

Mental Health Programmes and Animals

The benefits of pets are also obvious in mental health settings where people may feel psychologically or physically isolated from human–human attachments or relationships. Where others may be perceived to have given up on an individual, companion animals can provide a sense of being needed, a purpose to get up in the morning, a sense of daily routine. The impact of caring for an animal can be enormous—psychologically, emotionally, socially, and physically (Parshall, 2003).

For example, a randomized controlled trial with persons with schizophrenia and other serious psychiatric disorders found that only those who worked with farm animals for 12 weeks, in addition to receiving standard psychiatric care, gained significant improvement in coping, confidence, and quality of life (Berget, Ekeberg, & Braastad, 2008). In another study, older patients with schizophrenia benefited from animal-assisted therapy over a one-year period (Barak, Savorai, Mavashev, & Beni, 2001). Although the sample size (N = 10 in each group) was small, on a measure for adaptive social function the treated group showed significant gains which extended to other activities of daily living. (Barak et al., 2001).

Forensic Settings

The role of companion animals with respect to rehabilitation has been extended to forensic settings. Trials with prisoners with various criminal backgrounds serving in correctional facilities have indicated promising findings, suggesting that companion animals can play a significant role in the rehabilitation of this population. By being responsible for a pet, prisoners' self-efficacy and regard for others can increase (Hines, 1983). In another study, female prison inmates experienced improvements in depressed mood when training dogs (Walsh & Mertin, 1994).

One example of such a programme, Puppies Behind Bars, incorporates animals into rehabilitation efforts. Animals from rescue shelters receive supervised training from inmates to become service animals for people with disabilities, including combat veterans with PTSD and traumatic brain injuries. The programme decreases prison violence and contributes to better morale within the prison system (Turner, 2007).

Older Adults in Nursing Homes and Companion Animals

Recent advances in the pet therapy literature and the acknowledgement of the important therapeutic benefit that companion animals can have on emotional well-being and social support in older age have led to an increased number of aged care facilities incorporating companion animals, in some manner, into their facility. In one study conducted in a long-term residential facility with older adults, animal-assisted therapy was as effective as recreational activities ($d = 0.00$) in promoting positive social interaction behaviours (Bernstein, Friedmann, & Malaspina, 2000). Some nursing homes have welcomed visits from animal-assisted therapy organizations, have allowed residents or family to bring in a pet, or considered the use of robotic animals. Interestingly, companion animals in nursing homes are not just limited to domestic animals. In addition to dogs, cats, fish, and birds, recently, some nursing homes have acquired llamas, donkeys, and even goats.

Companion animals have proven effective when used therapeutically with persons with dementia. For example, there is evidence that the presence of a dog can increase pro-social behaviours when the animal is available temporarily or permanently for patients with Alzheimer's disease (Batson, McCabe, Baun, & Wilson, 1998). Moreover, while medication has a role in the management of problematic behaviours associated with dementia, there has been a growing call to focus on psychosocial methods as alternative or supplemental interventions, given the potential for adverse side effects of medication. Kanamori and colleagues (2001) documented the impact of AAT involving either a dog or cat in interactions with patients in a dementia day respite programme. Although activities of daily living remained unchanged for both the AAT and control groups, participants in the AAT programme experienced significant improvements in psychiatric symptoms and behaviours after three months compared to a matched control group within the facility. These improvements included decreases in aggressiveness ($p = 0.045$) and anxiety ($p = 0.004$), as well as caregiving burden ($p = 0.047$), which accounted for the improvement in overall behaviour scores.

In nursing homes where behavioural and mood problems can be prevalent in people with dementia and severe cognitive decline but staff may be hesitant to bring animals in for fear of burdening staff, inadvertent harm to residents, or even harm to the animal, robotic animals have been shown to be beneficial. Mechanical dogs such as AIBO that perform most of the actions of real dogs, robotic cats that purr and meow, and even robotic ponies have been trialled in aged care facilities with promising results. The benefits are similar to real animals in that residents display improvements in mood, social interaction, and emotional well-being, and reductions in loneliness, anger, and behavioural problems (Filan & Llewellyn-Jones, 2006). These robotic animals may be useful, in a similar manner, as an adjunctive approach to treating children with developmental problems such as autism and Asperger's syndrome, where they too may have a lack of emotional regulation and an incomplete understanding of how to appropriately interact with real animals.

However, the relative benefits of living versus artificial or mechanical companion animals, in a therapeutic sense, is still a topic of research. For example, Greer, Pustay, Zaun, and Coppens (2001) documented the effect of toy versus live cats on communication in a small group of older women with dementia. In this study living cats stimulated more communication both during their presence and immediately afterwards than did the toy animals.

Finally, the benefits of animals in long-term care settings can go beyond influencing interpersonal or behavioural variables, and impact more basic parameters. In one intriguing study, Edwards and Beck (2002) introduced specially designed aquaria into the dining areas of three special care units (SCU). Two facilities were treatment (fish tank introduced) and one was a control (scenic ocean picture), later crossing over to the treatment condition. In all facilities, food intake in residents with Alzheimer's disease was measured by weighing food consumed in meals and weighing residents. The results demonstrated that the scenic picture had no effect on food intake or resident weight in the control group. When aquaria were present in the dining room, however, residents ate more of their meals and gained weight. Staff reported that agitated residents were calmer when contemplating the aquaria, while those who were usually lethargic remained more alert and attentive. These effects were maintained throughout the eight-week study period. The authors also noted that aquaria served as a focal point of social interactions between residents and visitors. Increased food intake improved the health of residents and saved money as there was less need for nutritional supplements.

Pets and Grief

From a developmental perspective, the after-effects of human grief in response to losing a family member or friend can be long lasting, and are well documented, including, but not limited to, depression, anxiety, social withdrawal, and behavioural disturbances. Given the importance and role that pets play in the familial system, it is not surprising that losing a pet can also be one of the most traumatic experiences in life, and this experience appears to be no less significant for children, adults, or older adults. In fact, the grief experienced from the loss of a pet has been likened to that resulting from the loss of a significant human (Archer & Winchester, 1994) because an attachment bond has been broken.

The grief process for pets follows the same typical course of numbness, shock, and disbelief, followed by feelings of guilt and blame, sadness, anger, anxiety, and depression. There is also a preoccupation with the animal lost, such as thoughts, memories, and even flashbacks. As time goes by though, the grief process follows that of grieving for a human in that there is an acceptance of the loss, with an eventual openness to the prospect of getting another pet (Sharkin & Knox, 2003).

However, children compared to adults and older adults may differ in the way they process grief regarding the death of a pet. Children are at an earlier developmental stage compared to adults and older adults, therefore they have not yet consolidated a firm understanding of the meaning of pet loss. Children may still show the same patterns of grief for a pet that is not coming back; however, they may not understand why the pet is no longer there, and expect it to come back. This can be contrasted with adults, where the loss of a pet may signal getting a new pet for companionship. Thus, pet bereavement is an important topic of clinical interest that can go relatively unacknowledged in the community. Underestimating the significance and impact of pet bereavement has the potential to result in substantial unresolved grief for the individual or family involved. This again highlights the power of the human–animal relationship.

Conclusions

The benefits that pets and companion animals can provide across the lifespan are enormous. The above review has considered the human animal bond from a developmental perspective, reporting on a range of different populations and settings where the effects of companion animals across a variety of variables have been investigated. Moreover, age does not discriminate as to the effects of companion animals. They offer love and affection that is unconditional and non-judgemental, particularly in times where human–human contact is not possible or avoided. Companion animals offer non-judgemental and unconditional affection, and offer an opportunity for touch, for shared emotional displays, and for caring. These acts are important for all age groups, provide opportunities for positive interaction with another being, and offer an outlet for nurturing, making individuals feel needed. Enhancement of self-esteem, attitudes, and emotional security can all flow from having companion animals. In considering the extant literature from a developmental perspective, it is clear that the human–animal bond has a unique relationship and powerful influence across the lifespan.

References

Allen, K. M., Blascovich, J., & Mendes, W. B. (2002). Cardiovascular reactivity in the presence of pets, friends, and spouses: The truth about cats and dogs. *Psychosomatic Medicine, 64,* 727–739.

Anderson, K. L., & Olson, M. R. (2006). The value of a dog in a classroom of children with severe emotional disorders. *Anthrozoos, 19,* 35–49, Australian.

Anderson, W. P., Reid, C. M., & Jennings, G. L. (1992). Pet ownership and risk factors for cardiovascular disease. *The Medical Journal of Australia, 157,* 298–301.

Archer, J., & Winchester, G. (1994). Bereavement following death of a pet. *British Journal of Psychology, 85,* 259–272.

Barak, Y., Savorai, O., Mavashev, S., & Beni, A. (2001). Animal-assisted therapy for elderly schizophrenic patients: A one-year controlled trial. *American Journal of Geriatric Psychiatry, 9*, 439–442.

Barker, S., & Dawson, K. (1998). The effects of animal-assisted therapy on anxiety ratings of hospitalized psychiatric patients. *Psychiatric Services, 49*, 797–801.

Batson, K., McCabe, B., Baun, M. M., & Wilson, C. (1998). The effect of a therapy dog on socialization and physiological indicators of stress in persons diagnosed with Alzheimer's disease. In C. C. Wilson & D. C. Turner (Eds.), *Companion animals in human health* (pp. 203–215). London: Sage.

Beck, A. M. (2005). Review of pets and our mental health: The why, the what, and the how. *Anthrozoos, 18*, 441–443.

Beck, L., & Madresh, E. A. (2008). Romantic partners and four-legged friends: An extension of attachment theory to relationships with pets. *Anthrozoos, 21*, 43–56.

Begley, S., Contreras, J., & Hays, R. (2006). Mummified dogs: Best friends forever. *Maclean's, 119*(41), 31.

Berget, E., Ekeberg, O., & Braastad, B. (2008). Animal-assisted therapy with farm animals for persons with psychiatric disorders: Effects on self-efficacy, coping ability, and quality of life: A randomized controlled trial. *Clinical Practice and Epidemiology in Mental Health, 4*. doi:10.1186/1745-0179-4-9.

Bernstein, B., Friedmann, E., & Malaspina, A. (2000). Animal-assisted therapy enhances resident social interaction and initiation in long-term care facilities. *Anthrozoos, 13*, 213–224.

Brickel, C. M. (1985). Initiation and maintenance of the human-animal bond: Familial roles from a learning perspective. In M. B. Sussman. Pets and the family, *Marriage and Family Review, 8*(3/4), 34–41

Brown, S. E. (2007). Companion animals as self-objects. *Anthrozoos, 20*, 329–343.

Bryant, B. K. (1982). Sibling relationships in middle childhood. In M. E. Lamb & B. Sutton-Smith (Eds.), *Sibling relationships: Their nature and significance across the lifespan* (pp. 87–122). Hillsdale, NJ: Lawrence Erlbaum.

Cain, A. O. (1983). A study of pets in the family system. In A. H. Katcher & A. M. Beck (Eds.), *New perspectives on our lives with companion animals* (pp. 351–359). Philadelphia: University of Pennsylvania Press.

Charnetsky, C. J., Riggers, S., & Brennan, F. (2004). Effect of petting a dog on immune system functioning. *Psychological Reports, 3*, 1087–1091.

Cohen, S. P. (2002). Can pets function as family members? *Western Journal of Nursing Research, 24*, 621.

Companion Animal Inc. (2006). *Contribution of the pet care industry to the Australian economy*. Sydney: BIS Shrapnel.

Coren, S. (2002). *The pawprints of history: Dogs and the course of human events*. New York: Free Press.

Davis, J. H., & Juhasz, A. M. (1985). The pre-adolescent pet bond and psychosocial development. *Marriage and Family Review, 8*, 79–94.

Dembicki, D., & Anderson, J. (1996). Pet ownership may be a factor in the improved health of the elderly. *Journal of Nutrition for the Elderly, 15*, 15–31.

Edwards, N. E., & Beck, A. M. (2002). Animal-assisted therapy and nutrition in Alzheimer's disease. *Western Journal of Nursing Research, 24*, 697–712.

Euromonitor International (2008, November) Consumer lifestyles in China. Retrieved from http://www.portal.euromonitor.com/

Euromonitor International (2009, December). Consumer lifestyles in Argentina. Retrieved from http://www.portal.euromonitor.com/

Filan, S. L., & Llewellyn-Jones, R. H. (2006). Animal-assisted therapy for dementia: A review of the literature. *International Psychogeriatrics, 18*, 597–611, doi:10.1017/S1041610206003322.

Friedmann, E., Katcher, A. H., Lynch, J. J., & Thomas, S. A. (1980). Animal companions and one-year survival of patients after discharge from a coronary care unit. *Public Health Report, 95*, 307–312.

Friedmann, E., Katcher, A. H., Thomas, S. A., Lynch, J. J., & Messent, P. R. (1983). Social interaction and blood pressure: The influence of companion animals. *Journal of Nervous and Mental Disease, 171*, 461–465.

Friedmann, E., & Thomas, S. (1995). Pet ownership, social support, and one-year survival after acute myocardial infarction in the cardiac arrhythmia suppression trial (CAST). *American Journal of Cardiology, 76*, 1213–1217.

Friedmann, E., & Tsai, C. C. (2006). The animal-human bond: Health and wellness. In A. Fine (Ed.), *Animal-assisted therapy: Theoretical foundations and practice guidelines* (pp. 95–117). San Diego, CA: Academic Press.

Geisler, A. (2004). Companion animals in palliative care: Stories from the bedside. *American Journal of Hospice and Palliative Care, 21*, 285–288.

Gillum, R. F., & Obisesan, T. O. (2010). Living with companion animals: Physical activity and mortality in a U.S. national cohort. *International Journal of Environmental Research and Public Health, 7*, 2452–2459, doi:10.3390/ijerph7062452.

Greer, K. L., Pustay, K. A., Zaun, T. C., & Coppens, P. (2001). A comparison of the effects of toys versus live animals on the communication of patients with dementia of the Alzheimer's type. *Clinical Gerontologist, 24*, 157–182.

Grier, K. (2006). *Pets in America: A history*. New York: Harvest Book; Harcourt.

Hafen, M., Rush, B., Reisbig, A., McDaniel, K., & White, M. (2007). The role of family therapists in veterinary medicine: Opportunities for clinical services, education, and research. *Journal of Marital and Family Therapy, 33*, 165–176.

Headley, B. (1998). Health benefits and health cost savings due to pets: Preliminary estimates from an Australian national survey. *Social Indicators Research, 47*, 233–243, doi:10.1023/A:1006892908532.

Headley, B., & Grabka, M. (2007). Pets and human health in Germany and Australia: National longitudinal results. *Social Indicators Research, 80*, 297–311.

Hines, L. M. (1983). Pets in prison: A new partnership. *California Veterinarian, 5*, 7–17.

Hines, L. (2003). Historical perspectives on the human-animal bond. *American Behavioral Scientist, 47*, 7–15.

Jalongo, M. R. (2005). What are all these dogs doing at school? Using therapy dogs to promote children's reading practice. *Childhood Education, 81*, 152–158.

Jalongo, M., Astorino, T., & Bomboy, N. (2004). Canine visitors: The influence of therapy dogs on young children's learning and well-being in classrooms and hospitals. *Early Childhood Education Journal, 32*, 9–16.

Jessen, J., Cardiello, F., & Baun, M. (1996). Avian companionship in alleviation of depression, loneliness, and low morale of older adults in skilled rehabilitation units. *Psychological Reports, 78*, 339–348.

Johnson, R. A., & Meadows, R. L. (2002). Older latinos, pets and health. *Western Journal of Nursing Research, 24*, 609–620.

Kaminsky, M., Pellino, T., & Wish, J. (2002). Play and pets: The physical and emotional impact of child-life and pet therapy on hospitalized children. *Children's Health Care, 31*, 321–335.

Kanamori, M., Suzuki, M., Yamamoto, K., Kanda, M., Matsui, Y., Kojima, E., et al. (2001). A day care program and evaluation of animal-assisted therapy (AAT) for the elderly with senile dementia. *American Journal of Alzheimer's Disease and Other Dementias, 16*, 234–239.

Katcher, A. H., & Teumer, S. (2006). A 4-year trial of animal-assisted therapy with public school special education students. In A. H. Fine (Ed.), *Handbook on animal-assisted therapy* (pp. 153–177). New York: Elsevier.

Katcher, A. H., & Wilkins, G. G. (2000). The centaur's lessons: Therapeutic education through care of animals and nature study. In A. H. Fine (Ed.), *Handbook on animal-assisted therapy* (pp. 153–177). New York: Elsevier.

Katz, J. (2003). *The new work of dogs: Tending to life, love, and family*. New York: Villard Books.

Limond, J., Bradshaw, J., & Cormack, K. F. (1997). Behavior of children with learning disabilities interacting with a therapy dog. *Anthrozoos, 10*, 84–89.

Martin, F., & Farnum, J. (2002). Animal assisted therapy for children with pervasive developmental disorders. *Western Journal of Nursing Research, 24*, 657–671.

McNicholas, J., Collis, G. M., Gilbey, A. P., & Seghal, J. (2004). *Beneficial effects of pet ownership on child immune function.* Paper presented at the 10th International Conference on Human-Animal Interactions, Glasgow, Scotland, October 2004.

McNicholas, J., Gilbey, A., Rennie, A., Ahmedzai, S., Dono, J. A., & Ormerod, E. (2005). Pet ownership and human health: A brief review of evidence and issues. *British Medical Journal, 331*, 1252–1254.

Melson, G. F. (2001). *Why the wild things are: Animals in the lives of children.* Cambridge, MA: Harvard University Press.

Melson, G. F. (2003). Child development and the human-companion animal bond. *Animal Behavioral Scientist, 47*, 31–39.

Mueller, K. (2004). A critical analysis: Animal therapy with children and adolescents. Unpublished Masters Thesis.

Mugford, R. A., & M'Comisky, J. G. (1975). Some recent work on the psychotherapeutic value of caged birds with old people. In R. S. Anderson (Ed.), *Pet animals and society.* London: Balliere-Tindall.

Nagengast, S. L., Baun, M. M., Megel, M., & Leibowitz, J. M. (1997). The effects of the presence of a companion animal on physiological arousal and behavioral distress in children during a physical examination. *Journal of Pediatric Nursing, 12*, 323–330.

Nathanson, D. E., Castro, D., Friend, H., & McMahon, M. (1997). Effectiveness of short-term dolphin-assisted therapy for children with severe disabilities. *Anthrozoos, 10*, 90–100.

Norris, P. A., Shinew, K. J., Chick, G., & Beck, A. M. (1999). Retirement, life satisfaction, and leisure services: The pet connection. *Journal of Park and Recreation Administration, 17*, 65–83.

Ownby, D. R., Johnson, C. C., & Peterson, E. L. (2002). Exposure to dogs and cats in the first year of life and risk of allergic sensitization at 6 to 7 years of age. *Journal of the American Medical Association, 288*, 963–972.

Pachana, N. A., Ford, J. H., Andrew, B., & Dobson, A. J. (2005). Relations between companion animals and self-reported health in older women: Cause, effect or artifact? *International Journal of Behavioral Medicine, 12*, 103–110.

Parshall, D. P. (2003). Research and reflection: Animal-assisted therapy in mental health settings. *Counselling and Values, 48*(1), 47–57.

Podbercek, A. L., Paul, E. S., & Serpell, J. A. (2000). *Companion animals and us.* Cambridge: Cambridge University Press.

Prothmann, A., Bienert, M., & Ettrich, C. (2006). Dogs in child psychotherapy: Effects on state of mind. *Anthrozoos, 19*, 265–277.

Raina, P., Waltner-Toews, D., Bonnett, B., Woodward, C., & Abernathy, T. (1999). Influence of companion animals on the physical and psychological health of older people: An analysis of a one-year longitudinal study. *Journal of the American Geriatrics Society, 47*, 323–329.

Serpell, J. A. (1991). Beneficial effects of pet ownership on some aspects of human health. *Journal of the Royal Society of Medicine, 84*, 717–720.

Serpell, J. A. (2002). Anthropomorphism and anthropomorphic selection: Beyond the "cute response". *Society & Animals, 10*, 437–454.

Serpell, J. A. (2008). *In the company of animals: A study of human-animal relationships.* Cambridge: Cambridge University Press.

Sharkin, B. S., & Knox, D. (2003). Pet loss: Issues and implications for the psychologist. *Professional Psychology: Research and Practice, 34*(4), 414–421.

Siegel, J. M. (1990). Stressful life events and use of physician services among the elderly: The moderating role of pet ownership. *Journal of Personality and Social Psychology, 58*, 1081–1086.

Siegel, J. M. (1993). Companion animals: In sickness and in health. *Journal of Social Issues, 49*, 157–167.

Siegel, J. M., Angulo, F. J., Detels, R., Wesch, J., & Mullen, A. (1999). AIDS diagnosis and depression in the Multicenter AIDS Cohort Study: The ameliorating impact of pet ownership. *AIDS Care, 11*, 157–170.

Spence, L. J., & Kaiser, L. (2002). Companion animals and adaptation in chronically ill children. *Western Journal of Nursing Research, 24*(6), 639–656.

Terra Noticias (2008, May 6). Los animales de compañia estan presentes en 6 de cada 10 hogares. Retrieved from http://noticias.terra.es/2008/genteycultura/0306/actualidad/los-animales-de-compania-estan-presentes-en-6-de-cada-10-hogares.aspx

Triebenbacher, S. (1998). Pets as transitional objects: Their role in children's emotional development. *Psychological Reports, 82*, 191–200.

Turner, W. (2007). The experience of offenders in a prison canine program. *Federal Probation, 71*, 38–43.

Van Houtte, B. A., & Jarvis, P. A. (1995). The role of pets in preadolescent psychosocial development. *Journal of Applied Developmental Psychology, 16*, 463–479.

Virues-Ortega, J., & Buela-Casals, G. (2006). Psychophysiological effects of human-animal interaction: Theoretical issues and long-term interaction effects. *Journal of Nervous and Mental Disease, 194*, 52–57.

Walsh, F. (2003). *Normal family processes: Growing diversity and complexity* (2nd Ed.). New York: Guilford Press.

Walsh, F. (2009). Human-animal bonds I: The relational significance of companion animals. *Family Process, 48*, 462–480.

Walsh, F. (2009a). Human-animal bonds II: The role of pets in family systems and family therapy. *Family Process, 48*, 481–499.

Walsh, P. G., & Mertin, P. G. (1994). The training of pets as therapy dogs in a women's prison: A pilot study. *Anthrozoos, 7*, 124–128.

Walter-Esteves, S., & Stokes, T. (2008). Social effects of a dog's presence on children with disabilities. *Anthrozoos, 21*, 5–15.

Wells, D. L. (2009). The effects of animals on human health and well-being. *Journal of Social Issues, 65*, 523–543.

Wood, L. J., Giles-Corti, B., Bulsara, M. K., & Bosch, D. A. (2007). More than furry companion: The ripple effect of companion animals on neighborhood interactions and sense of community. *Society and Animals, 15*, 43–56.

Zasloff, R. L., & Hart, L. A. (1999). Animals in elementary school education in California. *Journal of Applied Animal Welfare Science, 2*, 347.

Chapter 10
Pet Ownership and Health

Judith M. Siegel

Overview

The relationship between naturally occurring pet ownership and health, both phys-ical and mental, is reviewed. Key methodological issues are discussed at the outset and the emphasis of the review is on recent literature. Collectively, the body of work is inconsistent, with some studies showing profound benefits of pet ownership, some showing no advantage, and others demonstrating poorer health outcomes among pet owners relative to non-owners. What may be most useful to researchers and prac-titioners at this juncture is not *whether* pet ownership facilitates good health, but *under what circumstances* might pet ownership facilitate it. Accordingly, this review describes some of the circumstances in which pet ownership appears to act as a moderator variable in regard to health, and incorporates theoretical approaches that provide a context for understanding the relationship. Recommendations for future research include focusing on quality of life, recruiting ethnically diverse samples, and enlarging the policy applications of the work.

Pet Ownership and Health

The relationship between pet ownership and health has received considerable scrutiny yet the question of whether humans achieve a health benefit from own-ing pets has not been answered definitively. Most of the *review* articles on this topic conclude that, on balance, ownership is beneficial, even while citing methodologi-cally strong studies that yield no advantage or demonstrate worse health for those with pets than those without (i.e., Barker & Wolen, 2008; Knight & Edwards, 2008; Siegel, 1993).

Addressing the link between pet ownership and health raises a number of ques-tions that cloud our interpretation of the data. Foremost among them is the fact that researchers study naturally occurring pet ownership—that is, individuals self-select

J.M. Siegel (✉)
Department of Community Health Sciences, School of Public Health, University of California,
Los Angeles, CA, USA
e-mail: jmsiegel@ucla.edu

C. Blazina et al. (eds.), *The Psychology of the Human–Animal Bond*,
DOI 10.1007/978-1-4419-9761-6_10, © Springer Science+Business Media, LLC 2011

into pet ownership. Random assignment to owner and non-owner groups would be neither feasible nor ethical. Individuals and families decide to incorporate a pet into their lives for a variety of reasons that may be related to structural factors, such as income, or personality factors, such as sociability. Many of these factors, in turn, are related to health status. In fact, the association of income with health is among the most robust in the epidemiological literature. Furthermore, some people who would like to self-select into ownership are unable to have one because of their living situation, health status, or wishes of household members. Studies that include statistical controls for demographic and other differences between owners and non-owners strengthen the inferences that can be drawn.

Studies of naturally occurring pet ownership leave open the issue of causal ordering. It is not only highly plausible that pet ownership promotes good health but also reasonable that health status influences ownership. The latter yields two possibilities as well. If sick people cannot take care of pets, they would be less likely to have them and an observed relationship between ownership and good health would be inflated. Alternatively, if sick people acquire a pet for companionship, to reduce isolation, and as a means of coping with illness, they would be more likely to own a pet and it would appear that ownership is associated with poor health. Prospective studies of initially healthy populations are in the best position to address this question.

These issues are raised at the outset of this chapter to raise sensitivity to the complexity of studying pet ownership and health. What may be most useful to researchers and practitioners at this juncture is not *whether* pet ownership facilitates good health, but *under what circumstances* might pet ownership facilitate it. The review presented here concentrates on recent literature, describes some of the circumstances in which pet ownership appears to act as a moderator variable in regard to health, and incorporates theoretical approaches that provide a context for understanding the relationship. Pet ownership would be considered a moderator variable if it affects the direction or strength of a relationship between a predictor variable and a health outcome (Baron & Kenny, 1986). For example, in a study of older persons, the accumulation of life events was associated with greater number of doctor contacts for persons who did not own pets, but not for pet owners. Pet ownership moderated the impact of life events on use of physician services.

This chapter is not intended as an exhaustive review of the many published studies, but several in-depth literature reviews are cited, some of which provide complete data from Medline or other searchable databases. The emphasis is on naturally occurring pet ownership and does not include the literature relevant to the use of pets in a therapeutic context (e.g., animal-assisted therapy, service animals, and pets as detectors of disease).

Physical Health

The most dramatic demonstration of the impact of pet ownership on health comes from studies of survival following a cardiac event. Over a 30-year period, there have been three carefully conducted longitudinal studies of hospitalized patients. The first found greater longevity for heart attack survivors who owned pets than those who did not (Friedmann, Katcher, Lynch, & Thomas, 1980). The authors replicated their findings regarding survival in the subsequent cardiac arrhythmia suppression trial, with the greatest benefit conferred by dog ownership. This effect was independent of physiologic status and other psychosocial factors, including social support (Friedmann & Thomas, 1995). Additional analyses of these data suggested that the survival advantage may have been due to differences in cardiac autonomic modulation, as indicated by higher heart rate variability among pet owners (Friedmann, Thomas, Stein, & Kleiger, 2003). Reduced heart rate variability is associated with cardiac disease and mortality and is an independent predictor of mortality following a heart attack.

In 2010, a third study was published that addressed this issue (Parker et al., 2010). The participants were consecutive patients admitted over a two-year period for acute coronary syndrome (heart attack or unstable angina) and the outcome variable was mortality or hospital readmission during the one- to 12-month follow-up period. In contrast to the previous studies, pet owners, especially those with cats, fared more poorly than non-owners. They were more likely to be readmitted or die from cardiac events. In multivariate models, the effect of pet ownership was independent of demographic factors and measures of health status, including physical exercise. The authors discussed the prior studies at length but were unable to identify specific factors leading to the divergent results.

Research on pet ownership and physiological indices (e.g., blood pressure, heart rate) has produced inconsistent results, as well. Procedures, settings, and outcomes are more varied than in the work on cardiovascular mortality discussed above, making it even more difficult to reconcile conflicting results. In an unusual study, in that it involved random assignment, stock brokers with hypertension either adopted a cat, a dog, or no pet, simultaneously with starting medication to control blood pressure (Allen, Shykoff, & Izzo, 2001). At the outset of the study, all participants had agreed to adopt a pet if they were assigned to that experimental intervention. Smaller stress-related increases in blood pressure were subsequently noted in the pet owners compared to non-owners. In a laboratory study, pet owners and non-owners participated in stressful tasks while their heart rate and blood pressure were being monitored (Allen, Blascovich, & Mendes, 2002). In addition to lower levels at baseline, pet owners were less physiologically reactive to the laboratory stressors and the cardiovascular indices returned to baseline levels more quickly than they did among the non-owners. Comparisons among different experimental conditions (completing the tasks in the presence of pets, friends, or spouses) showed that the least arousal occurred in the presence of pets. It is interesting to note that for the most challenging laboratory task, pet owners showed the highest level of physiological reactivity (interpreted as most stressed) with their spouse present.

A study among older persons incorporated a mailed questionnaire with a clinic visit, during which blood pressure was assessed (Wright, Kritz-Silverstein, Morton, Wingard, & Barrett-Connor, 2007). Pet owners had lower systolic blood pressure, but once age and other potential confounding variables were included in the analyses, there were no differences between pet owners and non-owners. This held for systolic and diastolic blood pressure, or derivative measures, including pulse pressure, mean arterial pressure, and risk of hypertension. Other research demonstrated higher diastolic blood pressure among pet owners than non-owners, despite greater engagement in mild physical activity among the pet owners (Parslow & Jorm, 2003a). In this sample, pet owners had higher body mass index and were more likely to smoke than non-owners, variables that were statistically controlled in the blood pressure analyses. A 2006 literature review on the psychophysiological effects of human–animal interaction reached the conclusion that despite the variability in findings, companion animals may have a salutary effect on blood pressure, especially in instances where an animal was adopted as a therapeutic intervention (Virues-Ortega & Buela-Casal, 2006).

Studies of pet ownership and use of health services are useful from a public health perspective in that potential cost savings in medical expenditures associated with pet ownership can be estimated. A one-year longitudinal study of Medicare enrollees in an Health Maintenance Organization (HMO) showed that pet owners contacted the doctor less often than non–pet owners (Siegel, 1990). Moreover, pets, especially dogs, appeared to buffer the impact of stress on health. The accumulation of stressful life events was associated with increased doctor contacts among non–pet owners but had no effect on doctor contacts for dog owners. Demographic factors and health status at baseline were statistically controlled.

Pursuing the notion of cost saving, data were collected from a national, stratified sample of Australians, age 16 years and older (Headey, 1999). Pet owners made fewer visits to the doctor and were less likely to be taking medication for heart problems or sleep. Extrapolating to the population, the author estimated a potential savings of 988 million dollars. A later study of doctor contacts, also conducted in Australia, sampled older persons exclusively (age 60–64) (Parslow, Jorm, Christensen, Rodgers, & Jacomb, 2005). In contrast to the two studies showing lower service use among pet owners, there was no difference in health service use as a function of pet ownership. Several of the indices in this study pointed to poorer health among pet owners. They reported more depressive symptoms and used more pain medication than non-owners and, if they were also female and married, they had worse physical health than non-owners.

Several of the studies on pet ownership and health have used self-report symptom, activity, or illness checklists as the outcome measure, often yielding subscales for both physical and mental health. For example, a nationally representative sample of the Swedish population found better general health, but poorer mental health, when comparing pet owners with non-owners (Müllersdorf, Granström, Sahlqvist, & Tillgren, 2010). Among older Canadian adults (age 65 or older), deterioration over a one-year period in ability to perform day-to-day activities was slower among pet owners than non-owners (Raina, Waltner-Toews, Bonnett, Woodward, & Abernathy, 1999). Pet ownership did not influence change in psychological well-being. Other investigations find no association of pet ownership and self-reported health, including a study of patients with chronic fatigue syndrome (Wells, 2009) and a study of older adults that assessed attachment to pet as well as pet ownership (Winefield, Black, & Chur-Hanson, 2008). All of these studies noted sociodemographic differences between owners and non-owners, but only some of them controlled for these differences when determining if pet ownership was associated with health status.

An oft cited explanation for any health benefit associated with pet ownership is the potential for greater physical exercise among owners, if the pet is a dog. On a population level, physical activity is positively associated with cardiovascular health and negatively associated with body mass index. Here, too, the findings regarding pet ownership have been contradictory, perhaps because different breeds of dogs require greater or lesser exercise, and this has not been taken into account in the research. Several studies demonstrated more walking among dog owners (Thorpe et al., 2006; Yabroff, Troiano, & Berrigan, 2008), but did not document that activities with dogs were of sufficient intensity to be considered health enhancing. An Internet-based study in Japan included the well-validated International Physical Activity Questionnaire, which assessed different levels of physical activity, including heath enhancing (Oka & Shibata, 2009). Dog owners had higher levels of physical activity than owners of other pets or non-owners, but only 30% of the dog owners met the criteria for vigorous (e.g., health enhancing) activity. One study noted a correlation between degree of overweight in dogs and their owners, a finding that could be accounted for by the amount of time the dog was being walked (Nijland, Stam, & Seidell, 2010).

Most of the research on pet ownership and physical health is aimed at addressing whether pets enhance health. A smaller body of work looks at the potential for ill health among those living with pets, usually in regard to owners (or family members) who have allergies or are immunologically compromised, and thus at greater risk for animal-transmitted infections. Findings are difficult to interpret because many people with allergies avoid having pets, and recall errors are significant (Bertelsen et al., 2009). Testing whether early exposure to pets is protective for children who eventually develop asthma or allergies is not feasible in observational studies because of the tendency in these families to avoid pets (Svanes et al., 2006). One study using data from the third National Health and Nutrition Examination survey showed that pet ownership was an independent predictor of asthma and/or wheezing among US adults (Arif, Delclos, Lee, Tortolero, & Whitehead, 2003). Indoor air pollutants were not a predictor. A review of the literature on pet bird ownership and respiratory illness concluded that there is little consensus regarding a hypothesized link (Gorman et al., 2009). In regard to immunocompromised persons, exposure to most pet species is not risky if guidelines for hygienic practices are followed (Hemsworth & Pizer, 2006). Beyond animal bites or scratches, other researchers have raised the possibility that humans may avoid medical care because they fear being hospitalized and unable to care for their pet (McNicholas et al., 2005), or may act inappropriately in an emergency evacuation situation out of concern for their pet (Heath & Champion, 1996).

Psychological Health

The reliance on descriptive data collected from convenience samples is, if anything, more common in the studies on psychological than physical health. Several investigations described in the previous section on physical health also assessed psychological health. These studies are not reviewed again here. In the aggregate, some of the research suggests that pet ownership is beneficial for mental health (Budge, Spicer, Jones, & St. George, 1998), some studies show no relation (Parslow & Jorm, 2003b), and others suggest that pets are deleterious for mental health (Parslow et al., 2005).

The presumed mechanism for the salutary effect of pets is that they function in a similar manner to human attachments and supports (Pachana, Ford, Andrew, & Dobson, 2005). The benefits of close relationships among humans are well documented in the research literature. They have been shown to reduce mortality and morbidity from a variety of conditions, especially cardiovascular disease (Uchino, 2008), and contribute to overall psychological well-being (Seeman, 1996). The data are robust that social isolates fare poorly, but are less clear in regard to an accumulated benefit associated with increasing network size. A single close and dependable relationship may be sufficient to experience the benefits. In addition, human social relationships have been shown to buffer stress, such that the negative impact of stress on health is ameliorated among humans with adequate level of support.

There have been a number of typologies offered to differentiate among types of human social support. For example, support can be: *emotional*, involving the expression of empathy, caring, reassurance, and trust; *informational,* referring to the provision of relevant information intended to help the individual cope with current difficulties; or *instrumental*, involving the provision of material aid, such as financial assistance or help with daily tasks (Cohen, 2004). One of the lessons from the social support literature is that support is most effective when the type of support that is offered meets the aroused need. For example, a person who needs instrumental support, such as a ride to a chemotherapy appointment, may find that receiving emotional support, in the form of expressions of love and affirmation, does little to ease the psychological burden of having cancer.

When looking for parallels in the human–pet literature, it is apparent that pets could provide neither informational nor instrumental support. The primary avenue would be emotional support. It follows, then, that individuals benefitting most from pets should be those for whom companionship needs are most pronounced. This has been shown among people living alone (Goldmeier, 1986; Kiel, 1998; McHarg, Baldock, Headey, & Robinson, 1995) and persons who rate their human social support as inadequate (Siegel, Angulo, Detels, Wesch, & Mullen, 1999). In the later case, pets buffered (or moderated) the relationship between symptoms of AIDS and psychological distress, especially when human ties were lacking. Similarly, a study of older women showed that attachment to pets mediated the relationship between loneliness and poor health (Krause-Parello, 2008). The term *mediation*, rather than *moderation*, is appropriate here in that attachment to one's pet accounted for the relation between the loneliness and health (Baron & Kenny, 1986). Still, inconsistencies in the literature exist in that some studies have found that those who appeared to benefit most from pet ownership, in terms of psychological health, were those with strong social ties (Wells & Rodi, 2000). Contrary findings emerged too when considering whether pet attachment and human attachment are related. They have been shown to be uncorrelated constructs that acted independently on psychological state (Winefield et al., 2008) and inversely related (Stallones, Marx, Garrity, & Johnson, 1990), suggesting that stronger ties with pets are formed when bonds with humans are more limited. Disentangling the multiple social influences on psychological well-being remains a challenge because most people with pets live with other people and households with pets, usually contain children, as well.

Also in the realm of potential psychological benefits of animal companionship is that pets provide nonjudgmental acceptance and love (Soares, 1985). A study described in the preceding section "Physical Health" showed that for an intellectually challenging task, presumably when evaluation apprehension would be highest, pet owners were most physiologically aroused in the presence of their spouses, and least aroused in the presence of their pets (Allen et al., 2002). Thus, in some circumstances, pets are calming and reassuring, even beyond what an intimate human partner could provide. A distinction drawn between companionship and social support emphasized the daily benefits to well-being fostered by companionship, in contrast with the stress buffering effects of social support (McNicholas et al., 2005). According to this line of thought, animals are not a replacement for human social support, but may be more advantageous in some contexts, such as the one described above. These authors noted, in addition, that relationships with pets were less likely than close relationships with humans to involve burnout, fluctuations, or concern about stability.

Other studies have addressed the role of pets as a social lubricant that may increase human social interaction and promote psychological well-being. Pet owners with serious mental illness demonstrated higher community integration than similar individuals without pets (Zimolag & Krupa, 2009) and pet ownership was associated with a higher level of social capital and civic engagement (Wood, Giles-Corti, & Bulsara, 2005). It has been shown, however, that the impact on social networks was minimal from the superficial social interaction that accrued to dog owners (Collis, McNicholas, & Harker, 2003).

In a review of the benefits of human–companion animal interaction, covering 129 peer-reviewed published studies (Barker & Wolen, 2008), the authors addressed the inconsistencies and methodological shortcomings in the database. Nonetheless, they concluded that "seniors in nursing homes and those with Alzheimer's disease or dementia appear to benefit from both pet ownership [and animal-assisted activities] in the areas of mood, loneliness, social behaviors, and caloric intake" (p. 492).

Concluding Comments

We want to believe that pets are good for our health, and those who own pets strongly hold this belief. In a focus group study of people recruited from dog-walking sites, all of the participants endorsed that pets enhanced their health (Knight & Edwards, 2008). Still, it has been hard to demonstrate this empirically on a consistent basis. Some studies have looked for direct effects, that is, better health among owners than non-owners, while others have looked for indirect effects. In regard to the latter, this would occur when pets moderate the direct relationship between some sort of stressor (i.e., loneliness, negative life event) and a health outcome. Most likely, the stress buffering model will be more fruitful than the direct effects model in guiding future research in that it provides opportunities for identifying which stressors arouse which need, which needs can be satisfied by pets, and for whom. In other words, circumstances that arouse companionship needs may be ameliorated by pets, whereas life events that exacerbate financial strains may actually be compounded by the expense of providing for a household pet. Although this approach is methodologically and logistically complex, it may address the inconsistencies in the body of literature on pet ownership and health.

In regard to the "for whom," it is important to expand the populations sampled beyond non-Hispanic whites, as ethnic minorities have been included in this area of research with rare exception (Johnson & Meadows, 2002; Siegel, 1995). Data drawn from a multiethnic urban sample showed considerable variability as a function of race/ethnicity in the likelihood of owning a pet, and the nature of the relationship (in this study, adolescent's) to his/her pet (Siegel, 1995). White families were much more likely to own pets than either Latino, Asian, or African American families, but whites were also more likely to live in single family homes and had higher incomes. Likewise, white teens reported the highest level of attachment to their pets. Future research would benefit by utilizing diverse samples and by attempting to determine why the role of pets in the family is a culturally bound phenomenon. The potential for pets to buffer stress among populations other than non-Hispanic whites is worthy of exploration, given the relatively low cost of such an intervention.

A slightly different direction would be put less emphasis on health status (physical or mental) as the outcome variable and focus more on quality of life. Many of the noted benefits of pet ownership enhance quality of life, which in turn, can have a distal effect on health under some circumstances. Researchers and practitioners alike have assumed that the experience of bonding with a pet is a positive and beneficial one for children and adolescents, yet one would anticipate that the impact on health would be negligible when so many developmental processes are unfolding. Pets are never too busy for their owners, they take a subordinate role to children, they can be trusted to be consistent and not cause hurt, and they are unaware of human shortcomings (Davis & Juhasz, 1985). The down-the-road impact on health, even for older, vulnerable populations, may not be strong enough to detect statistically, but this should not negate the importance of the human–companion animal bond. A variety of measures have been developed to assess attachment to one's pet and they all show that the feelings that humans have for their pets are strong, they are tangible, and that pets are considered to be beloved family members.

Beyond the research arena, there are a number of policy-relevant implications of this body of work (Siegel, 1993). In times of fiscal constraint, local and state governments are unlikely to subsidize the needs of pet owners. A more modest proposal would be to enforce federal legislation that prohibits discrimination against pet ownership in public-assisted housing, and to inform elderly and other citizens of their rights in this regard. Additionally, community and volunteer organizations may play a constructive role in facilitating pet ownership among people who wish to own pets and, in certain cases, care for pets if the owner is temporarily or permanently unable to fulfill certain duties. Also, if previously understudied populations (i.e., ethnic minorities) are shown to benefit from animal companionship, program planners may want to think creatively about incorporating animals into community-based services and at recreational sites.

References

Allen, K., Blascovich, J., & Mendes, W. B. (2002). Cardiovascular reactivity and the presence of pets, friends, and spouses: The truth about cats and dogs. *Psychosomatic Medicine, 64*, 727–739.

Allen, K., Shykoff, B. E., & Izzo, J. L., Jr. (2001). Pet ownership, but not ACE inhibitor therapy, blunts home blood pressure responses to mental stress. *Hypertension, 38*, 815–820.

Arif, A. A., Delclos, G. L., Lee, E. S., Tortolero, S. R., & Whitehead, L. W. (2003). Prevalence and risk factors of asthma and wheezing among US adults: An analysis of the NHANES III data. *European Respiratory Journal, 21*, 827–833.

Barker, S. B., & Wolen, A. R. (2008). The benefits of human-companion animal interaction: A review. *Journal of Veterinary Medical Education, 35*, 487–495.

Baron, R. M., & Kenny, D. A. (1986). The moderator-mediator variable distinction in social psychological research: Conceptual, strategic and statistical considerations. *Journal of Personality and Social Psychology, 51*, 1173–1182.

Bertelsen, R. J., Carlsen, K. C., Granum, B., Carlsen, K. H., Håland, G., Devulapalli, C. S., et al. (2009). Do allergic families avoid keeping furry pets? *Indoor Air, 20*, 187–195.

Budge, R. C., Spicer, J., Jones, B., & St. George, R. (1998). Health correlates of compatibility and attachment in human-companion animal relationships. *Society and Animals: Journal of Human-Animal Studies, 6*, 219–234.

Cohen, S. (2004). Social relationships and health. *American Psychologist, 59*, 676–684.

Collis, G., McNicholas, J., & Harker, R. (2003). *Could enhanced social networks explain the association between pet ownership and health?* Unpublished paper, Department of Psychology, University of Warwick, Coventry, UK.

Davis, J. H., & Juhasz, A. M. (1985). The preadolescent/pet bond and psychosocial development. *Marriage and Family Review, 8*, 79–94.

Friedmann, E., Katcher, A. H., Lynch, J. J., & Thomas, S. A. (1980). Animal companions and one-year survival of patients after discharge from a coronary care unit. *Public Health Reports, 95*, 307–312.

Friedmann, E., & Thomas, S. A. (1995). Pet ownership, social support, and one-year survival after acute myocardial infarction in the Cardiac Arrhythmia Suppression Trial (CAST). *American Journal of Cardiology, 76*, 1213–1217.

Friedmann, E., Thomas, S. A., Stein, P. K., & Kleiger, R. E. (2003). Relation between pet ownership and heart rate variability in patients with healed myocardial infarcts. *American Journal of Cardiology, 91*, 718–721.

Goldmeier, J. (1986). Pets or people: Another research note. *Gerontologist, 26*, 203–206.

Gorman, J., Cook, A., Ferguson, C., van Buynder, P., Fenwick, S., & Weinstein, P. (2009). Pet birds and risks of respiratory disease in Australia: A review. *Australia New Zealand Journal of Public Health, 33*, 167–172.

Headey, B. (1999). Health benefits and health cost savings due to pets: Preliminary estimates from an Australian national survey. *Social Indicators Research, 47*, 233–243.

Heath, S. E., & Champion, M. (1996). Human health concerns from pet ownership after a tornado. *Prehospital and Disaster Medicine, 11*, 67–70.

Hemsworth, S., & Pizer, B. (2006). Pet ownership in immunocompromised children – a review of the literature and survey of existing guidelines. *European Journal of Oncology and Nursing, 10*, 117–127.

Johnson, R. A., & Meadows, R. L. (2002). Older Latinos, pets, and health. *Western Journal of Nursing Research, 24*, 609–620.

Kiel, C. (1998). Loneliness, stress, and human-animal attachment among older adults. In C. Wilson & D. Turner (Eds.), *Companion animals in human health* (pp. 123–134). Thousand Oaks, CA: Sage.

Knight, S., & Edwards, V. J. (2008). In the company of wolves: The physical, social, and psychological benefits of dog ownership. *Journal of Aging and Health, 20*, 437–455.

Krause-Parello, C. A. (2008). The mediating effect of pet attachment support between loneliness and general health in older females living in the community. *Journal of Community Health Nursing, 25*, 1–14.

McHarg, M., Baldock, C., Headey, B., & Robinson, A. (1995). *National people and pets survey.* Sydney: Urban Animal Management Coalition.

McNicholas, J., Gilbey, A., Rennie, A., Ahmedzai, S., Dono, J. A., & Omerod, E. (2005). Pet ownership and human health: A brief overview of evidence and issues. *British Medical Journal, 331*, 1252–1254.

Müllersdorf, M., Granström, F., Sahlqvist, L., & Tillgren, P. (2010). Aspects of health, physical/leisure activities, work and socio-demographics associated with pet ownership in Sweden. *Scandinavian Journal of public Health, 38*, 53–63.

Nijland, M. L., Stam, F., & Seidell, J. C. (2010). Overweight in dogs, but not in cats, is related to overweight in their owners. *Public Health Nutrition, 13*, 102–106.

Oka, K., & Shibata, A. (2009). Dog ownership and health-related physical activity among Japanese adults. *Journal of Physical Activities and Health, 6*, 412–418.

Pachana, N. A., Ford, J. H., Andrew, B., & Dobson, A. (2005). Relations between companion animals and self-reported health in older women: Cause, effect or artifact? *International Journal of Behavioral Medicine, 12*, 102–110.

Parker, G. B., Gayed, A., Owen, C. A., Hyett, M. P., Hilton, T. M., & Heruc, G. A. (2010). Survival following an acute coronary syndrome: A pet theory put to the test. *Acta Psychiatrica Scandinavica, 121*, 65–70.

Parslow, R. A., & Jorm, A. F. (2003a). Pet ownership and risk factors for cardiovascular disease: Another look. *Medical Journal of Australia, 179*, 466–468.

Parslow, R. A., & Jorm, A. F. (2003b). The impact of pet ownership on health and health service use: Results from a community sample of Australians aged 40 to 44 years. *Anthrozoös, 16*, 43–46.

Parslow, R. A., Jorm, A. F., Christensen, H., Rodgers, B., & Jacomb, P. (2005). Pet ownership and health in older adults: Findings from a survey of 2,551 community-based Australians aged 60–64. *Gerontology, 51*, 40–47.

Raina, P., Waltner-Toews, D., Bonnett, B., Woodward, C., & Abernathy, T. (1999). Influence of companion animals on the physical and psychological health of older people: An analysis of a one-year longitudinal study. *Journal of the American Geriatric Society, 47*, 323–329.

Seeman, T. E. (1996). Social ties and health: The benefits of social integration. *Annals of Epidemiology, 6*, 442–451.

Siegel, J. M. (1990). Stressful life events and use of physician services among the elderly: The moderating role of pet ownership. *Journal of Personality and Social Psychology, 58*, 1081–1086.

Siegel, J. M. (1993). Companion animals: In sickness and in health. *Journal of Social Issues, 49*, 157–167.

Siegel, J. M. (1995). Pet ownership and the importance of pets among adolescents. *Anthrozoös, 8*, 217–223.

Siegel, J. M., Angulo, F. J., Detels, R., Wesch, J., & Mullen, A. (1999). AIDS diagnosis and depression in the Multicenter AIDS Cohort Study: The ameliorating impact of pet ownership. *AIDS Care, 11*, 157–170.

Soares, C. J. (1985). The companion animal in the context of the family system. *Marriage and Family Review, 8*, 49–62.

Stallones, L., Marx, M. B., Garrity, T. F., & Johnson, T. P. (1990). Pet ownership and attachment in relation to the health of U.S. adults, 21 to 64 years of age. *Anthrozoös, 4*, 100–112.

Svanes, C., Zock, J. P., Antó, J., Dharmage, S., Norbäck, D., Wjst, M., et al. (2006). Do asthma and allergy influence subsequent pet keeping? An analysis of childhood and adulthood. *Journal of Allergy and Clinical Immunology, 118*, 691–698.

Thorpe, R. J., Kreisle, R. A., Glickman, L. T., Simonsick, E. M., Newman, A. B., & Kritchevsky, S. (2006). Physical activity and pet ownership in year 3 of the Health ABC study. *Journal of Aging and Physical Activity, 14*, 154–168.

Uchino, B. N. (2008). Understanding the links between social support and physical health: A life span perspective with emphasis on the separability of perceived and received support. *Perspectives in Psychological Science, 4*, 236–255.

Virués-Ortega, J., & Buela-Casal, G. (2006). Psychophysiological effects of human-animal interaction: Theoretical issues and long-term interaction effects. *Journal of Nervous and Mental Disease, 194*, 52–57.

Wells, D. I. (2009). Associations between pet ownership and self-reported health status in people suffering from chronic fatigue syndrome. *Journal of Alternative and Complementary Medicine, 15*, 407–413.

Wells, Y., & Rodi, H. (2000). Effects of pet ownership on the health and well-being of older people. *Australasian Journal on Ageing, 19*, 143–148.

Winefield, H. R., Black, A., & Chur-Hanson, A. (2008). Health effects of ownership of and attachment to companion animals in an older population. *International Journal of Behavioral Medicine, 15*, 303–310.

Wood, L., Giles-Corti, B., & Bulsara, M. (2005). The pet connection: Pets as a conduit for social capital? *Social Science and Medicine, 61*, 1159–1173.

Wright, J. D., Kritz-Silverstein, D., Morton, D. J., Wingard, D. L., & Barrett-Connor, E. (2007). Pet ownership and blood pressure in old age. *Epidemiology, 18*, 613–618.

Yabroff, K. R., Troiano, R. P., & Berrigan, D. (2008). Walking the dog: Is pet ownership associated with physical activity in California? *Journal of Physical Activity and Health, 5*, 216–228.

Zimolag, U., & Krupa, T. (2009). Pet ownership as a meaningful community occupation for people with serious mental illness. *American Journal of Occupational Therapy, 63*, 126–137.

Part III
Bereavement, Loss, and Disenfranchised Grief

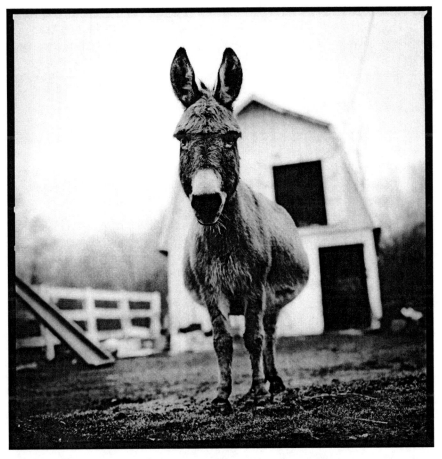

Dee Dee, Resident of Star Gazing Farm
A donkey that is a guardian to the sheep and goats. Her exact age is not known, but she is estimated to be in her late twenties or early thirties.

Chapter 11
Family-Present Euthanasia: Protocols for Planning and Preparing Clients for the Death of a Pet

Laurel Lagoni

Notes About Language

There is debate within the animal care community about continuing to use the words "pet" and "owner" within professional discussions, as they seem to diminish the mutually beneficial relationship known as the "human–animal bond." However, the author has chosen to use them for the purpose of this chapter as they remain the most common terms used by those in the veterinary medical community. The terms "pet" and "companion animal" are used interchangeably.

In this chapter, "companion animal euthanasia" refers to a humane method of terminating the life of an animal who is dearly loved, but has little or no hope for recovery. It does not refer to euthanasia that is performed for "convenience," "population control," or "public safety." The decision to perform "companion animal euthanasia" usually comes about due to an animal's severe injury, terminal illness, or deterioration due to the aging process. This type of euthanasia is usually deemed "justifiable" and is provided primarily for domesticated cats, dogs, birds, and small mammals. The methods and support protocols described in this chapter, as well as the issue of family presence, may differ when applied to horses, as well as food, zoo, wild, and shelter animals, even though these animals may also be held in high regard by the humans who care for them.

Overview

Anticipating the euthanasia of a beloved companion animal can be a nerve-wracking experience. This is especially true if owners or entire families wish to be present when their pets die.

While there is much written to help pet owners deal with grief *after* their pets die, there is very little information available to help them make necessary plans

L. Lagoni (✉)
World by the Tail, Inc., Fort Collins, CO 80525, USA; Argus Institute for Families and Veterinary Medicine, James L. Voss Veterinary Teaching Hospital, Colorado State University, Fort Collins, CO 80523, USA
e-mail: llagoni@comcast.net; www.veterinarywisdom.com

C. Blazina et al. (eds.), *The Psychology of the Human–Animal Bond*,
DOI 10.1007/978-1-4419-9761-6_11, © Springer Science+Business Media, LLC 2011

and to prepare themselves emotionally *before* the procedure of euthanasia. There are even fewer studies and published information about the interventions mental health practitioners can use to be of assistance to clients during this preparation and planning phase.

However, clinical experience shows that mental health practitioners are most helpful to clients when they themselves are well informed about the choices and decisions pet owners typically face prior to a pet's euthanasia. This chapter presents an applied, systematic overview of the various pet euthanasia–related issues that clinical experience has proven to be helpful for mental health practitioners to discuss with clients should the request for their guidance occur. In order to orient mental health practitioners, the chapter also describes what pet owners can expect to experience during the companion animal euthanasia procedure itself. Information about resources for after-death follow-up and pet loss support training programs is also included.

While relevant research is cited, companion animal euthanasia and the resulting human grief reaction is not an area of veterinary medicine or the human experience that has been frequently studied or documented. The overall theories and grief counseling techniques used to support pet owners have their genesis in the field of human loss and grief. The few articles and studies that exist on the topic of pet loss and grief were published, for the most part, in the late 1980s and early 1990s. Thus, the approach described in this chapter is largely drawn from the author's textbook entitled *The Human–Animal Bond and Grief* (Lagoni, Butler, & Hetts, 1994) and based on the author's clinical experience during her tenure as Director of the Argus Institute for Families and Veterinary Medicine at Colorado State University's James L. Voss Veterinary Teaching Hospital (1984–2004). The Argus Institute provides grief support for clients, as well as coursework and clinical experience for veterinary students, interns, residents, and faculty. The Argus Institute, one of the first clinical pet loss support programs in the nation, pioneered many of the practice tools and techniques that are routinely used today by veterinarians and mental health practitioners to facilitate and support pet owners through family-present euthanasia.

Family-Present Euthanasia: Protocols for Planning and Preparing Clients for the Death of a Pet

Anticipating and preparing for the euthanasia of a beloved companion animal can be a nerve-wracking experience for pet owners and members of the veterinary practice team alike. This is especially true if individuals or entire families wish to be present during the procedure when their pets die.

Mental health practitioners can play a vital role in guiding pet owners through their feeling grief after a pet has died (Toray, 2004). As the field of pet loss counseling evolves, mental health practitioners can also become a valued link between veterinarians and pet owners to ensure that pre-euthanasia communication between them is clear, complete, and timely, in terms of planning and preparing for a pet's death.

While the emotional impact of pet loss on human bereavement for both pet owners (Cowles, 1985; Gage & Holcomb, 1991; Gosse & Barnes, 1994; Planchon & Templer, 1996; Planchon, Templer, Stokes, & Keller, 2002; Weisman, 1991) and veterinary professionals (Fogle & Abrahamson, 1990; Hart, Hart, & Mader, 1990) has been studied, and much has been written in the popular literature about how pet owners can deal with grief *after* their pets die (Carmack, 2003; Kowalski, 2006; Sife, 1998), there is far less information available about how veterinarians or mental health practitioners can help pet owners cope with anticipatory grief and make necessary plans and preparations *before* the procedure of pet euthanasia (Barton Ross & Baron-Sorensen, 2007; Lagoni et al., 1994; Nakaya, 2005).

Research suggests that the experience of pet loss is emotionally painful for many people (Gage & Holcomb, 1991; Gosse & Barnes, 1994) and clinical experience has shown that the experience of euthanasia, especially when the procedure is *not* performed sensitively or skillfully, can complicate and exacerbate negative feelings associated with grief (Lagoni et al., 1994). It follows, then, that the assistance and support of well-informed and experienced mental health practitioners, both during anticipatory and post-death grief, may help mitigate many of the potentially negative effects of pet loss. Mental health practitioners can serve as preparatory resources for clients, teaming up, either formally or informally, with their clients' veterinarians. This role requires mental health professionals to be well informed about the medical and emotional realities of pet euthanasia (according to each individual veterinarian's beliefs and methods), as well as the numerous choices pet owners must navigate prior to the procedure.

This chapter presents an applied, systematic description of the conversations mental health practitioners can facilitate for clients in terms of the various decisions leading up to companion animal euthanasia. It also provides a guide for providing effective emotional support for pet owners throughout the companion animal euthanasia experience. Information about after-death grief support and resources that mental health practitioners can suggest or refer clients to for follow-up is also included.

Companion Animal Euthanasia in Today's Veterinary Medicine

The term "euthanasia" comes from the Greek "eu," meaning "good," and "thanatos," meaning "death." Used together, they qualify euthanasia as a "good death" (Fogle, 1981). Words such as humane, painless, and loving are also associated with "good death" or euthanasia. Yet, setting the more positive meaning aside, euthanasia is still, in reality, the purposeful act of terminating a life.

Most veterinarians accept the responsibility of providing their patients with a "good death" in order to spare them unnecessary pain and suffering. Indeed, veterinarians are the only medical doctors with the legal right to do so. Until the mid-1980s, most veterinarians thought of euthanasia as a somewhat routine, although emotionally uncomfortable, medical procedure and performed the "duty" in a sterile medical environment with no one, except perhaps another member of the veterinary team, present. Pet owner participation and presence at euthanasia was most often discouraged and even forbidden.

In this traditional model of veterinary euthanasia, the standard operating procedure was to talk about the process as little as possible, involve clients as little as possible, and get the deed over with as quickly as possible. Euthanasia was often referred to only indirectly or euphemistically ("disposed of," "put to sleep") and clients were encouraged to simply drop off their animals at their veterinary clinics so they wouldn't be burdened by the actual details of death. This method also allowed veterinarians to perform the procedure when it worked best for them, rather than at the time and place most suitable for their client. The common belief was that this impersonal, clinical approach to euthanasia was the best way to protect both clients and veterinarians from dealing with the negative emotions surrounding death (Garcia, 1986).

While this traditional paradigm probably worked for some pet owners and veterinarians, for others it created a different kind of emotional pain, leading to feelings of guilt, shame, depression, and unresolved grief (Hart & Hart, 1987). The traditional model of euthanasia was particularly hard on veterinarians because it placed the bulk of the emotional burden on their shoulders. For example, veterinarians were usually the ones to decide *when*, *why*, *how*, and *where* animals should die. In addition, veterinarians usually refrained from formally acknowledging their patients' deaths and from contacting their clients afterward. Thus, the traditional model forced everyone to grieve in isolation and, in general, didn't allow either veterinarians or clients to experience "closure" regarding the loss. Many veterinarians resented this overwhelming responsibility and, even though they colluded with it, many clients resented the fact that they had little control over what happened to their own animals (Lagoni et al., 1994).

In the late 1980s and early 1990s, due primarily to the rapidly emerging fields of veterinary oncology and veterinary grief counseling, veterinary medicine began to see companion animal euthanasia in a new light. This shift in attitude was reinforced by a 1999 Veterinary Market Study that stressed the "recognition of the human–animal bond as an important determinant of a successful practice." (Brown & Silverman, 1999) Today, most veterinarians realize that few other medical procedures can have as great an impact on them, their staff members, their clients, and the quality of their veterinarian–client relationships as euthanasia. This is due to the fact that, when euthanasia is performed well, it can soothe and reassure all involved that the decision to end an animal's life was the right one, thus bonding clients to the veterinary practice with gratitude. However, when euthanasia is done poorly, meaning thoughtlessly or without compassion and sensitivity, it can deepen, complicate, and prolong grief, thus damaging and even ending the client–veterinarian relationship due to a client's resentment and anger (Lagoni et al., 1994).

The modern approach to pet euthanasia takes into account such factors as job satisfaction, client loyalty, business success, and more positive grief outcomes for clients may all be somewhat linked to the veterinary team's ability to perform companion animal euthanasia in an emotionally sensitive way (Lagoni et al., 1994). This connection has helped evolve the procedure into more than a dreaded medical task. Today, euthanasia is most often viewed by veterinary professionals as a privilege and by pet owners as a gift: a gift that can be bestowed upon beloved animals who may be suffering or who have little or no hope for recovery. In recent decades, the procedure of companion animal euthanasia has evolved from an emotionless medical procedure to an oftentimes spiritual ceremony, with entire families in attendance and with emotional responses treated with respect and reverence by all involved.

With this modern paradigm for companion animal euthanasia in mind, progressive veterinarians, animal health technicians, and grief counselors from across the country have worked together to create and perfect euthanasia protocols that have the patients', clients', veterinarians', and veterinary staff members' emotional comfort and well-being in mind. These multidisciplinary teams of professionals have considered many variables, including the attitudes of those involved in the euthanasia process, the physical surroundings and emotional ambience of the euthanasia site, and the combination of drugs and methods used to induce peaceful and painless death. How veterinarians and mental health practitioners can best work together, as clinical team members, in order to prepare clients to face the circumstances surrounding the euthanasia procedure have also been discussed.

The modern standard operating procedure for companion animal euthanasia is the opposite of the former, more traditional paradigm. In the modern model, it is more common for veterinarians and clients to discuss the details surrounding euthanasia together, directly, and at length. It is also common to set aside as much time as possible for the procedure, to involve clients in the process as much as possible, and to openly acknowledge the animals' deaths and to reminisce at length about them afterward. The modern paradigm is much more congruent with research conducted in the fields of death and dying and veterinary medicine regarding the links between positive grief outcomes and effective bereavement support techniques (Rando, 1984; Worden, 2008). For example, much more attention is paid today to the planning and preparation process prior to pet euthanasia in reference to classic studies showing that longer preparation time may diminish the intensity of grief reactions (Ball, 1977) and that anticipatory grief can act as a mitigating influence on post-death grief (Ball, 1977; Parkes, 1975). Recent research, as well as clinical experience, has shown that having a period of time for planning and preparing for a pet's death often minimizes the "regrets," the "what ifs," and the "if onlys" that inevitably plague pet owners if they haven't had, or taken, time to make conscious choices about how they want and need the experience surrounding their pet's death to unfold (Kellehear & Fook, 1997). Therefore, the modern paradigm for companion animal euthanasia is both a sensitive and pragmatic one and it is the one mental health practitioners should reference when preparing clients to face a pet's imminent death.

Helping Clients Move Through Choices Surrounding Companion Animal Euthanasia

As a mental health practitioner, it's important for you to understand that the modern paradigm of companion animal euthanasia is characterized by one key word: *choice*. In the modern paradigm, clients are given choices about as many details as possible, the emotional burdens are shared, and, within the context of their relationship, veterinarians and clients decide together about the *when*, *why*, *how*, and *where* of companion animal euthanasia.

When people are allowed to make conscious choices, they feel empowered (Gershon & Straub, 1989). Feeling empowered means they are more likely to make decisions that are right for them, thus feeling more positive about the experience overall. Clinical experience has shown that pet owners felt they had maintained their control, even when their pets ultimately died, if they were presented with options and choices to consider regarding *how* and *when* their pets died (Lagoni et al., 1994). Obviously, each client makes different choices. Some choose total involvement and orchestrate fairly complex euthanasia processes. Others choose minimal involvement, opting for only a good-bye hug as they leave their pet with their veterinarian.

Euthanasia is not a common, everyday experience for pet owners. In addition, many pet owners can only refer to a previous experience with pet euthanasia, which was most likely conducted within the context of the traditional paradigm. Thus, they may not realize that they *do* have choices. In order for pet owners to make wise and informed decisions, then, it can be very helpful for them to be provided with information and guided through the numerous decisions and choices they must make by those who are well informed about the procedure.

In the veterinary clinic, discussions about the choices and decisions related to euthanasia may take place over a period of days, weeks, or even months as pet owners bring their pets in for treatment for chronic or terminal illness. On the other hand, euthanasia-related discussions might be collapsed into a matter of hours or even minutes in cases of acute illnesses or traumatic injuries. The same scenario may apply to you, the mental health practitioner, as you work with clients who are in the midst of anticipating a pet's impending death. Whatever the time frame you have to work with, the choices you present and the conversations you have with clients should cover the same basic topics that are universal to making arrangements for companion animal euthanasia. These topics include timing and presence during death, as well as several logistical considerations.

Timing

No doubt, clients, veterinarians, and mental health professionals struggle with the timing of euthanasia. In fact, there is no "perfect time" for the procedure to occur. Yet, there are signs and signals pet owners can look for that may alert them to the fact that a pet's death is near. During your consultations with clients, you can help them think through the "benchmarks" and "bottom lines" that will help them know that their pets are no longer happy or experiencing any quality of life. Examples of these benchmark events might include a pet's lack of interest in drinking or eating or in going for walks. It might also be the client's emotional agony that comes with watching a pet struggle to breathe or to get comfortable in bed. For many clients, the deciding "bottom line" is when their pet becomes incontinent, no longer has the inability to walk or to get up from the floor, or can no longer respond to its owner in ways it had before.

One profound technique mental health practitioners can use to aid clients during the decision-making process about euthanasia timing is to call upon the power of the human–animal bond. This can be done by reminding clients that the relationship they have always shared with their pet is still available to them and can still be a source of support. Remind clients that they have always been able to "communicate" with their pet and that, if they "talk" with their pet and gaze into their eyes, the pet will most likely "let them know what they want" and, thus, they can make the decision together.

It's also a good idea for mental health professionals to encourage clients to contact their veterinarians to clarify the medical facts pertinent to this discussion. For example, encourage clients to ask their veterinarians if there are specific medical signs like seizures, disorientation, or tenderness in the abdomen that they can watch for in their pets, as these are often signs that the time to consider euthanasia is approaching soon. Remind clients that it's a good idea to write down what the veterinarian tells them to look for, as well as to note any medical symptoms they may observe, so they can consciously track their pet's diminishing quality of life. Knowing what to look for and honestly acknowledging what is actually occurring by recording it in a journal or on a calendar can help clients feel more accepting about their pet's impending death.

Presence During Death

When it's time for euthanasia, it's normal for those who've loved a pet to want to "be there" for the pet, just as the pet was always there for them. Family-present euthanasia provides the opportunity to say good-bye to a companion animal, not only before or after death, but also at the moment that death occurs.

Without question, it is emotionally painful for pet owners to watch their dearly-loved companion animals die. However, clinical experience shows that *not* being present when companion animals die potentially increases feelings of pain and distress (Lagoni et al., 1994). It also shows that being present when a beloved pet dies may facilitate the acceptance of the reality of death and the resolution of the loss and the grieving process just as it does when a human loved one dies (Rando, 1991).

Although being present may have value, encouraging clients to be present must be done with care. As a mental health practitioner, you should never aggressively attempt to convince your clients to be present during euthanasia. Some clients very clearly decide to leave their animals in their veterinarians' hands to be euthanized. Others choose to be nearby, but not witness the actual procedure, perhaps viewing the body and saying good-bye after death has occurred. Most veterinarians still consider these options to be acceptable and clients should not be deterred from these options, providing their choices are informed ones.

Some pet owners want to be present or feel they "should" be present at euthanasia, but doubt their abilities to do so. They may have been told by well-meaning friends that they "shouldn't put themselves through that" or they may fear that death is too upsetting to see based on experiences with previous pet euthanasia. These kinds of misconceptions about euthanasia are damaging to the field of veterinary medicine, as well as to pet owners themselves. They imply that the methods used for euthanasia are insensitive, inhumane, and difficult to witness. It's important for pet owners to know that, with rare exception, companion animal euthanasia today is facilitated in peaceful, painless ways, with skilled and sensitive attention paid to the people involved, as well.

In order for your clients to decide whether or not they wish to be present during their pet's euthanasia, they need information about what the actual euthanasia procedure entails. Since each veterinarian performs the procedure in a way that is unique to him or her and the particular clinic within which they practice, this discussion must begin with your client's veterinarian. It would be a big mistake for you or any mental health professional to attempt to describe any of the methods used for euthanasia without first talking to the veterinarian who will perform the procedure. However, it is appropriate for you, as a professional guiding your client through the decision-making process, to help clients identify the questions they wish to ask during a euthanasia planning session with their veterinarian. The most important questions you should encourage your clients to ask include the following:

- *"Can I be present?"*
  Although this is the twenty-first century, there are still "old school" veterinarians who operate from the traditional paradigm for pet euthanasia and discourage or even refuse to offer "family-presence" during euthanasia. This attitude can actually be a relief for some clients as it takes the pressure off them to deal any further with the details of their pet's death. However, for the majority of today's pet owners, this difference of opinion may spur them to seek out another veterinarian to perform the procedure. If this is the case, you can assist your clients at this time by helping them explore other options for veterinary care, like veterinary hospice programs or veterinarians who offer mobile or home euthanasia services. These kinds of specialty practices and programs are becoming more and more prevalent, especially in larger cities (Bishop, Long, Carlsten, Kennedy, & Shaw, 2008).

- *"What will the actual euthanasia experience be like?"*
  Your client's veterinarian is the best source for detailed information about the process of euthanasia. An example of the explanation your client will most likely hear is as follows:

  > "Judy, I know how special Pepper is to you and to your family. He's very special to us, too. I want you to know that we are committed to making this experience as meaningful and as positive for you as possible.

Now, in order to decide whether or not you want to be with Pepper when he dies, you need some more information about the procedure. Would you like me to discuss that with you now?"

With the pet owner's permission, the veterinarian continues.

"The first thing I like to do after you arrive with Pepper is take him back to our treatment area, shave a small area of fur, and place an intravenous catheter in a vein, most likely in one of his rear legs. Using a catheter means I can administer the drugs more smoothly. It also means that I can accomplish what I need to do without interfering with your desire to pet or to hold Pepper's head and front paws.

After we place the catheter, Pepper will be brought back to you and you can have more time to spend with him, if you want that. Then, when we all agree that it's time to proceed, I'll begin the euthanasia process.

The method I use involves three injections. (Note: This method and the drugs used may vary from clinic to clinic.) The first is simply a saline solution flush so I'm sure that the catheter is working. The second is a barbiturate which will make Pepper feel very relaxed and sleepy. The third injection will be the euthanasia solution, which is an overdose of pentobarbital sodium. This injection is the one that will actually stop Pepper's heart and brain activity and ultimately cause his death. Judy, many people are surprised by how quickly death takes place using this method. All three injections will take place within a minute or two and death will occur in a matter of seconds after the final injection.

You should know that, although euthanasia is painless and peaceful, Pepper may urinate, defecate, twitch, or even sigh a bit. All of this is completely normal and to be expected. Pepper won't be aware of any of these behaviors and he won't feel any discomfort or pain. In addition, you should be aware that Pepper's eyes won't close when he dies. It takes muscles to close your eyelids and Pepper's muscles won't be able to do their job once he has been euthanized. Do you have any questions about any of this?"

If the pet owner expresses understanding, the veterinarian will conclude with information about how long the clients may stay with their pet's body and may even go on to discuss issues like body care or appointment availability.

In addition to gathering information about the procedure itself, your clients may also want to ask the following questions:

- *"Do you offer home euthanasia or must I bring my pet to the clinic?"*
More and more veterinarians are finding ways to accommodate their clients' wishes for euthanasia that takes place at a pet's own, familiar home. This can be especially desirable when a pet is very sick and might be made more uncomfortable during travel.

Recently, a few progressive veterinarians have dedicated their entire practices to providing home euthanasia. These veterinarians often work on a referral basis with other veterinary clinics which are unable, or unwilling, to offer such a service (Vaughan, 2004). Veterinary hospice programs are also growing in popularity and may be available to your clients (Bishop et al., 2008).

- *"How much time will I spend with my pet once we arrive at the clinic?"*
Many clients don't want to feel rushed through the last moments they have with their pets. On the other hand, some want the procedure done right away as they find a prolonged good-bye process too painful to bear. Clients should communicate clearly with their veterinarians regarding how much time they wish to spend

with their pets. Conversely, clients should ask their veterinarians about how much time they typically allow for family-present euthanasia.

- *"My children and other family members may want to be there, too. How many people can you accommodate in the space where the euthanasia will take place?"* Today, many clinics have "family comfort rooms" that are larger than a typical exam room and decorated more like a home environment. These rooms are often equipped with lowered lighting, distractions like toys or books for young children, and pads or blankets that can be placed on the floor so families can gather around a pet while the procedure takes place and they can say good-bye. Family comfort rooms are usually large enough to accommodate several people and are located in an out-of-the-way location so as not to interfere with the clinic's ongoing examination schedule.

    If the weather is acceptable, many veterinary clinics also have garden rooms outdoors where several people can be in attendance during a pet's euthanasia. Most veterinary staff members are happy to provide clients with a "preview" of the various locations available for euthanasia upon the client's request.

If children wish to be present, encourage clients to research how they can best prepare them to witness their pet's death. It's helpful to provide some education regarding how children of various ages comprehend and commonly react to pet loss and death, in general (Harvey, Butler & Lagoni, 1999). You may also suggest they bring a friend along who will supervise young children should they change their minds about being with their pet.

Logistics

The final set of choices mental health practitioners can help clients face are the logistical details of planning the actual euthanasia procedure. For example, pet owners must decide who else they may want to accompany them to the euthanasia. With proper preparation, for instance, children often choose to be present when their companion animals die. Clients may also wish to include other relatives, friends, or even ex-spouses, if they were close to their pet. Appropriate times and settings for the procedure must also be determined.

Appointment Times

It can be very helpful for mental health practitioners to help clients understand that, although it can be difficult, scheduling a definite time for euthanasia is often the most beneficial plan for everyone involved. This is often true because, if clients are reluctant to schedule an appointment time, preferring to leave the time to fate, there are several things that may go wrong, thus making their pet's death feel more like a negative experience. For example, their pet may die alone at home, perhaps with accompanying pain or struggle. Or your client's veterinarian may be out of town, unavailable, or simply unable to respond to your client's needs at the time when they are needed the most. Making an appointment ensures that your client's beloved companion animal will die in the way in which he or she has chosen, with all who wish to be there in attendance.

From a veterinarian's point of view, the ideal times for euthanasia appointments are the least busy parts of their days, such as early morning, over a lunch hour, the last appointment in the afternoon, or even in the evening after normal clinic hours. Regardless of the time chosen, your clients should expect to be given first priority over everything else, except medical emergencies, once they arrive at the clinic. They should also expect to be immediately escorted to wherever the euthanasia will take place.

Location

While most pet owners assume that their pets will be euthanized at their veterinarian's clinic, this isn't necessarily the case within the modern paradigm. Today, many veterinary clinics, especially large specialty or referral practices like university teaching hospitals, offer clients several options for where euthanasia can take place. These options may include a specially appointed "comfort room" or a secluded garden-like area outdoors. Some veterinarians offer to perform euthanasia at a client's home and some are even willing to travel to a pet's favorite place (e.g., a lake, mountain trail, or cabin in the woods).

With the rise of cemeteries and crematories dedicated to pets, a recent trend is toward euthanasias that take place on the cemetery/crematory grounds, followed immediately by a funeral for the pet and then either burial or cremation. Of course, a euthanasia that takes place in a location other than the veterinary clinic requires much more of the veterinarian's time and resources. Therefore, the fees charged for these services are usually higher than the standard costs for an in-clinic euthanasia appointment. As a mental health practitioner, you can help your clients explore which location they prefer, as well as whether or not they can afford to pay for their chosen option.

Procedural Details

Regardless of where and when pet euthanasia occurs, there are several procedural matters that you can help clients deal with beforehand, if possible. For example, most veterinarians require clients to sign a consent form prior to the procedure. Many also require payment before the euthanasia takes place. Some veterinarians allow clients to stop by their clinic and take care of these tasks the day before the procedure. Others may agree to FAX forms back and forth in order to obtain a client's signature and will accept a credit card payment via the telephone. Urge clients to contact their veterinary clinic if making these prior arrangements would be of help to them.

Day-of-Euthanasia Support

Occasionally, pet owners feel the need to plan an elaborate ceremony as part of their pet's euthanasia. For example, some may want a priest or other spiritual guide to give their pet "last rites" immediately following the death or to help their pet "cross the Rainbow Bridge." While some understanding and compassionate veterinarians do their best to accommodate these special requests, most find it too disruptive to their other clinic demands and will discourage such elaborate plans. As a mental health practitioner who is guiding your client toward a realistic view of the euthanasia process, encourage clients to check with their veterinarians to be certain their plans, elaborate or not, can be accommodated.

You can also help clients think about the plans they can put in place for their own support and comfort immediately following their pet's death. For example, will they want someone to drive them home? Will they want to spend time alone or be with family and friends? Will they want to arrange ahead of time to clear their schedule for that day and perhaps take additional days away from work?

Being present at a pet's euthanasia is usually exhausting. Even when clients are well prepared, most still feel the strong, spontaneous effects of grief, like shock and disbelief, once death has occurred. Help your clients think about what items they may want to bring with them to make the time after their pet's euthanasia more comforting and soothing for all involved. These might include bringing a favorite photo to keep with them, a meaningful prayer or poem to read throughout the day, soothing music, or a pet's favorite blanket or toy.

Memorializing

Mental health practitioners are often very helpful to clients who are deciding how they want to honor their pets' memories, as well as how they want to say good-bye to their pets, both prior to and following death. For example, many pet owners decide they want to make one final effort to engage in a favorite activity (hiking, visiting a park) with their pets. Others wish to take photos or make videos of their pets while they're going about their normal day-to-day routines, like sleeping in their favorite spots or eating their usual food. While these activities can be considered a way to memorialize pets, some pet owners want to go further, planning a funeral or ceremony for friends and family who knew the pet or creating a keepsake like a garden stepping stone or clay paw print that's personalized and unique to their pet.

Memorializing helps bring meaning to loss and helps draw closure to relationships (Rando, 1984). Yet, many pet owners don't think about how to memorialize without the expert guidance of a mental health practitioner or veterinarian. There are countless ways to memorialize companion animals. Websites and companies who provide pet memorials are listed in the Resources section of this chapter.

Body Care

It's helpful for mental health practitioners to facilitate decisions about a pet's body care prior to euthanasia because researching the option that is right for them can take time and patience, two qualities most grievers don't have *after* death has occurred. Encourage your clients to make informed decisions about body care by helping them research all of the options that are available to them in your area. This may require them to identify their options, visit pet crematory and/or burial facilities, and talk to their veterinarians to see who and which options their veterinarians recommend. The cost of each option should also be determined.

In most areas of the country, body care options for pets include individual or mass cremation, burial at home (where allowed) or in a pet cemetery, or general disposal (usually via rendering or disposition to a landfill). If your city doesn't have a crematory dedicated to pets, you might help your clients contact one of the human funeral homes in your town to ask if they are willing to handle pet cremations.

What Clients Can Expect to Experience During a Pet's Euthanasia

Most family-present euthanasia procedures are conducted by a team consisting of a veterinarian and a veterinary technician. This allows the technician to focus on the pet owner's emotional needs and the veterinarian to concentrate on the medical aspects of the euthanasia procedure.

If pet owners have elected to be present, the veterinarian may place an intravenous catheter in the rear leg of the animal. Catheters do not always improve the *medical* procedures involved with euthanasia; however, they are often an enhancement to the *emotional* side of euthanasia as they provide extra insurance that the drugs can be administered without the animal flinching or appearing to struggle. The placement of a catheter usually requires removing the animal from the euthanasia site and taking it to a treatment room where a small area of fur is shaved and the catheter is placed in a vein (Butler, Lagoni, Harvey, Withrow, & Durrance, 2001).

After the catheter has been placed and the animal has been returned to the euthanasia site, pet owners are usually given the opportunity to spend a short time alone with their companion animals. When everyone fees it is time to proceed, the veterinarian begins a series of injections, administering them quickly, with little or no lapse of time between them. Every veterinarian uses a slightly different technique and drug protocol, but, in general, the injections may include a saline flush to make sure the catheter is working properly, a barbiturate that helps the pet feel relaxed and induces a soothing plane of anesthesia, and finally, the lethal dose of euthanasia solution, which is commonly an overdose of sodium pentathol (Butler et al., 2001). While the veterinarian is performing the euthanasia, pet owners are usually standing or sitting near their pets, acutely focused on them, and petting or holding them and saying good-bye.

This method of performing euthanasia usually goes so quickly and smoothly that most pet owners don't realize that their pets have actually died. It's important for veterinarians, then, to use a stethoscope to listen for a final heartbeat and pronounce the animal dead. At this time, most owners may gasp, cry, sob, or sigh with relief. They often make remarks about how quickly death came and about how peaceful the experience was. Many owners appreciate the opportunity to talk a bit about their pets and to reminisce about the life that has just come to an end. Pet owners commonly review their pets' lives and share special or funny stories.

After-Death Follow-Up

After euthanasia, some pet owners want to leave the veterinary facility or site quickly, while others need more time alone with their pets. Many pet owners have invested a great deal in the physical and financial care of their companion animals and, even after death, their pets' bodies remain important to them. Sometimes, family members who have not been present at the euthanasia want to view their animal's body before it is buried or cremated. Many grief experts and classic studies agree that viewing a body after death may help people accept and integrate the reality that death has actually occurred (Rando, 1991; Glick, Weiss, & Parkes, 1974).

If clients wish to view a pet's body, mental health practitioners can encourage clients to ask the veterinarian about what they will see and about what will be acceptable for them to do. For example, depending on the situation, they may want to know if their pet's body will feel warm or cold, whether the eyes will be open or closed, and whether or not it is appropriate to touch or even hold their pet's body. They may also want to know about any wounds, bandages, shaved areas, or surgical incisions they may see on their pet's body.

In the case of emergency or sudden death, it's not uncommon for clients to ask a supportive helper (e.g., family friend, mental health practitioner) to accompany them while they view their pet's body. If you are a mental health practitioner who has been asked to accompany your client and provide support, you should lead the way into the viewing room and make the first move toward touching, petting, and talking to the animal. After you have spent some time talking with and listening to your client as you view the pet, ask your clients if they would like some time alone. If the answer is yes, you should leave the room, telling your client how soon you plan to return.

When clients wish to view a pet's body, veterinarians can be asked to position the body so it will be pleasing for them to see. One way this can be achieved is to curl the body slightly inside a casket or box, with the head and limbs tucked into a "sleep-like" position. Positioning bodies is especially important if animals are to be placed into a casket or other container for burial or transport at a later time. This is vitally important if a veterinarian has agreed to keep an animal's body in a cooler until a later time when other family members can view it or pick it up. This is a detail that most veterinarians and pet owners don't think ahead about and in which mental health practitioners like you can play a useful role. You can suggest that your clients either request this type of body placement from their veterinarians or provide a casket or container of some kind so the veterinarian can accommodate this preference.

Grief Following Pet Loss

As you begin to play a more active role in your clients' experiences with pet loss, you may find that most people know very little about coping effectively with grief. In addition, you may find that what your clients do know, or think they know, is generally inaccurate.

Many grief experts have observed that what people say and do during bereavement is based primarily on the myths and misinformation about grief that are passed along in families from generation to generation (James & Cherry, 1988). One of the most prominent of these myths is the belief that the "best" way to handle loss is to stay strong and composed while grieving. Another is the belief that staying busy and keeping one's mind off thoughts of the loss is the "best" way to feel better and to recover more quickly. However, research and clinical experience suggest that these methods can actually prolong the grieving process and, in some cases, may even cause grief to become complicated or pathological (Rando, 1993). In order to avoid reinforcing the myths and misinformation, then, it's important for you, as a skilled mental health practitioner, to become knowledgeable about the normal, healthy grieving process, as well as the grief support techniques that have been shown to be most helpful to pet owners. There are many credible books on the market about loss and grief and, more specifically, about pet loss and grief that discuss these techniques. Some suggested titles can be found in the Resource section of this chapter.

In general, clinical experience (Lagoni et al., 1994) has shown that it's most helpful for mental health practitioners to:

- *Contact your client* following a pet's death with a telephone call, condolence card, or both. You might also make note of the date and remember the one-year anniversary with a second card or note.
- *Avoid using euphemisms* like "put to sleep" during follow-up consultations. Using words like "died" and "dead" help clients accept the reality of loss.
- *Listen to your client's story.* It's rare for pet owners to find anyone who is willing to listen to the entire saga of their pet's diagnosis, treatment, and death. Doing so provides a chance for you to normalize your clients' experience with grief and reassure them about their decision to euthanize.
- *Facilitate any follow-up conversations* your client may need to have with a veterinarian, crematory, etc., in order to reconcile any misunderstandings or to clarify any questions that may be nagging at them and preventing them from moving through grief in a healthy manner.

- *Assess which clients may be more at-risk* for abnormal or complicated grief reactions (McCutcheon & Fleming, 2001) and *refer them to other mental health practitioners or grief support resources*, like pet loss support groups in your area, as appropriate.

As a trusted mental health practitioner, you should also refrain from suggesting that your clients simply "move on" and adopt another pet. While this often seems like the obvious solution to a client's feelings of loneliness and grief, adopting a new pet too soon can interfere with the healing process of grieving and create complications in terms of the bonding process. It can also be viewed as trivializing the value and worth of a pet who has recently died.

Conclusion

Obviously, the family-present euthanasia procedures and support protocols discussed in this chapter represent the ideal. However, with forethought, organization, and interdisciplinary team cooperation and coordination, it *is* possible to implement them.

During conversations with your clients, it's important to remember that the veterinarian who will ultimately perform your client's pet's euthanasia *must* be consulted about any specific plans or requests your client may have, as there are sometimes circumstances that call for modifications. For example, veterinarians often have difficulties placing a catheter in the veins of very old or ill cats. Veterinarians may also have cases where clients themselves have special needs or have animals that are considered to be nontraditional pets. Large animals, like horses and llamas, require some special preparation and techniques, yet clients are often given the option of being present at euthanasia.

When family-present euthanasia is well planned and sensitively conducted, it can engender tremendous loyalty and gratitude for the veterinarians and mental health practitioners who helped clients prepare and cope. When clients make informed choices, have their emotional needs met, and witness their pets' deaths, while feeling supported by people who love and care about them, they can be emotionally at peace with an otherwise sad and painful experience.

General Sources About Providing Pet Loss Support

Barton Ross, C., & Baron-Sorensen, J. (2007). *Pet loss and human emotion: A guide to recovery*. New York: Routledge.

Carmack, B. J. (2003). *Grieving the death of a pet*. Minneapolis, MN: Augsburg Fortress.

Cornell, K. K., Brandt, J. C., & Bonvicini, K. A. (Eds.) (2007, January) *Veterinary clinics of North America: Effective communication in veterinary practice* (Vol. 37, No. 1). Philadelphia: W. B. Saunders Co.

Durrance, D., & Lagoni, L. (2010). *Connecting with clients: Practical communication for 10 common situations*. Lakewood, CO: AAHA Press.

Gage, M.G., & Holcomb, R. (1991). Couples' perception of stressfulness of death of the family pet. *Family Relations, 40*, 103–106.

Lagoni, L. (1997). *The practical guide to client grief: Support techniques for 15 common situations*. Lakewood, CO: AAHA Press.

Lagoni, L., Butler, C., & Hetts, S. (1994). *The human–animal bond and grief*. Philadelphia: W.B. Saunders Co.

Nakaya, S. F. (2005*). Kindred spirit, kindred care: Making health decisions on behalf of our animal companions*. Novato, CA: New World Library.

Odendaal, J. (2002). *Pets and our mental health: The why, the what, and the how*. New York: Vantage Press.

Sife, W. (1998). *The loss of a pet: A guide to coping with the grieving process when a pet dies*. New York: Macmillan Publishing.

Books About Providing Pet Loss Support for Helping Professionals

Barton Ross, C., & Baron-Sorensen, J. (2007). *Pet loss and human emotion: A guide to recovery* (2nd Ed.). New York: Routledge.

Carmack, B. J. (2003). *Grieving the death of a pet*. Minneapolis, MN: Augsburg Fortress.

Cornell, K. K., Brandt, J. C., Bonvicini, K. A. (Eds.). (2007, January). *Veterinary clinics of North America: Effective communication in veterinary practice* (Vol. 37, No. 1). Philadelphia: W. B. Saunders Co.

Durrance, D., & Lagoni, L. (2010). *Connecting with clients: Practical communication for 10 common situations* (2nd Ed.). Lakewood, CO: AAHA Press.

Lagoni, L. (1997). *The practical guide to client grief: Support techniques for 15 common situations*. Lakewood, CO: AAHA Press.

Lagoni, L., Butler, C., & Hetts, S. (1994). *The human–animal bond and grief*. Philadelphia: W.B. Saunders Co.

Odendaal, J. (2002). *Pets and our mental health: The why, the what, and the how*. New York: Vantage Press.

References

Ball, J. F. (1977). Widows grief: The impact of age and mode of death. *Omega, 7*, 307–333.

Barton Ross, C., & Baron-Sorensen, J. (2007). *Pet loss and human emotion: A guide to recovery*. New York: Routledge.

Bishop, G. A., Long, C. C., Carlsten, K. S., Kennedy, K. C., & Shaw, J. (2008). The Colorado State University pet hospice program: End-of-life care for pets and their families. *Journal of Veterinary Medical Education, 35*, 525–531.

Brown, J. P., & Silverman, J. D. (1999). The current and future market for veterinarians and veterinary medical services in the United States: Executive summary. *Journal of American Veterinary
Medical Association, 215*(2), 161–183.

Butler, C., Lagoni, L., Harvey, A., Withrow, S., & Durrance, D. (2001). A bond-centered approach
to diagnoses, treatment and euthanasia. In S. Withrow & G. MacEwen (Eds.), *Small animal
clinical oncology*. Philadelphia: W.B. Saunders.

Carmack, B. J. (2003). *Grieving the death of a pet*. Minneapolis, MN: Augsburg Fortress.

Cowles, K. U. (1985). The death of a pet: Human response to the breaking of the bond. In
M. B. Sussman (Ed.), *Pets in the family* (pp. 135–148). New York: Haworth.

Fogle, B. (1981). Attachment-euthanasia-grieving. In B. Fogle (Ed.), *Interrelations between people
and pets* (pp. 331–343). Springfield, IL: Charles C. Thomas.

Fogle, B., & Abrahamson, D. (1990). Pet loss: A survey of the attitudes and feelings of practicing
veterinarians. *Anthrozoos, 3*, 143–150.

Gage, M. G., & Holcomb, R. (1991). Couples' perception of stressfulness of death of the family
pet. *Family Relations, 40*, 103–106.

Garcia, E. (1986). Pet loss considered from the veterinary perspective. *The Latham Letter, 7*(2),
10–13.

Gershon, D., & Straub, G. (1989). *Empowerment: The art of creating your life as you want it*.
New York: Dell Publishing.

Glick, I. O., Weiss, R. S., & Parkes, C. M. (1974). *The first year of bereavement*. New York: Wiley.

Gosse, B. H., & Barnes, M. B. (1994). Human grief resulting from the death of a pet. *Anthrozoos,
7*, 103–112.

Hart, L. A., & Hart, B. L. (1987). Grief and stress from so many animal deaths. *Companion Animal
Practice, 1*, 20–21.

Hart, L. A., Hart, B. L., & Mader, B. (1990). Humane euthanasia and companion animal death:
Caring for the animal, the client and the veterinarian. *Journal of the American Veterinary
Medical Association, 197*, 1292–1299.

Harvey, A., Butler, C., & Lagoni, L. (1999). Children and Pet Loss, Part I, Kids Grieve, Too.
Veterinary Technician, 20(5), 283–286

James, J. W., & Cherry, F. (1988). *The grief recovery handbook: A step-by-step program for moving
beyond loss*. New York: Harper & Row.

Kellehear, A., & Fook, J. (1997). Lassie come home: A study of "lost pet" notices. *Omega, 34*,
191–202.

Kowalski, G. (2006). *Goodbye friend: Healing wisdom for anyone who has ever lost a pet*. Novato,
CA: New World Library.

Lagoni, L., Butler, C., & Hetts, S. (1994). *The human–animal bond and grief*. Philadelphia: W.B.
Saunders.

McCutcheon, K. A., & Fleming, S. J. (2001). Grief resulting from euthanasia and natural death of
companion animals. *Omega, 44*, 169–188.

Nakaya, S. F. (2005). *Kindred spirit, kindred care: Making health decisions on behalf of our animal
companions*. Novato, CA: New World Library.

Parkes, C. M. (1975). Unexpected and untimely bereavement: A statistical study of young Boston
widows and widowers. In B. Schoenberg, I. Gerber, A. Wiener, D. Kutscher, D. Peretz, &
A. Cam (Eds.), *Bereavement and it's psychological aspects*. New York: Columbia University
Press.

Planchon, L. A., & Templer, D. I. (1996). *The correlates of grief after death of pet. Anthrozoos, 9*,
107–113.

Planchon, L. A., Templer, D. I., Stokes, S., & Keller, J. (2002). Death of a companion cat or dog
and human bereavement: Psychosocial variables. *Society & Animals, 10*, 93–105.

Rando, T. A. (1984). *Grief, dying, and death: Clinical interventions for caregivers*. Champagne,
IL: Research Press Company.

Rando, T. A. (1991). *How to go on living when someone you love dies*. New York: Bantom.

Rando, T. A. (1993). *Treatment of complicated mourning*. Champagne, IL: Research Press.

Sife, W. (1998). *The loss of a pet: A guide to coping with the grieving process when a pet dies.* New York: Howell Book House.

Toray, T. (2004). The human–animal bond and loss: Providing support for grieving clients. *Journal of Mental Health Counseling, 26,* 244–259.

Vaughan, D. (2004). Home euthanasia a valuable service. Veterinary Practice News (online). Retrieved July 10, 2010, from http://www.veterinarypracticenews.com

Weisman, A. D. (1991). Bereavement and companion animals. *Omega, 22,* 241–248.

Worden, W. J. (2008). *Grief counseling and grief therapy: A handbook for the mental health practitioner.* New York: Springer Publishing Company, Inc.

Resources

Cards, Memorials, Counselors and Information

World by the Tail, Inc.
"caring for people who care for pets"
126 West Harvard Street, Suite 5
Fort Collins, CO 80525
1-888-271-8444
info@wbtt.com
www.veterinarywisdomforpetparents.com

> Up-to-date referrals, resources, consultation, and products for pet parents and mental health professionals who provide pet loss support.
> VeterinaryWisdom® Support Center
> Free instant downloads about pet loss
> Dana Durrance, M.A., veterinary grief counselor
> Condolence cards
> ClayPaws® paw print kits and other pet tribute products

Argus Institute
Colorado State University
James L. Voss Veterinary Teaching Hospital
300 West Drake, Fort Collins, CO 80525
1-970-297-4143
argus@colostate.edu
www.argusinstitute.colostate.edu/whatnow.htm

> What Now booklet for grieving pet owners
> Clinical Service providing client grief support
> Pet Hospice Program

Marty Touseley, certified hospice bereavement counselor
www.griefhealing.com

> Supportive information and "A Different Grief: Coping with Pet Loss", a 24-lesson e-course for pet parents who've lost a pet. Supplemental material for supporting grieving children is also available.

Center for Loss and Life Transition
www./centerforloss.com

> When Your Pet Dies: *A Guide to Mourning, Remembering, and Healing* by be-
> reavement expert Dr. Alan Wolfelt

Pet Loss/Grief Support & Training

Argus Institute
Colorado State University
James L. Voss Veterinary Teaching Hospital
300 West Drake, Fort Collins, CO 80525
1-970-297-4143
argus@colostate.edu
www.argusinstitute.colostate.edu

> Veterinary communication/grief support curriculum and trainings
> FRANK: Veterinarian-Client Communication Initiative (workshops and trainings
> with CE credits available)

World by the Tail, Inc.
"caring for people who care for pets"
126 West Harvard Street, Suite 5
Fort Collins, CO 80525
1-888-271-8444
info@wbtt.com
www.veterinarywisdom.com

> Up-to-date referrals, resources, consultation, and products for pet parents and
> veterinary professionals who provide pet loss support.
> VeterinaryWisdom® Resource Center
> Dana Durrance, M.A., veterinary grief specialist and practice consultant

Association for Pet Loss and Bereavement (APLB)
www.aplb.org

> National organization providing training and "certification" for pet loss support
> counselors. The Association's website offers information, counselor referrals,
> and online forums/support for pet owners.

Center for Loss and Life Transition
www./centerforloss.com

> Directed by bereavement expert Dr. Alan Wolfelt, the center offers a "Pet Loss
> Companioning" Certification Program, as well as books and information about
> pet loss.

Canadian Centre for Pet Loss Bereavement
www.petlosssupport.ca

A national free public service website offering support, information, and training in pet loss counseling.

Institute for Healthcare Communication, Inc.
555 Long Wharf Drive, 13th Floor
New Haven, CT 06511-5901
Ph: 800-800-5907 or 203-772-8280
FAX: 203-772-1066
Email: info@healthcarecomm.org
www.healthcarecomm.org

A nationally accredited, not-for-profit organization that trains physicians and, in recent years veterinarians, throughout North America in effective communication skills. The veterinary communication training initiative is funded by a grant from Bayer Animal Health.

Association for Death Education and Counseling (ADEC)
111 Dear Lake Road, Suite 100
Deerfield, IL 60015
847-509-0403
www.adec.org

A national membership association providing certification and distance learning programs, as well as resources, information, and an annual conference.

Professional Veterinary Organizations that Address Pet Loss Issues

American Veterinary Medicine Association (AVMA)
ww.avma.org (search pet loss)

Written Guidelines for Pet Loss Support Services and Veterinary Hospice Programs Brochures about Pet and Equine Euthanasia

American Animal Hospital Association (AAHA)
www.aaha.org

Training materials for veterinary professionals and books/pamphlets for veterinary clients

American Association for Human–Animal Bond Veterinarians (AAH-ABV)
http://aah-abv.org/net/home
(for membership and contact information)

Provides education, research, and support to enhance veterinarians' ability to create positive and ethical relationships among people, animals, and their environments.

Association for Veterinary Family Practice (AVFP)
www.avfp.org
(for membership and contact information)

Offers online and on-site (UC-Davis) coursework in the emerging specialty of Veterinary Family Practice. Topics include pets in families and society and the clinical skills needed to care for both patients and clients.

International Association for Animal Hospice and Palliative Care (IAAHPC)
620 W. Webster Avenue
Chicago, IL 60614
www.iaahpc.org

An interdisciplinary organization dedicated to promoting comfort-oriented nursing and medical for companion animals as they near the end of their lives and as they die.

International Conference on Communication in Veterinary Medicine (ICCVM)
www.iccvm.com
iccvm@bayleygroup.com
(for registration and conference information)

The purpose of this conference is to promote the development of veterinary communication research and education

International Society for Anthrozoology (ISAZ)
www.isaz.net
(for membership and contact information)

Promotes the scientific and scholarly study of human–animal interactions. Also publishes the Anthrozoos journal and offers professional meetings and conferences worldwide.

Delta Society: *the human–animal health connection*
www.deltasociety.org
(for membership and contact information)

Improves human health through service and therapy animals

Chapter 12
Life After Loss: Psychodynamic Perspectives on a Continuing Bonds Approach with "Pet Companion"

Christopher Blazina

Life After Loss: Psychodynamic Perspectives on a Continuing Bonds Approach with Pet Companions

As evident in the chapters that make up this anthology, there has been an evolving perspective in the field of mental health regarding pet loss as a significant clinical matter. Attachment and loss issues related to a pet companion seem to have gained greater awareness, if not acceptance, in some parts of society, based on the recent volume of journal articles, book chapters, and books written for a professional audience. In order to provide the best therapeutic care, various clinical and research approaches may be reexamined in light of those working with pet-related issues.

One goal of this chapter is to review theories that we will place under the broad category of psychodynamic/psychoanalytic theory (e.g., ego psychology, attachment theory, self-psychology). A psychodynamic perspective is argued to be pertinent for understanding the significance of the human–animal bond. In particular, how grief work may lead to achieving an ongoing bond with the pet companion that has passed. Research suggests that a high percentage of owners endorse an amicable, if not familial, sentiment toward pets. In research studies, between 87 and 99% of pet owners defined their pets as being *like a friend or family member* (Cain, 1983; Voith, 1985). Given that there may be a deep sense of attachment, one may also expect one's grief upon loss of a pet to be substantial (Field, Orsini, Gavish, & Packman, 2009). When losing a pet, the intensity and duration of some pet owners' mourning mirrors or even surpasses the grief experienced when losing a human companion (Gosse & Barnes, 1994; Planchon & Templer, 1996; Quackenbush, 1982; Wrobel & Dye, 2003). Therefore, theoretical consideration for attachment and loss regarding a pet companion is of clinical importance.

The chapter's examination includes the recent shift from the earlier Freudian (1917) grief work assumptions emphasizing detachment and withdrawal to that of

C. Blazina (✉)
Department of Psychology, Tennessee State University, Nashville, TN 37209, USA
e-mail: christex01@msn.com

C. Blazina et al. (eds.), *The Psychology of the Human–Animal Bond*,
DOI 10.1007/978-1-4419-9761-6_12, © Springer Science+Business Media, LLC 2011

more contemporary focus, centering upon continuity with the lost loved one. The argument posed is that a *continuing bonds* approach will be most effective in dealing with various losses, including those involving a pet companion. The phrase *continuing bonds* was coined by Klass, Silverman, and Nickman (1996) stressing that the importance of an ongoing relationship with the deceased is a normative part of bereavement. While others in the psychoanalytic field have emphasized the importance of continuity in the process of bereavement (e.g., Bowlby, 1969/1982, 1980; Gaines, 1997; Hagman, 1995, 2001; Kaplan, 1995; Parkes, 1970, 2009; Parkes & Weiss, 1983), the phrase *continuing bonds is* utilized as the umbrella term for various works consistent with the current bereavement literature (see Field, Orsini, Gavish, & Packman, 2009). When possible, themes of the current bereavement literature are interfaced with psychodynamic perspectives in order to inform research and practice.

Finally, it is also argued in this chapter that clinical implications derived from psychodynamic theory will be of assistance in forming a continuing bond with a pet companion, thereby allowing the connection established in life to be sustained in a meaningful way after the pet's passing. To date, only one empirical study has been conducted, considering the significance of continuity and the loss of pet companions (Field, Gao, & Paderna, 2005; Field, Orsini, Gavish, & Packman, 2009). Field et al. suggested that forming a continued bond represented an adaptive component of grief. Within the clinical realm, there is strong relevance for utilizing a continuing bonds approach concerning pet loss, but this topic has largely remained unexplored. In this chapter, pertinent clinical implications are addressed that include a pet companion as a *significant object*, internalization and integration of the pet object, and the import role of context in research and clinical work. Each topic has direct application for the grieving client's ability to sustain a sense of continuing bonds with a pet companion.

The Standard Psychoanalytic Model of Mourning

Hagman (1995, 2001) suggested that the *standard psychoanalytic model of mourning* has until recently still been defined by Freud's 1917 work "Mourning and Melancholia" and a relatively few other of his writings. Some have suggested (Furman, 1974) that Freud's intention was not to set up a formal model of mourning; though, for almost a century, many have taken aspects of his writing to guide how we view grieving. Freud's writings are influenced by the drive theory (1920), which emphasizes homeostasis and a return to psychic equilibrium when we are disrupted by a significant loss. Successful bereaved from this perspective entails reviewing one's relationship with the loved one, and then subsequently discharging related feelings associated with loss, allowing the bereaved to withdraw psychic investment in the lost love object one memory at a time. It is through the painful process of decathexis (detachment) that one attempts to return to a premorbid level of functioning. With this type of approach grief work mourning is completed when all ties to the loved one have been severed, homeostasis has been restored, and there is the possibility of loving another.

Later in 1926, Freud wrote in "Inhibition, Symptoms, and Anxiety" of the extreme painfulness that accompanies mourning, and now this reaction is also placed within the context of the psychic economy that pushes for a return to homeostasis. Again, there is a press for preloss functioning, as one attempts to discharge feelings onto the now-departed target. Since the departed is no longer available, one makes these attempts with no real avail. In order for one to find relief, Freud argues, one must find a substitute target(s) on which to redirect these reactions. The substitute target is often the surviving members upon whom the lost other's memories can be pressed. According to the hydraulic nature of Freudian emotion, including dealing with grief, the mourner can utilize the proxy in order to release pent-up feelings as well as revive the memory of the lost loved one.

In Freud's other significant contribution on the topic, he suggests in "The Ego and the Id" (1923/1960) the possibility of identification as a method for grief resolution: "It may be that this identification is the sole condition under which the Id can give up its object" (p. 425). Abraham (1927/1960) would also build upon these thoughts, suggesting that the lost loved one is temporarily drawn (introjected) into the psyche, "Its main purpose to preserve the person's relation with the lost object" (p. 435) until grief subsides.

From the perspective of the standard model, forms of identification that lingered too long were seen as representing still-unresolved grief work and/or the subsequent use of defenses that might lead to melancholia or depression (Gaines, 1997). Helene Deutsch's 1937 article "Absence of Greif" expresses how "... the process of mourning must be carried to its completion... the attachments are unresolved as long as the affective process of mourning has not been accomplished" (pp. 16–17). Her contribution adds to the standard model by emphasizing the importance of the expression of grief symptoms to loosen the bond; to not do so is the hallmark of pathological or complicated bereavement.

The continuing importance of the role of detachment is seen in more contemporary times. In *Psychoanalytic Terms and Concepts* (Moore & Fine, 1991), object loss in the external world is equated with ego loss in the internal world, making the task of grief work to mend the psyche through slowly giving up the temporarily internalized representation of the other. "Mourning is... the mental process by which man's psychic equilibrium is restored following the loss of a meaningful love object..." The work of mourning includes three successive, interrelated phases... (1) Understanding, accepting and coping with the loss... (2) The mourning proper which involves withdrawal of attachment to and identification with the lost object... (3) Resumption of emotional life in harmony with one's level of maturity, which frequently involves establishing new relationships (Moore & Fine, 1991, p. 122).

While the standard psychoanalytic model places an emphasis upon detachment and the eventual relinquishment of the lost love object, other theories within the psychodynamic/psychoanalytic tradition place an emphasis upon continuity. Attachment theory, object relations, and self-psychology all highlight ways of maintaining and/or reestablishing a new tie with the deceased (Baker, 2001; Hagman, 1995). The continued bond is not viewed in pathological terms, but rather a part of the normative grief work leading to various forms of intrapsychic repair, or even, transformation. From a psychodynamic perspective, one may internalize the lost object, identify with some aspects of him or her, and even incorporate some former role the loved one played as a self-object. Issues of attachment then loss related to each theory will be reviewed in the following sections.

Continuity in Psychodynamic Theory: Attachment Theory

Bowlby (1969/1982, 1980) suggested that, much like our nonhuman counterparts, humans are biologically predisposed toward making connections with others, especially the caregiver. Attachment is sought for its own sake, irrespective of potential positive gratification (counter to Freud's (1920) drive theory model outlined in *Beyond the Pleasure Principle*). The *attachment figure* represents someone to whom we have formed an emotional and psychological bond and who is integral in supplying certain basic psychological experiences such as a *safe haven* to return to in times of distress and *safe base,* the means to explore the world (Bowlby, 1969/1982, 1980). Confirmation for the establishment of the bond, and the subsequent transformation into an attachment figure, is also seen through *proximity seeking*, and then, distress at being apart. Bowlby (1969/1982, 1980) argued it is the attachment bond formed in infancy that provides the foundation and template for relating to the world to others and will guide relationship behavior throughout life.

From the attachment bond, one begins to develop an *internal working model* with a more systemized view of how one perceives self, others, and the world (Bowlby, 1969/1982, 1980). The working model forms the foundation for expectations of relationships throughout adolescence and into adulthood. It is a set of rules guiding thoughts, actions, and feelings in the relational context. That is, the individual will begin forming expectations for the way others will treat them, especially significant others (Ainsworth, 1979; Bartholomew & Horowitz, 1991; Hazan & Shaver, 1987). The prospect of regarding self and others shape the structure of one's *Attachment style*: the predominate style of relating. Attachment styles are formed in infancy and operate throughout the life span with consistency, unless altered by other relationships and life occurrences such as unresolved loss, trauma, and striving for secure attachments (Bowlby, 1969/1982, 1980).

There are several unique perspectives that shed light on attachment theory; each proposes various ways to classify attachment styles, strategies, or defenses (e.g., Ainsworth, 1979; Bartholomew & Horowitz, 1991; Bowlby, 1969/1982; Fonagy, 2001; Hazan & Shaver, 1987; Main, 2000; Main, & Solomon, 1986; Mikulincer & Shaver, 2003; Mikulincer & Shaver, 2007; Wallin, 2007). A comprehensive review is beyond the scope of this chapter. However, the field focused initially upon categories of attachment and then, later, also included a continuum of attachment styles emphasizing how each individual has his or her own unique configuration based upon avoidance and anxiety. The terms *secure, anxious,* and *avoidant styles* are used in this chapter, though it is acknowledged other terms are used by theorists and researchers in their investigations. An individual may look at the self and others in a positive or negative way; he or she will believe the world is safe and consistent (secure attachment style), unpredictable in terms of safety (anxious attachment style), or potentially dangerous (avoidant attachment style).

The utilization of defense mechanisms is also incorporated into the internal working model and attachment style (Ainsworth, 1979; Bartholomew & Horowitz, 1991; Main, 2000; Main, & Solomon, 1986; Wallin, 2007). While the primary need is to connect, as a defense, the infant simultaneously may learn to prepare himself/herself for rejection. For example, the dismissing behavior of avoidant child is a defensive maneuver developed to avoid the pain of experiencing rejection for seeking proximity and attention from the caregiver when the infant is in distress. As with any attachment figure, separations and reunions carry the potential to evoke one's style of attaching. Avoidant attachment style has become particularly skilled at masking the stress of the events. In this case, the child shows an almost blasé attitude toward the caregivers' whereabouts when apart and likewise upon reuniting. This may appear outwardly as having a strong sense of self-confidence; however, the child has actually learned to disguise vulnerability and presentation of distress in order to preserve a tie with the caregiver (Ainsworth, 1979; Bartholomew & Horowitz, 1991; Bowlby, 1969/1982, 1980; Wallin, 2007). The stoic appearance is a defense mechanism. By denying their need for close relationships, avoidances circumvent the attachment behaviors during infancy that led to rejection, anxiety, and negative consequences. The child learns to use repression and compartmentalization in relation to needs experienced and expressed.

The anxious attachment–styled child experiences an inconsistent style of parenting, which leads to difficult separations from his or her caregiver, characterized by protest and despair (Ainsworth, 1979; Bartholomew & Horowitz, 1991; Bowlby, 1969/1982, 1980; Wallin, 2007). The child develops the defensive style of becoming preoccupied with the caregiver's whereabouts, allowing for an illusionary internal sense of control over the inconsistency of care. Reunions are often marred by angry feelings that are not easily soothed, perceiving separation as potential abandonment. As we will see, attachment styles guide forming bonds, as well as, the difficulty in sustaining them after a loss has occurred.

The best possibility is when we have experienced basic features of attachment with caregivers (and other attachment figures), which allows a secure style of relating to emerge (Ainsworth, 1979; Bartholomew & Horowitz, 1991; Bowlby, 1969/1982, 1980; Wallin, 2007). *The secure attachment style* is thought to develop within the context of a relationship with a caregiver that is characterized by an ability to read the child's responses and, then, respond in sync with them. The long-term impact of a responsive, warm caregiving relationship is that it allows the child's internal working model to develop a faith in one's own worthiness and others' trustworthiness. We do not feel that attachment figures will abandon us in our hour of need nor do we have to take on the persona of total self-sufficiency, fearing others may get too close and then later exploit this very private information. With these more secure assumptions in place, one is allowed to more easily access our own inner worlds, as well as journey comfortably into the experience of others.

Attachment Theory: Phases of Grief and Searching after Loss

Bowlby and Parkes (1970) suggested that a series of phases regarding grief. The phases of grief consist of (a) numbness, (b) yearning and searching, (c) disorganization and despair, and (d) reorganization. Bowlby suggested that each phase had its own distinctiveness. Numbness was the initial shocked state of being after the loss. Helping cushion the blow is the numb sensation, without which, we might be overwhelmed. *Yearning and searching* phase was characterized by acute distress that follows a loss and can be expressed through crying loudly, anger, anxiety, and the investigation of sights and sounds that may announce the return of the lost loved one. Bowlby concludes that this phase is about trying to protest loud and long enough in hopes of reestablishing a connection with the lost one. The next phase involves d*isorganization and despair,* which is a form of helplessness that nothing can be done to ignite a reunion with the lost loved one. Disorganization occurs as the result of life feeling out of sorts and unrecognizable without the presence of the one that has been lost. Being in the disorganized phase can affect eating, sleeping, and play. The world feels poorer for the loss, and aspects of living that used to give us pleasure, now do not. Finally, in the *reorganization* phase, one comes to terms with the reality of the loss and forms a new type of connection with the lost loved one, thus preserving the bond.

If we follow the observations of Bowlby and Parkes (1970) concerning the loss of someone to whom we have become attached, there are a few points to be noted in terms of *searching*. Searching is a key concept as it emphasizes the hope for continuation of the relationship with the departed (Bowlby, 1980; Parkes, 1970, 1986, 2009; Parkes & Weiss, 1983). The individual is of two minds shortly after a loss occurs. One part attempts to accept that the circumstances are real but painful, while the other protests the loss. Anger and frustration push the person forward through perceived and real barriers that keep one apart from the lost attachment figure. While some consciously pursue the loved one, others attempt to stifle the search. Even in these situations, one can track the lost loved one in unconscious or disguised ways. In either case, therein begins a restless search for signs indicating the hoped-for appearance of the significant other. Parkes (1986) argues that the mourner constructs a "perceptual set" or mental map based upon familiar places, sights, and sounds related to the loved one. By following the map and attending to its clues, we think perhaps this will eventually lead to a reunion. To facilitate a rejoining, we search for hints in the well-known places in the outer world. The trouble is one can become focused upon the signs pertaining to the lost loved often to the exclusion of other indicators that state the search will not lead to the hoped-for results.

Attachment Style and Grief

We can shed light upon process of individual grief patterns by interfacing the *searching* component that was just reviewed (Bowbly & Parkes, 1970; Parkes, 1986) with consideration for particular attachment styles. The internal working model supplies instructions for sustaining bonds as well as dealing with separations (both temporary and permanent) (Field & Sundin, 2001; Parkes, 2009; Parkes & Weiss, 2003; Stroebe, Schut, & Stroebe, 2005). In the day-to-day encounters, old defensive styles of relating (or nonrelating) are called upon to guide, even protect, us in the course of normal separations and reunions. However, there is a bigger challenge when the loss of a loved one is permanent. A permanent loss represents the ultimate frustration. Under the conditions of loss, old directions for handling pain related to frustration and separation have the potential for getting reactivated for each of the attachment styles.

Avoidant individuals will try to push the pain away, staying busy and trying not to let the loss land on them (Bowlby, 1980; Parkes, 2009). In many cases, they verbalize to themselves or others that the best way to grieve is to just "move on." However, even with this approach there is often a breaking point of stress where avoidant styles give way temporarily to moments of vulnerability that can be surprising both to the person and to those around them. Avoidant styles can result in a grief reaction sometimes long after the actual loss. Because there may be some need to initially distance from the pain, avoidant style people may more readily show their grief through somatic sensations, that is, they have body aches and pains. This becomes their method for disguising and expressing loss. Whereas avoidant styles try to keep focused on anything but the loss, ambivalent styles are often characterized by becoming preoccupied with the lost loved one (Bowlby, 1980; Parkes, 2009). They let others know in their words and actions that they are pining, that it hurts, and that their sole focus is the departed. The searching for the lost loved one discussed previously is actively dialed up for some ambivalent styled persons. This is the continuation of the style of attachment they learned but now being applied to dealing with loss. Part of the way they have learned to ward off anxiety related to abandonment is keeping the loved one front and center in their mind. When the other to whom they have become so devoted moves off the center stage of awareness, ambivalent styles may protest, sometimes loudly. For ambivalent styles, grief reactions can also be prolonged and complicated. Ambivalent-styled person maintain a tunnel vision regarding the lost loved one. The loss may dominate their thoughts, feelings, and interactions with others. They may rarely take a break from this aspect of mourning. At one level, they may hope that if the protest is intense enough they can magically evoke the powers to bring the loved one back. Secure attachment style may fare better than the rest in cases of attachment and loss, but they too go through the normal process of grief (Bowlby, 1980; Parkes, 2009). After all, loss is a universal experience in terms of its difficulties. Where the secure style is at an advantage is having more positive experiences and psychological resources at hand when facing loss. Ironically though, they may be at a disadvantage in not having to experience the levels of chronic frustration the insecure attachment styles have. Dealing with the ultimate disappointment such as the permanent loss of a loved one can be a new experience, one for which the secure type may initially find themselves not fully equipped. Their internal working model has told them that others will respond and be in sync with their needs. In this case, the loved one is not able to do this. The secure style is challenged to stretch and grow in the area of frustration tolerance while maintaining some of their overall positive outlook toward the world.

Attachment Theory and Pet Loss

In this section, concepts from the attachment theory emphasizing continuity are applied to pet loss. Bowlby's (1969/1982, 1980) attachment theory has supplied the theoretical underpinnings for pets' importance in much of the current research literature (Sharkin & Knox, 2003). Bowlby's theory has provided a heuristic to examine both the attachment bond between owner and pet companion (e.g., safe base, safe haven, proximity seeking) and the resulting experience of grief after loss has occurred. Kobak (2009) suggests pet companions, specifically a dog, can serve as an attachment figure, though special attention needs to be given to further define the nature of attachment across the life span with both people and pets. Kurdek (2008, 2009) argued that pet companions can meet various attachment figure criteria. Kurdek (2008) had college students compare their sense of attachment with their pets to that of their mother, father, siblings, friends, and significant others. For instance, secure base was the most salient feature for mothers, fathers, and friends. Secure base and proximity seeking were the most important attachment features for siblings, and for significant others, all four characteristics attachment figure criteria (i.e., secure base, proximity seeking, separation distress, and safe haven) were equally important. The most important of the four attachment features for dog owners was the secure base and the proximity maintenance; that is, they enjoyed having their dogs near them and saw them as a dependable source of comfort that aided in exploring the world. Other studies report inconclusive results when comparing pet and human companions in terms of attachment-related issues. Kurdek (2010) found in his sample of adult subjects that they were less securely attached to dog companions than to people. While Beck and Madresh (2008) found that subjects reported more secure attachment to their pets than to romantic partners and family members. Field et al. (2009) suggested that the strength of attachment to one's pet companion, not the security of the bond, was the most influential factor when predicting intensity of grieving for a pet. While the area of attachment is in need of further research to give clarification upon these matters, we can still derive clinical implications from the manner in which attachment and pet companions intersect.

As with other attachment figures that have been lost, clinicians should be aware of the client's potential searching behavior for their pet companion. Cowles (1985) found that searching behavior was common after the death of a pet companion. The clinician should then be aware of *how* the client searches based upon one's attachment style. Within the attachment theory paradigm, one may consider how one's attachment style impacts one perception on pet loss (Field et al., 2009). Following the familiar attachment and loss patterns reviewed above, clinicians will want to be aware that avoidant styles may have more difficulty engaging the emotional aspects of grief. They may instead, manifest their symptoms in the form of somatic complaints such as pain, chest aches, and so on. Anxiously styled persons may pine for the lost one in intense and often uninterrupted ways. The secure style, while faring better, may struggle with a new type of developmental challenge of not having the lost one be attuned to his or her needs. In terms of comparing the three styles, the ambivalent styles may show the most outward signs of searching, the avoidant ones to show the least, and the secure to be somewhere in the middle. In trying to understand the bereavement reactions, regardless of attachment style, pet owners feel the pain of loss and press for reunion.

Self-Psychology

From a self-psychology perspective, a self-object is a quintessential other that provides emotional and psychological resources for enhancing one's sense of well-being. For some, the resource (i.e., self-object) meets desired, if not essential, psychological needs. Kohut (1971) suggested that the psychological function of a "self-object" is to supply certain psychological needs one has yet to master obtaining for oneself. The self-object can appear in various forms and supply a variety of psychic needs, not all of them regressive in nature. These can include soothing in moments of distress, mirroring one's accomplishments, and acknowledging one's lovability. Kohut (1984) emphasized the lifelong need for self-objects as the individual can neither thrive nor survive without them. Kohut's self-psychology focus emphasizes the function this important other plays. When one loses the object associated with one's ideal psychological state of well-being, that is, the supplier of certain emotional needs, the psychic pipeline of essential resources is severed. The result can be a sense of loss for both the object itself and the needs that were being fulfilled.

In terms of dealing with the loss of a self-object, Hagman (1995, 2001) utilized Kohut's (1971) notion of *transmuting internalization,* in which the self-object function is gradually incorporated. Kohut (1971) proposed the concept of *optimal frustration* in which the individual internalizes the essential function of the other in his or her absence. Kohut likened the optimal frustration progression to mourning, as the tie with the other is slowly reworked over time. If the self-object is not present, then, in a form of resolution or desperation, he or she gradually and painfully accepts the reality of the loss, while also attempting to drawn into the psyche the function of the other. Later others (Hagman, 1995, 2001; Stolorow, Brandchaft, & Atwood, 1987) make note that it is the attuned response to the frustrating absence of the self-object that allows for the essential other to be internalized, not the absence itself per se. As Hagman (1995, 2001) notes, this shift in theory holds significant implications not only for the normal developmental process of internalizing the self-object but also in dealing with its permanent loss through death. The key to transmuting internalization is an attuned environment to the innately difficult situation of the absence of the other. The empathic stance of another allows the loss to be more manageable, and, therefore, the self and the reestablishment of the bond to the other can both be restored.

The nature of the self-object (i.e., archaic versus mature) also has an impact upon loss (Hagman, 1995, 2001; Kohut, 1971, 1977, 1984). The archaic version speaks to more primitive needs that are associated with the formative years and is subject to many of the developmental challenges that go with that critical period. This includes perceiving the essential other as an extension of self, not having developed appropriate expectations, or boundaries, that go with the recognition of the other as their own person and not ours to possess. By contrast, the individual who has a mature self-object has a better appreciation of the more relational context that goes with a grown-up perspective of another. We can draw from the essential function the self-object performs in a more measured way of connection. As Kohut notes, the need for self-object is prevalent throughout the life span, but in the case of the mature self-object one has a better sense of self and other in this context.

Self-Psychology and Pet loss

From a self-psychology perspective, a pet owner can experience a pet companion as a resource for enhancing one's emotional or psychological sense of well-being (Brown, 2004, 2007). The human–animal bond allows for a sense of social related-ness and belonging. One may turn to pets to fill a range of roles from companion to child substitute. The relatedness encompassed within human–animal compan-ionship may in turn foster an individual's ability to connect with others in more appropriate ways by increasing self-cohesion and esteem (Brown, 2004, 2007). Pet companionship may also serve as a source of emotional sustenance for those who have no or limited connection (both physical and emotional) with people (e.g., Brown, 2004, 2007; Sharkin & Bahrick, 1990).

Just as connections with pets can foster well-being, the loss of a pet can lead to significant distress for their owners. In keeping with Brown (2004, 2007), it is suggested that a pet owner can view his or her pet companion as a self-object. The owner begins to recognize the pet companion as being responsible for fueling some needed or desired emotional sustenance. One may increase the likelihood of deeper bonds of attachment to one's pet, or even experience them as a friend or family member, when they are felt to be suppliers of certain sine qua nonpsychological requirements. To lose an essential self-object, then, is to disrupt the delivery of psy-chic support, which naturally produces the feeling of loss and grief. Likewise this may lead to further complications when a human companion does not fully compre-hend the significance of the loss, potentially leading to a form of complicated grief. Adding to the intricacy, the nature of the self-object (i.e., archaic versus mature) may also have an impact upon the perceived loss of the pet companion. That is, the types of needs met may influence the perceived meaning of the relationship. For instance, one may expect greater disruption in the self when the pet companion is seen as an archaic object meeting essential needs that were not before met by others.

Object Relations Theory

This section will provide a brief review of concepts taken from object relations the-ory, ones that may be applicable for the continuing bonds approach, especially as it relates to pet loss. As with previous sections, this is a concise summary of the theory. Object relations theory provides various ways to conceptualize the object or person; these may include a mental representation of the whole person, part of the person, and how the self is seen in relation to the object (Horowitz, 1987, 1988; Kernberg, 1976). In various object relations theories, the good object facilitates the individual's growth and development. The object can be in the external world, such as a person, but emphasis is also placed upon drawing an object into the internal world, becoming internalized as a mental representation of the other (Sandler & Rosenblatt, 1962). Fairbairn (1952) is credited for developing the first "pure object relations" theory. That is, Fairbairn envisioned a rather dramatic shift from the traditional psychoanalytic perspective of the day, which emphasized gratification of needs as the basis for forming bonds. Instead, Fairbairn suggested we are driven to form and sustain emotional connection with others, for its own sake. Fairbairn argued for the internalization of only bad objects as a defense against unsatisfying relations in the outer world. Klein (1940/2002) suggested the important task of integrating often divergent and conflicted perceptions of others (i.e., both good and bad objects) into a more complete and integrated picture. Likewise, Mahler et al. (1975) emphasized how the child works toward *object constancy*, ushering in a more mature and integrated picture of the gratifying and frustration aspects of all caregivers.

In terms of object loss, Melanie Klein (1940/2002) conceived mourning as a process of "reparation." Klein often envisioned the psychic worlds filled with intense and destructive fantasies under normal conditions, but in the case with mourning, the psychic material/dynamics are unleashed further by the sense of loss. The process of mourning includes reestablishing a positive internal relationship with the lost object. Also, according to Klein (1940/2002), the loss of an important love object in adulthood leads to a reactivation of earlier developmental struggles, intense fantasies that he or she is bereft of good internal objects, and stirring of intense primitive feelings of guilt, persecution, and punishment. Mourning restores and repairs the lost and damaged "good object," re-creating internally what was felt to be lost externally (Segal, 1974). However, the result of the mourning process is more than a simple restoration of the internal world. Klein (1940/2002) suggested the person is enriched by gaining a better ability to appreciate other people and experiences in one's life. There also results "a deepening in the individual's relation to his inner objects," which includes both an increased trust in those objects and a greater love for them because they survived and "proved to be good and helpful after all" (Klein, 1940/2002, p. 360).

The process of separation–individuation (Mahler et al., 1975) also plays a key role in how the individual responds to loss, both the numerous minilosses that accompany growing up and permanent loss of a loved one (Bloom-Feshback & Bloom-Feshback, 1987). Separation–individuation consists of the ongoing act of coming together, being separate, and, then, reuniting. The connect-then-separate experiences promote the internalization of a caregiver in order to deal with a state of disequilibrium that accompanies being apart (Kernberg, 1976; Mahler et al., 1975; Sandler & Rosenblatt, 1962). The individual slowly begins to draw into the psyche the loving and soothing aspects of the caregiver. With more internalization goes the capacity for extended periods of separation. When there is a permanent object loss, such as in the case of death, part of the grief work involves learning to access the internal representation as a source of connection and soothing. In a similar vein, Rubin (1984, 1985) described ways in which bereaved individuals maintain ongoing internal relationships with love objects after their death. Mourning is interpreted as a process of inner transformation of both self and object images. The internal relationship serves as a sustaining presence for the bereaved individual. Marwit and Klass (1996) studied the responses of university students who had experienced a significant loss in hopes of discerning how the role of the deceased continued to play in their lives. Four roles emerged: (a) the deceased acted as a role model; (b) provided a source of situation-specific guidance; (c) assisted in clarifying values; and (d) provided feelings of comfort or happiness. Baker (2001) described markers for determining the health associated with the internalization of a lost loved one: (1) The degree to which the bereaved individual is preoccupied with images and memories of the deceased; (2) A realistic mixture of both positive and negative qualities, reflecting the real person who has died; (3) The way the memories of the deceased are experienced (intrusive versus voluntarily accessed);. (4) Rubin's (1984) notion that memories of the deceased should evoke a sense of well-being rather than dysphoria or threat, and (5) Memories of the deceased should be experienced as fluid, open to change in step with the individual's own development (Rubin, 1984).

Object Relations Theory and Pet Loss

Pets have been noted as a type of transitional object for children (Noonan, 2008; Triebenbacher, 1998) and as a linking object (Volkan, 1981) to the departed. A transitional object helps the child deal with the inevitable frustrations of growing up, whereas a linking object helps preserve the connection to a person who is deceased. However, besides being seen as a potential therapeutic aid under certain circumstances (e.g., assist the elderly) (Levenson, 1969), there is limited mention of a pet companion as an object in its own right to internalize or integrate. In fact, Roth (2005) notes that in the psychoanalytic literature, there is a tendency to diminish the role of human–pet connection and to even pathologize it. While there is a dearth of object relations theory and research attending to human–animal, many of the previously reviewed themes lend themselves well to the continuing bonds approach regarding pet loss. The pet is perceived as a good object, facilitating growth and sense of well-being. Likewise, a pet, or mental representations of the pet, can be potentially internalized, acting as a role model, source of soothing, and so on. One may also strive to have an integrated perspective of the pet (addressed further in section below). Perhaps, many of Baker's (2001) and Rubin's (1984) guidelines for healthy internalizations may also be applicable. The internalized representation is fluid and open to change over time and with grief work. The hoped-for end of grieving may include how one can voluntarily call upon the recollection, evoking well-being not conflict and a sense of painful intrusion.

Psychodynamic Theory Applied to the Loss
of a Pet Companion

Having completed a brief review of attachment theory, self-psychology, and object relations, and how each may make specific contributions to understanding pet loss, what follows is a synthesis of these various contributions as it pertains to specific clinical issues. This by no means is an exhaustive list of considerations. In fact, one goal of this section is to spur on further discussion. However, with that said, the hope is to provide some assistance to the client working toward a continued bonds goal. We should begin thinking of a pet companion in terms of being a *significant object.* That is, the pet can take on various noteworthy roles and meanings, many that are better understood by exploring various psychodynamic themes (e.g., pet as an attachment figure, self-object, good object). While not every pet is transformed into a significant object, those that do may understandably assume an importance in an individual's life. We strive to help a client better understand the psychological significance and, in doing so, work toward forming a continued bond.

Layers of Loss

Melanie Klein (1940/2002) and Bowlby (1960) discussed how losses in adulthood are particularly challenging when the current lost object took over an essential psychic role of another from an earlier time, such as a caregiver. However, we can also expand the significance of the lost love object to include adult friends, family, romantic partners, and pet companions in the role of a significant object, as well. For the person experiencing a pet companion as an attachment figure, a good object, or self-object (i.e., pet as a significant object), the psychological importance may seem similar to the contributions and connections of other generative persons (or pets) from the past. In this case, one object may have picked up in some ways where the other(s) left off. However, even with the perceived similarity with former relations, the client may experience the pet companion as a unique relationship in its own right. The pet companion is not only a generative presence like other important objects but also has his or her own distinctive contribution in one's psychic landscape. Part of grief work is to recognize the distinguishing role(s), while simultaneously integrating the experience into one's general relational frame of reference regarding the viability of self, others, and the world, as reasonably fulfilling. If there is a history of secure, satisfying relations, one might expect the client to approach loss with more potential resources in hand, although he or she may still need assistance working toward forming a continuous bond in the ways discussed below.

For others with differing developmental histories, the pet companion may have offset certain needs that were never fulfilled in childhood or the ensuing years. In this case, the pet served in part a compensatory function, making up for prior deficits. That is, the pet companion played a central role as a significant object, laying down the fundamental relational tracks for the better. In the best situation, the pet companion altered one's internal psychic space regarding the world, relationships, and self for the better. The psychoanalytic concept of mental representation (e.g., Sandler & Rosenblatt, 1962) is similar to the concept of the internal working model in attachment theory, or, in self psychology terms, the pet companion has become integrated through transmuting internalization. To use an attachment theory phrase (see Wallin, 2007 for discussion), See Main & Goldwyn, the pet has helped the individual achieve an *earned sense of secure attachment*. When the transformation of the inner world occurs in the context of the pet companion, the clinical issue of continuing bonds is particularly important. Part of the clinician's focus may be to ensure that a continued bond with the pet companion is maintained, in order to draw from the powerful relationship in both the current grief work and future connections (people and pets). However, to accomplish these tasks, there may be certain obstacles with which to contend.

Fairbairn (1952) discussed how children go to great lengths to preserve a perception of some goodness about the world when growing up in dire familial circumstances. To not preserve hope in this manner means developing skewed relational perceptions, rigid defenses, and even extinguishing the expectancy of having any satisfying relations. For those who view the connection with the pet companion as a tether to such hope, he or she may be in danger of feeling their world has become bereft of any goodness. This situation can lead to a forked road: one path leads to utilizing the continued bond with the pet companion as a means to improving relation standing and attachment style, while the other to a regression to an earlier pre-pet companion perception of viewing and relating to self and others in skewed ways. To prevent a permanent regression, one may include under the category of "losses needed to be grieved" not only the death of the current significant object but also the conflicted feelings now reawakening concerning other relationships from a different time, to use Fairbairn's words, *the return of the bad objects* (1952). The client may feel psychologically separated from the significant object and, as a consequence, feel at the mercy of old conflicts now resurfaced or those that were previously held in check by the presence of the pet companion now set loose. The work at preserving the bond may then consist of dealing with various layers of loss, issues related to the now-deceased pet and less than satisfying objects from a different time. The clinician may help the client better understand which loss he or she is grieving at any given moment and work toward integrating the various divergent experiences into a meaningful whole.

In the best of conditions, the resurgence of unresolved layers of conflict and grief can provide another opportunity for making peace with the past. The old issues that are prompted can be worked through and then reframed, as yet another part of the legacy a pet companion can bestow. This would seem to be another pivot clinical place in terms of acknowledging the reality of the loss, but also working toward the preservation of the pet companion bond. If the bond to the pet companion is not preserved, clients may feel at the mercy of previous experiences that were damaging. That is, one is left to contend with the residual from previously unsatisfying connection(s), but, now, without the access to the pet companion.

Attunement

Those in the mental health profession have long noted that "attunement" is a quintessential psychological need. Psychoanalysts such as John Bowlby (1969/1982, 1980), Donald Winnicott (1971), Margret Mahler et al. (1975), Heinz Kohut (1971, 1977, 1984), and Daniel Stern (1985) all draw upon various notions of attunement in the development of self. To be attuned means to be in sync with the other, both in thought and deed. For instance, Winnicott (1971) argues that caregivers need to be aware of a child's earliest expressions of authentic personality. A caregiver's attunement helps the child's "true self" continue to grow. While attunement has been a particular focus for the health and welfare of infants and children, this same concept is important for adults. Attunement is a necessary part of vibrant adult interactions that range from good friends and romantic partners to the healing power of the therapeutic relationship. In terms of the latter, psychoanalyst Heinz Kohut (1959) suggested that one aspect of attunement, empathy, was the major tool of psychoanalysis. While this concept has varying definitions and subtle nuances, we refer to it as being in sync with how another thinks or feels and responding in kind in both verbal and nonverbal ways.

Attunement has direct implications for a wide variety of issues within the clinical settings, including recognizing its importance as a fundamental quality strengthening the human–animal bond and how the clinician helps the client deal with pet loss. Attunement provides the psychological sense of accompaniment as one explores thoughts and feelings (Winnicott, 1971) or, as argued here, in the case of a pet owner and companion, a psychological witness/participant in one's life events. The dynamic of attunement manifests in observable ways as owners and pets interact and react to one another in greeting, saying good bye, and interacting variedly throughout the course of the day. It is argued, in a dyad (or perhaps even in a larger group that makes up a family), that these shared experiences based upon attunement with a pet companion promote a sense of positive well-being and interpersonal functioning. It is suggested that issues of attachment to animal companions are actually built in part upon the more fundamental psychological experiences of an attuned relationship. Human beings experience strong emotional bonds to their animal companions in part because they are, as Bowlby (1969/1982) and Fairbairn (1952) would argue, fundamentally driven toward connection. But, in addition, the attachment with another, in this case to a pet companion, forms as a result of interactions with another that are perceived as being attuned, provide psychological accompaniment, in nonverbal ways.

Attunement plays a central role in the therapist–client dyad as well. To *understand and explain,* as Kohut (1971, 1977, 1984) would argue, is a quintessential tool for the clinician aiding the client's recognition and subsequent integration of an object in one's life. It is important to explore and recognize the personal meaning attached to the loss of a pet companion. This issue may be more challenging for some clients, as pet loss may not be considered justifiable grounds for a period of bereavement by the immediate surroundings that include family, friends, and culture. Even with the advent of the popular "pet lover memoir," the loss of a beloved pet still often falls under the category of "disenfranchised grief" (Meyers, 2002; Sharkin & Bahrick, 1990; Stewart, Thrush, & Paulus, 1989). Disenfranchised grief is a loss that is not viewed as valid in society's eyes Doka (1989). Consequently, one of the possible impacts for those that grieve is not receiving the proper support, potentially leading to a complicated mourning process. However, even a well-meaning other who knows that a pet companion was important may not know exactly for what reasons. One result of disenfranchised grief is mourners misunderstand at a profoundly deep and personal level. In some cases, this leads to a breakdown of dialogue with the outside world. The bereaved avoids the topic with others for fear of further misunderstandings. The net effect is that personal material becomes even more private, feeling locked away from view.

Part of the attuned work of the clinician is helping client find the words to construct and tell his or her own narrative, in this case, a *pet story:* the ways a pet companion impacted one's life and had meaning. Those that work from a constructionist perspective, especially concerning loss (e.g., Neimeyer, 2001; Neimeyer & Mahoney, 1995; Neimeyer & Raskin, 2000; Rosen & Kuehlwein, 1996), have recognized the personal meaning attributed to one's own phenomenal experience. In lieu of a fixed *truth* concerning an event, there are instead, subjective alternative constructions. Neimeyer (2001) comments on a *relational constructivist view,* where we are shaped by attachments and subsequent losses we sustain. The loss prompts the revision of our life story along many potential lines of meaning. One may be informed by the constructivist perspective when working with a clients' interpretation of a significant attachment and subsequent loss of a pet companion. The relational constructivist interfaces with the psychodynamic practitioner in terms of the common goal of uncovering the personal meaning imbued upon the relationship with the pet companion. Constructing the narrative is also, in a way, a symbolic form of *searching* for the continuation of the relationship with the departed, in the spirit of Bowlby (1969/1982, 1980) and Parkes (1970, 2009). The search may involve working with various psychodynamic themes suggested in this chapter. One may investigate the self-objects role(s) that may have transformed in-step with one's own life changes. It can also include telling how a successful recalibration of the internal working model took place as a result of a trusting attachment figure or good object within our psychic realm. Ultimately, writing a pet story also includes a final chapter, detailing how the client learns to call upon the continued bond for remembrance, comfort, and connection. The use of the narrative technique may be ultimately used to integrate and preserve the bond with a pet companion.

Contextual Consideration

In the broader cultural context, there is a current shifting of the family structure seen in the US and in many industrial countries abroad. It has been suggested that this increasing investment and reliance on pets for companionship and social support is due to recent demographic and social changes such as smaller family size, increased longevity, and higher incidences of relationship breakdown (Endenburg, 2005). Pets can impact the functioning of a family system in terms of interaction and coping (Albert, & Bulcroft, 1988; Sharkin & Knox, 2003). Triebenbacher (2000) suggested pets can serve as substitutes for absent family members who are no longer physically or emotionally in the family. Pets can also play pivotal roles during difficult or stressful periods, as in the case of illness, death of a family member, or separation or divorce (Cain, 1983). Salmon and Salmon (1983) indicate that dogs satisfy the needs of widowed and divorced people in the changing family network. For all these reasons and more, the death of a pet can be very stressful for families (Gage & Holcomb, 1991), resulting in a sense of familial disruption and functioning (Carmack, 1985; Sharkin & Knox, 2003).

From these contextual perspectives, certain clinical implications related to attachment and loss come into focus. For instance, once it was common (in the US) for multiple generations to live in or nearby the same home so that in a single broad stroke one could be witness to the assortment of goings-on that occurred across the life span. This might include couples forging new relationships, newborns entering the world, individuals in their prime, as well as those transitioning to the later years. But the multiple-generations-in-one-space approach has been replaced with a shrinking nuclear family impacting issues of attachment. We may make more demands on those few connections in our inner circle (people and pets) and feel the stakes are even higher when faced with a potential loss. For some, pet companions have assumed the role of family members, placing a greater emphasis upon the role(s) he or she plays in our lives. It makes sense that another consequence of cultural shifts may be to compartmentalize death and loss, keeping both issues at a safe distance. It is also important to be aware of differences in cultural norms around grief, loss, death, and the role of animals, as these various dynamics impact the family unit.

One unique feature of the most popular pet companion connections (i.e., dog and cat) is that the length of the relationship is vastly shorter than what could be that of a human family member or friend. We have the potential to experience the full life cycle of the pet companion from infancy, adolescence, adulthood, and old age (see Chapter 8, *Pachana et al.*). In seeing the complete cycle we are reminded of not only our own developmental challenges (previous or current) but also those of others who may be in our life. The meaning of our relationship with our pet companion may also shift in step with our own developmental needs as well as that of the pet companion. A pet that is the cuddly child substitute may give way to become protector in adulthood, and/or companion when our adult relationships fail, and then, finally, in his or her old age challenge our generative needs to take care of an elderly relation. A pet companion can have many lives in the context of our own. He or she may serve multiple psychological roles, some of which we are not aware of until a loss has occurred. The challenge then is to integrate the various and sundry chapters of a pet companion life into our own personal narrative.

Conclusion

There is a real need to have a better understanding of the nature of grief work, for what may seem to some as is a new postmodern love object, the pet companion. When working with a client who has grief and loss issues regarding a pet companion, one can draw from psychodynamic-based therapies, adding to our understanding certain contextual notions. First, we need to recognize that the loss is legitimate. When a pet is psychologically transformed into a significant object that is perceived as a friend or family member, guidelines for a continued bonds approach may be applied.

We also need to remove barriers that block preservation of the connection, such as conflicted or guilty goodbyes. Research does suggest there are effects associated with the various forms of pet loss, such as euthanasia and, also, relinquishment of the pet companion under unfavorable circumstances (see Chapter 16, Sharkin & Ruff). Rando (1993) coined the phrase, a *haunting loss*, one that intrudes upon the survivor, sometimes resulting in dysfunction or despair. A haunting loss may also be experienced by an owner when a pet has been transformed into a significant object, and the ending was less than satisfactory. To remedy the potential for this type of experience, one may help clients be aware of various issues in a preemptive manner, taking necessary steps when loss is looming. Psycho-education about loss may be an important role for the therapist. However, this work understandably also occurs for many after the fact. Other barriers to consider after the loss include the presence, or resurgence, of archaic psychological conflicts that a significant object helped offset. Clients should be encouraged to sort through thematic issues of attachment and loss concerning relationships from the formative years and beyond, as this also gives a new contextual meaning to the importance of the pet companion.

Another aspect to consider is what has been referred to in the bereavement literature as *posttraumatic growth* (Calhoun & Tedeschi, 1999; Tedeschi & Calhoun, 1995; Tedeschi, Park, & Calhoun, 1998). We become a little wiser and perhaps even a better person because we have taken a closer look at the meaning of things, reprioritizing our life. From a psychodynamic perspective posttraumatic growth may include not only a sense of continuity with a lost object but also the potential to integrate the various seemingly divergent experiences of self-other within the context of the human–animal bond. Our relationship with important objects, Schafer (1968) argues, is *a permanent one*. Objects may be revised, embraced fully, distanced from, and, even better, integrated, but they do not disappear. When we consider a pet companion as not just a pet but as a significant object, many of these same considerations may apply.

One unique feature of the human–animal bond is the potential for many significant pet companions over the life time, each carrying their own meaning. We can explore in future studies the impact of repeated losses and attempts to keep the various bonds unbroken. Do we become more skilled at developing a sense of continuity the *next time*, or do we shy away from future attachments (people and pets) because the inevitability of loss may feel underscored? Research with human companions suggests post traumatic growth is in some ways paradoxical (Calhoun & Tedeschi,

1999). Having experienced significant loss, some individuals may have a heightened sense of vulnerability to subsequent ones (Janoff-Bulman, 1992), while at the same time he or she may view themselves as stronger and more capable (Tedeschi, & Calhoun, 1995). Exploring the future of the human–animal bond will need to be based on striving for continuity after not just one loss but many. There remain many unanswered questions about how finding a continued bond with a lost pet companion, and the experience, may prepare one in dealing with other losses.

A continued bond approach may involve work in both the inner and outer worlds. Therapists may help clients with the process of internalization through exploring the various ways the pet companion was important and may take up residence within our inner landscape. The actual integration of the loss leading to the eventual continuing bond may be assisted through telling the *pet story*, that is, weaving together the various meanings and roles one has imbued onto the pet companion over the course of the relationship. The outer world work may involve telling the narrative to another, as well as acting from it. That is, various types of personal memorials may be constructed. One may even find inspiration in prosocial forms of remembering, working toward a cure or cause associated with the lost pet companion. Utilizing the aforementioned techniques and theoretical considerations adds to the psychodynamic dialogue addressing the significance of the human–animal bond. Matters of importance include attachment as well as why it is we grieve when the pet companion is gone. Having a fuller understanding as to the meaning of the connection begins the journey toward keeping the bond unbroken.

References

Abraham, K. (1927/1960). A short history of the development of the libido. In D. Bryan & A. Strachey (Eds.), *Selected papers of Karl Abraham* (pp. 418–503). New York: Brunner/Mazel. (Original work published 1927)

Ainsworth, M. (1979). Infant–mother attachment. *American Psychologist, 34*, 932–937.

Albert, A., & Bulcroft, K. (1988). Pets, family, and the life course. *Journal of Marriage and Family, 50*, 543–552.

Baker, J. E. (2001). Mourning and the transformation of object relationships evidence for the persistence of internal attachments. *Psychoanalytic Psychology, 18*(1), 55–73.

Bartholomew, K., & Horowitz, L. (1991). Attachment styles among young adults: A test of a four-category model. *Journal of Personality and Social Psychology, 61*(2), 226–244.

Beck, L., & Madresh, E. A. (2008). Romantic partners and four-legged friends: An extension of attachment theory to relationships with pets. *Anthrozoös, 21*(1), 43–56.

Bloom-Feshback, J., & Bloom-Feshback, S. (Eds). (1987). *The psychology of separation and loss.* New York: Jossey-Bass.

Bowlby, J. (1960). Separation anxiety. *International Journal of Psychoanalysis, 41*, 89–113.

Bowlby, J. (1969/1982). *Attachment and loss: Vol. 1. Attachment,* 2nd ed. New York: Basic. (Original work published 1969)

Bowlby, J. (1980). *Attachment and loss, Vol. 3. Loss: Sadness and depression.* New York: Basic Books.

Bowlby, J., & Parkes, C. M. (1970). Separation and loss within the family. In E. J. Anthony (Ed.), *The child in his family.* New Work: Wiley.

Brown, S. E. (2004). The human–animal bond and self psychology: Toward a new understanding. *Society & Animals, 12*(1), 67–86.

Brown, S. E. (2007). Companion animals as self-objects. *Anthrozoos, 20*(4), 329–343.

Cain, A. O. (1983). A study of pets in the family system. In A. H. Katcher & A. M. Beck (Eds.), *New perspectives on our lives with companion animals* (pp. 72–81). Philadelphia: University of Pennsylvania Press.

Calhoun, L., & Tedeschi, R. G. (1999). *Facilitating posttraumatic growth: A clinicians guide.* Mahwah, NJ: Erlbaum.

Carmack, J. (1985). The effects on family members and functioning after death of a pet. *Marriage and Family Reviews, 8,* 149–161.

Cowles, K. V. (1985). The death of a pet: Human responses to the breaking of the bond. *Pets and the Family, 8,* 135–161.

Deutsch, H. (1937). Absence of grief. *Psychoanalytic Quarterly, 6,* 12–22.

Doka, K. J. (1989). *Disenfranchised grief: Recognizing hidden sorrow.* Lexington, MA: Lexington.

Endenburg, N. (2005). The death of a companion animal and bereavement. In F. H. de Jonge & R. van den Bos (Eds.), *The human–animal relationship: Forever and a day* (pp. 110–122). Assen: Royal Van Gorcum.

Fairbairn, W. R. D. (1952). *An object relations theory of personality.* New York: Basic books.

Field, N. P., Gao, B., & Paderna, L. (2005). Continuing bonds in bereavement: An attachment theory based perspective. *Death Studies, 29,* 1–23.

Field, N. P., Orsini, L., Gavish, R., & Packman, W. (2009). Role of attachment in response to pet loss. *Death Studies, 33,* 334–355.

Field, N. P., & Sundin, E. C. (2001). Attachment style in adjustment to conjugal bereavement. *Journal of Social and Personal Relationships, 18,* 347–361.

Fonagy, P. (2001). *Attachment theory and psychoanalysis.* New York: Other Press.

Freud, S. (1920). Beyond the pleasure principle. *Standard Edition of the Complete Works of Sigmund Freud, 18,* 3–64.

Furman, E. (1974). *A child's parent dies: Studies in childhood bereavement.* New Haven, CT: Yale University Press.

Gage, M.G., & Holcomb, R. (1991). Couples perception of stressfulness of death of the family pet. *Family Relations, 40,* 103–106.

Gaines, R. (1997). Detachment and continuity: The two tasks of mourning. *Contemporary Psychoanalysis, 33,* 549–571.

Gosse, G. H., & Barnes, M. J. (1994). Human grief resulting from the death of a pet. *Anthrozoos, 7*(2), 103–112.

Hagman, G. (1995) Death of a self object: Towards a self psychology of the mourning process. In A. Goldberg (Ed.), *Progress in self psychology* (Vol. 11, pp. 189–205). Hillsdale, NJ: Analytic Press.

Hagman, G. (2001). Beyond decathexis: Toward a new psychoanalytic understanding and treatment of mourning. In R. A. Neimeyer (Ed.), *Meaning reconstruction & the experience of loss* (pp. 13–31). Washington, DC: American Psychological Association.

Hazan, C., & Shaver, P. (1987). Romantic love conceptualized as an attachment process. *Journal of Personality and Social Psychology, 52,* 511–524.

Horowitz, M. J. (1987). *States of mind.* New York: Plenum.

Horowitz, M. J. (1988). *Introduction of psychodynamics.* New York: Basic Books.

Janoff-Bulman, R. (1992). *Shattered assumptions: Towards a new psychology of trauma.* New York: Free Press.

Kaplan, L. (1995). *No voice if wholly lost.* New York: Simon & Schuster.

Kernberg, O. F. (1976). *Object relations theory and clinical psychoanalysis.* New York: Jason Aronson.

Klass, D., Silverman, P., & Nickman, S. L. (Eds.). (1996). *Continuing bonds: New understandings of grief.* Washington, DC: Taylor & Francis.

Klein, M. (1940/2002). Mourning and its relation to manic-depressive states. In *Love, guilt and reparation and other works, 1921–1945* (pp. 344–369). New York: Free Press.

Kobak, R. (2009). Defining and measuring of attachment bonds: Comment on Kurdek (2009). *Journal of Family Psychology, 23*(4), 447–449.

Kohut, H. (1959). Introspection, empathy, and psychoanalysis: An examination of the relation-ship between mode of observation and theory. In P. H. Ornstein (Ed.), *The search for the self* (pp. 205–232). New York: International Universities Press.

Kohut, H. (1971). *The analysis of the self.* New York: International Universities Press.

Kohut, H. (1977). *The restoration of the self.* New York: International Universities Press.

Kohut, H. (1984). *How does analysis cure?* Chicago: University of Chicago.

Kurdek, L. (2008). Pet dogs as attachment figures. *Journal of Social and Personal Relationships, 25*(2), pp. 247–266.

Kurdek, L. (2009). Pet dogs as attachment figures for adult owners. *Journal of Family Psychology, 23,* 439–446.

Levenson, B. M. (1969). *Pet oriented child psychotherapy.* Springfield, IL: Charles Thomas.

Mahler, M., Pine, F., & Bergman, A. (1975). *The psychological birth of the human infant.* New York: Basic Books.

Main, M. (2000). The organized categories of infant, child, and adult attachment: Flexible versus inflexible attention under attachment-related stress. *Journal of the American Psychoanalytic Association, 48,* 1055–1096.

Main, M., & Solomon, J. (1986). Discovery of a new, insecure-disorganized/disoriented attachment pattern. In M. Yogman & T. B. Brazelton (Eds.), *Affective development in infancy* (pp. 95–124). Norwood, NJ: Ablex.

Marwit, S. J., & Klass, D. (1996). Greif and the role of the inner representation of the deceased. In D. Klass, P. R. Silverman, & S. L. Nickman (Eds.), *Continuing bonds* (pp 297–309). Washington, DC: Taylor & Francis.

Meyers, B. (2002). Disenfranchised grief and the loss of an animal companion. In J. K. Doka (Ed.), *Disenfranchised grief: New directions, challenges, and strategies for practice* (pp. 251–264). Lexington, MA: Lexington Books.

Mikulincer, M., & Shaver, P. R. (2003). Attachment theory and affect regulation: The dynam-ics, development, and cognitive consequences of attachment related strategies. *Motivation & Emotion, 27*(2), 77–102.

Mikulincer, M., & Shaver, P. R. (2007). *Attachment in adulthood: Structure, dynamics, and change.* New York: Guilford Press.

Moore, B. E., & Fine, B. D. (1991). *Psychoanalytic terms and concepts.* New Haven, CT: Yale University Press.

Neimeyer, R. A. (2001). The language of loss: Grief therapy as a process of meaning reconstruc-tion. In R. A. Neimeyer (Ed.), *Meaning reconstruction & the experience of loss* (pp. 261–292). Washington, DC: American Psychological Association.

Neimeyer, R. A., & Mahoney, M. J. (1995). *Constructivism in psychotherapy.* Washington, DC: American Psychological Association.

Neimeyer, R. A., & Raskin, J. (Eds.). (2000). *Constructions of disorder.* Washington, DC: American Psychological Association.

Noonan, E. (2008). People and pets. *Psychodynamic Practice, 14*(4), 395–407.

Parkes, C. M. (1970). "Seeking" and "finding" a lost object: Evidence from recent studies of the reaction to bereavement. *Society of Science & Medicine, 4,* 187–201.

Parkes, C. M. (1986). *Bereavement* (2nd ed.). London: Tavistock.

Parkes, C. M. (2009). *Love and loss: The roots of grief and its complications.* New York: Routledge.

Parkes, C. M., & Weiss, R. S. (1983). *Recovery from bereavement.* New York: Basic Books.

Parkes, C. M., & Weiss, R. S. (2003). *Recovery from bereavement.* New York: Basic Books.

Planchon, L. A., & Templer, D. I. (1996). The correlates of grief after death of a pet. *Anthrozoos, 9,* 107–113.

Quackenbush, J. (1982). The social context of pet loss. *The Animal Health Technician, 3*(6), 333–337.

Rando, T. A. (1993). *Treatment of complicated mourning.* Champaign, IL: Research press.

Rosen, H., &Kuehlwein, K. (Eds.). (1996). *Constructing realities.* San Francisco: Jossey Bass.

Roth, B. (2005). Pets and psychoanalysis: A clinical contribution. *Psychoanalytic Review, 92,* 453–467.

Rubin, S. S. (1984). Mourning distinct from melancholia: The resolution of bereavement. *British Journal of Medical Psychology, 57,* 339–345.

Rubin, S. S. (1985). The resolution of bereavement: A Clinical focus on the relationship to the deceased. *Psychotherapy, 22,* 231–235.

Salmon, P. W., & Salmon, I. M. (1983). Who owns who? Psychological research into the human–pet bond in Australia. In A. Katcher & A. Beck (Eds.), *New perspectives on our lives with companion animals* (pp. 245–265). Philadelphia: University of Pennsylvania Press.

Sandler, J., & Rosenblatt, B. (1962). The concept of the representational world. *Psychoanalytic Study of the Child, 17,* 128–145.

Schafer, R. (1968). *Aspects of internalization.* New York: International Universities Press.

Segal, H. (1974). *Introduction to the work of Melanie Klein* (2nd ed.). New York: Basic Books.

Sharkin, B. S., & Bahrick, A. S. (1990). Pet loss: Implications for counselors. *Journal of Counseling and Development, 68,* 306–308.

Sharkin, B. S., & Knox, D. (2003). Pet loss: Issues and implications for the psychologist. *Professional Psychology: Research and Practice, 34*(4), 414–421.

Stern, D. (1985). *The interpersonal world of the infant: A view from psychoanalysis and developmental psychology.* New York: Basic Books.

Stewart, C. S., Thrush, J. C., & Paulus, G. (1989). Disenfranchised bereavement and loss of a companion animal: Implications for caring communities. In K. Doka (Ed.), *Disenfranchised grief: Recognizing hidden sorrow* (pp. 147–159). Lexington, MA: Lexington Books.

Stolorow, R., Brandchaft, B., & Atwood, G. (1987). *Psychoanalytic treatment: An intersubjective experience.* Norvale, NJ: Jason Aronson.

Stroebe, M., Schut, H., & Stroebe, W. (2005). Attachment in coping with bereavement: A theoretical integration. *Review of General Psychology, 9*(1), 48–66.

Tedeschi, R., Park, C., & Calhoun, L. (Eds.). (1998). *Posttraumatic growth: Positive changes in the aftermath of crisis.* Mahwah, NJ: Erlbaum.

Tedeschi, R. G., & Calhoun, L. G. (1995). *Trauma and transformation: Growing in the aftermath of suffering.* Sage, CA: Thousand oaks.

Triebenbacher, S. L. (1998). Pets as transitional objects: Their role in children's emotional development. *Psychological Reports, 82,* 191–200.

Voith, V. L. (1985). Attachment of people to companion animals. *Veterinary Clinics of North America: Small Animal Practice, 15,* 289–295.

Volkan, V. (1981). *Linking objects and linking phenomena.* New York: International.

Wallin, D. J. (2007). *Attachment in psychotherapy.* New York: Guilford.

Winnicott, D. W. (1971). *Playing and reality.* Middlesex: Penguin Books.

Wrobel, T. A., & Dye, A. L. (2003). Grieving pet death: Normative, gender, and attachment issues. *Omega, 47*(4), 385–393.

Chapter 13
Death of a Companion Animal: Understanding Human Responses to Bereavement

Helen L. Davis

Death of a Companion Animal: Understanding Human Responses to Bereavement

The best test of any relationship's significance in a person's life is, perhaps, what happens when it comes to an end. Although losing a pet has been likened to losing a valued possession or occupation (e.g., Parkes, 1971), current evidence suggests that an owner's response to pet death usually has more in common with bereavement following the death of a beloved human than with the loss of a possession (Archer & Winchester, 1994). Grief is a normal response to the death of a beloved other and has been characterised as progressing through a series of stages or phases from initial shock, numbness, and denial, occurring even when the death is expected, to a range of intense emotional reactions that may include anger and guilt, to depression and helplessness, where a person may become withdrawn, to a stage of dialogue and bargaining, where the bereaved person may begin to reach out to others, want to tell their story, and struggle to find meaning in what happened. The final stage involves acceptance of the loss and moving on (Kübler-Ross, 1969). The nature of response to pet death seems to follow this pattern, though being on average less extremely distressing and less prolonged (Archer & Winchester, 1994; Gerwolls & Labott, 1994). People vary considerably in how they manifest their grief. Nevertheless, some bereaved persons may find their response severely debilitating and protracted and may even become suicidal (Archer & Winchester, 1994). This is termed *complicated* or *pathological* grief (Williams & Mills, 2000).

Much research into people's response to the death of a companion animal has been concerned with identifying the factors that predict who is likely to experience extreme or pathological grief (e.g., Davis, Irwin, Richardson, & O'Brien-Malone, 2003; Field, Orsini, Gavish, & Packman, 2009; Gerwolls & Labott, 1994; McCutcheon & Fleming, 2001; Planchon, Templer, Stokes, & Keller, 2002). Although some level of grief is common among owners who have lost a pet and

H.L. Davis (✉)
Murdoch University, Perth, Australia
e-mail: hdavis@murdoch.edu.au

C. Blazina et al. (eds.), *The Psychology of the Human–Animal Bond*,
DOI 10.1007/978-1-4419-9761-6_13, © Springer Science+Business Media, LLC 2011

may be significant and enduring for 20–30%, pathological grief responses occur relatively rarely (Luiz Adrian, Deliramich, & Frueh, 2009). Predicting the extent of grief is no mean feat, given that bereaved owners' responses (or lack thereof) may surprise even themselves (Davis et al., 2003). Investigating predictors may be useful to some extent in helping practitioners to forecast who is at risk of extreme grief and in allocating resources accordingly, but it leaves open the question of *why* so much variation exists among individuals in their response to companion animal death. The question also arises as to whether high levels of grief are best thought of as pathological, implying an abnormal, unhealthy response, or as a normal response to the loss of an extremely important relationship.

In this chapter, we will briefly review the objective human and animal factors that predict the extent of a grief response, as well as the factors that bereaved animal owners themselves report as helpful or unhelpful in coping with grief. We will note that objective factors alone are not highly predictive of distress levels. We will argue that the psychological meaning of the person's relationship with their companion animal needs to be addressed in order to understand what exactly people lose when their companion animal dies. Attachment theory goes some way towards addressing this, but has been criticised for ignoring other kinds of affectional bond between humans and animals (Kobak, 2009). As a more generalised alternative, Fiske's (1991, 1992) theory of social models will be outlined and examined for its potential in helping us to understand human–animal relationships and the variety of people's responses when they end.

What Predicts Extreme Grief?

Human Factors

Various demographic factors of animal owners have been examined in relation to predicting the magnitude of grief responses. Although age has shown significant associations with grief in several studies, the findings are not entirely consistent with each other. For example, McCutcheon and Fleming (2001) report that younger adults are more susceptible to intense grief than older owners, whereas Quackenbush and Glickman (1983) found that young adults suffered lesser grief than either adolescents or adults over the age of 40. Still other researchers have found that age does not predict extent of grief (Davis et al., 2003; Gosse & Barnes, 1994).

In contrast to the mixed findings on age, gender emerges consistently as a risk factor, with females reporting more extreme grief responses than males (Davis et al., 2003; Gosse & Barnes, 1994; McCutcheon & Fleming, 2001; Planchon & Templer, 1996; Quackenbush & Glickman, 1983) and being more likely than males to seek support services (Turner, 1997). This is consistent with females' general tendency to report stronger negative (and also positive) emotions than males (Diener, Suh, Lucas, & Smith, 1999). Nevertheless, it is unclear whether bereaved female animal owners experience more extreme grief than their male counterparts, or whether they are simply more ready to report it. For example, when faced with problems, males and females show some characteristic differences in their use of coping strategies.

Females are more likely than males to seek social support (Forbes & Roger, 1999), and males are more likely than females to suppress their emotions as a way of coping (John & Gross, 2007). A further possibility described later in this chapter is that gender differences may exist in the kind of relationship that people form with their companion animals.

Animal owners' social environment also seems to affect their response to companion animal death. Owners who live alone are more susceptible to extreme grief (Davis et al., 2003; McCutcheon & Fleming, 2001), as are those who report having little social support available (Field et al., 2009), and other stressful life events occurring around the same time as the animal's death (Gosse & Barnes, 1994; Sanders, 1988). Having no children is a risk factor (Gosse & Barnes, 1994; Quackenbush & Glickman, 1983), as is dissatisfaction with one's children (Weisman, 1990).

Animal Factors

Stallones (1994) reports that the loss of a dog is more likely to evoke extreme grief than the death of other animals, but Davis et al. (2003) failed to replicate this finding. Other factors, such as the length of time that the person has owned the animal (Davis et al., 2003; Quackenbush & Glickman, 1983) and whether the person owns other companion animals, are sometimes found to be associated with the extent of the person's grief response, but not consistently (Gerwolls & Labott, 1994; Gosse & Barnes, 1994).

Situational Factors

The suddenness of the animal's death has been investigated as a predictor of grief response, but findings have been mixed (Gerwolls & Labott, 1994; Planchon et al., 2002). Similarly, having one's animal euthanised has been found in some studies to be associated with less grief (McCutcheon & Fleming, 2001; Planchon et al., 2002), whereas Davis et al. (2003) found that euthanasia was a relatively strong predictor of a greater grief response. Table 13.1 summarises the research literature on factors predicting an extreme grief response.

Factors that Help and Hinder with Coping

Davis et al. (2003) invited bereaved pet owners from a range of religious and nonreligious backgrounds to describe any factors around the time of death that made coping easier or more difficult. Some of the frequently cited difficulties included missing the routines that the owner had with the animal, being reminded of the animal on seeing its things, and having no one sympathetic to talk to about their experience. Some of the frequently reported helpful factors were getting a new pet soon after the death, having a ceremony or creating a memorial for their animal, showing respect

Table 13.1 Risk factors investigated as predictors of extreme grief

Factor type	Factor	Research findings on risk
Human	Age	Inconsistent—possible increased risk for adolescents and older adults
	Gender (female)	Greater risk
	Living alone	Greater risk
	No children	Greater risk
	Less social support	Greater risk
Animal	Type of animal	Inconsistent—possibly greater for dogs
	Length of ownership	Inconsistent
	Close relationship	Greater risk
	Other animals owned	Inconsistent
Situational	Sudden death	Inconsistent
	Euthanasia	Inconsistent
	Other stressors	Greater risk

by veterinarians and others for the individuality of their animal and specialness of their relationship with it, believing in an afterlife for their animal, and, among members of some religions, receiving teachings about the value of animals and accepting loss and letting go. Nevertheless, as this study focused on the spontaneous responses of a select sample of individuals, we would need a more comprehensive survey of these factors in the wider population before they can be declared generally helpful or harmful.

To summarise these findings, a number of factors emerge as significant predictors of the extent of an owner's grief at the death of their companion animal, and there are some common themes in the kinds of factors that make losing a beloved pet easier or harder. However, the amount of variability in grief response predicted by any of these factors is generally modest, many of the factors are not consistent in their effects across different methodologies and different populations, and indeed sometimes reverse the direction of their effect. Even where predictors are relatively consistent (e.g., gender differences), they bring us no closer to understanding why particular kinds of people might be prone to pathological grief while others experience little or no emotional reaction. It may be suggested that to understand the emotional response, we need to take seriously and understand clearly the nature of the relationship between human and animal.

Relationship Factors

Several studies report that owners with a close relationship to their animals are at greater risk of an extreme grief response (Gerwolls & Labott, 1994; Gosse & Barnes, 1994; Planchon et al., 2002), as are those who treat their animals as a surrogate relative (Keddie, 1977). Furthermore, there is overlap between the demographic characteristics associated with greater grief and those associated with stronger attachment—being female, older age, lack of children, not being married, smaller households, and smaller social circles (Johnson, Garrity, & Stallones, 1992).

Recently, attention has turned to taking a more theoretically based approach to studying the human–animal bond. Specifically, attachment theory (Ainsworth, Blehar, Waters, & Wall, 1978; Mikulincer & Shaver, 2003) has been recruited to aid our understanding of relationships with pets (Kurdek, 2008, 2009). While measures of pet attachment tend to use the term informally and measure strength of attachment quantitatively, Ainsworth's theory defines attachment by four necessary features: proximity maintenance (seeking to remain close to the attachment figure), separation distress (emotional distress when separated from the attachment figure), secure base (feeling confident to explore new things and take on challenges in the presence of the attachment figure), and safe haven (turning to the attachment figure for reassurance in times of danger or distress). Ainsworth identified four categories of attachment style in infants, based on how they responded to separation and reunion with their caregiver during a stressful situation.

Attachment theory has been extended to describe adult love relationships, and here too, four qualitatively different styles emerge: *secure* (i.e., comfortable being emotionally close, not fearful of rejection or abandonment) and three *insecure* styles: *preoccupied* (i.e., jealous and anxiously clinging), *dismissing avoidant* (i.e., avoiding emotional closeness because others are deemed untrustworthy), and *fearful avoidant* (i.e., avoiding closeness because of anxious distrust of others and feelings of personal inadequacy) (Bartholomew & Horowitz, 1991). Recently, several papers have been published showing qualitative similarities between attachment to pets and attachment to family members and romantic partners. Some studies report that adults show less-secure attachment to dogs than to other people (Kurdek, 2008), while others more provocatively report that they show more secure attachment to their companion animal than to human partners or relatives (Beck & Madresh, 2008; Kurdek, 2009). It has been argued that *security* of attachment to one's pet, rather than strength of attachment, might be an important predictor of grief at pet loss. Field et al. (2009) report moderate correlations between extent of grief and measures of anxious and avoidant insecurity of pet attachment.

Researchers have also investigated how social support from other human relationships might affect the association between pet attachment and grief. For example, insecure attachment to one's pet might be indicative of general problems with attachment, predicting poor adaptation to bereavement. Alternatively, secure attachment to pets may compensate for insecure attachment to other humans, amplifying the effects of pet death (Field et al., 2009). Beck and Madresh (2008) report only modest correlations between insecurity of attachment measures for pets and partners, suggesting no great consistency in the security of attachment across human and animal relationships. In contrast, Field et al. (2009) found that insecurity in pet attachment was associated with lower levels of human social support and with more grief at pet loss. This latter result is more consistent with the *pervasive relationship difficulty* interpretation rather than the *compensation* interpretation. Nevertheless, these findings describe on-average trends rather than demonstrating that pets cannot compensate for deficits in human relationships.

Notwithstanding the growing interest in the importance of pet attachment security, Kobak (2009) raises some concerns about the validity of applying the term *attachment* indiscriminately to human–animal relationships. As well as identifying some methodological problems in studies likening human attachment to pet attachment, he makes the more fundamental point that attachment in its original sense is just one type of affectional bond found in humans that, while clearly evident in infants, is much less central to older children's and adults' relationships. He argues that other types of bond, such as caregiving or friendship bonds, might better describe the human–animal bond in the majority of cases. In the following section, an alternative taxonomy of relationships will be explored, which arguably incorporates attachment but extends to qualitatively different forms of affectional relationship. The usefulness of this taxonomy to understanding human–animal relationships is then discussed.

Four Models of Sociality

Fiske (1991, 1992) proposes that all human social relationships can be categorised into one of four basic relational models. Given the grandeur of this claim, we might well expect that this set of relational models would be able to accommodate human–animal relationships too. These models describe the nature of the relationship between individuals, aid in interpreting people's experience within the relationship, help to direct appropriate behaviour within the relationship, define what behaviours are relevant and irrelevant to the relationship, and endow socially related events and objects with meaning. According to Fiske, humans are intrinsically, as distinct from instrumentally, motivated to form relationships that conform to each of these models (although this is not inconsistent with relationship members deriving benefits from belonging). Table 13.2 summarises the models' characteristics most relevant to human–animal relationships. The models are discussed here in order of complexity, which also seems to correspond to the age at which children begin to use them, and may also correspond to the relative frequency with which they can be seen in animal species, with the simpler models being more widespread.

Communal Sharing

This is the simplest of the four models. It typifies categorical, in-group–out-group relationships where in-group members are strongly bonded and focus their attention upon what they have in common rather than their differences. Communal sharing groups are also exclusive, contrasting themselves with out-group members. This model can involve as few as two group members, or many more. Characteristics of this model include the great importance of physical closeness and contact, with separation or loss being highly distressing. Material resources in a communal sharing relationship are seen as owned by all members. Physical objects and places can

Table 13.2 Summary of Fiske's (1992) four proposed social models

Domain	Communal sharing	Authority ranking	Equality matching	Market pricing
Nature of relationship	Categorical, "us and them"	Hierarchical	Equal individuals	Rational, proportional
Motivation	Intimacy	Power	Wish for equality	Achievement
Resource distribution	Communal ownership, free access to group members	Superiors have more and better resources than inferiors	Distributed exactly equally among individuals	Distributed in proportion to contribution or need
Decision making	Group consensus	Superiors make decisions and inferiors abide by them	Democratic voting or equal chance (e.g., lottery)	Cost-benefit analysis, or let market decide
Interpretation of misfortune	Stigmatisation, or shared suffering	Punishment for wrongdoing	"Things even out in the long run."	Calculable risk
Moral ideology	Kindness, generosity	Superiors protect inferiors, inferiors obey and show loyalty	Justice as strict equality	Greatest good for the greatest number
Physical objects	Keepsakes	Status symbols	Tokens of equality	Commodities for trade
Age of emergence in humans	Infancy	3 years	4 years	9 years
Evidence in animal species	Yes	Yes	Possibly among chimpanzees	No

come to be so closely associated with group members and their relationship that they take on a deep significance as keepsakes, or the family home. Misfortune, as well as resources, is shared: When one member suffers, all suffer. Alternatively, the victim of misfortune may be stigmatised and cut off from the group. Group members make decisions based on consensus. The central motivation of people in a communal sharing relationship is intimacy and the desire to belong (cf. Harlow & Zimmerman, 1959). The traits most morally valued within this type of relationship are kindness, caring and generosity. Fiske argues that people commonly use their most strongly identified communal sharing relationships as a way of defining their sense of self. These relationships are often idealised as eternal and supported by enactive, sensorimotor rituals. In Western cultures, communal sharing relationships are not only commonly found in romantic and mother–infant dyads but also apply to cultural groups. This social model is also central to most religions, where the unity of all humanity, or living creatures, or members of the religious in-group, is a recurrent theme. Humans first show behaviours consistent with the communal sharing model during infancy, and it also seems, according to Fiske, to reemerge as particularly important during adolescence. An attachment relationship, in Ainsworth's original sense, would be a classic example of a communal sharing relationship, but Fiske also gives examples of less-intense relationships that are structurally similar, such as sharing CDs with housemates.

Authority Ranking

This is the label Fiske applies to relationships that involve asymmetrical, hierarchically ordered social relationships. This model focuses on the differences in status between individuals. Those of higher status have the right to more and better resources than those of lower status. They also have the right to make decisions and control the actions of lower-status individuals. Higher-ranked members have the right to mete out punishment to lower-ranked members, but not vice versa. Within this social model, physical objects are treated as symbols of status or prestige, and places are viewed as part of the higher-ranking individual's territory. The moral imperatives for a lower-ranked member are obedience and loyalty to the higher-ranked member. Conversely, higher-ranked members have the moral obligation to protect and sustain the lower-ranked members under their control—and indeed, the loyalty of lower-ranked individuals may be contingent upon higher-ranked individuals fulfilling this obligation. Individuals in authority ranking relationships are argued to gain a sense of identity from whom they have authority over, and to whom they defer, and derive self-worth from the extent to which they are a beneficent or powerful leader, or a loyal follower. The power motivation is argued to be central to the authority ranking relationship. First signs of using authority ranking social models emerge around age three in humans. Authority ranking relationships are commonly seen in Western society between parents and their children and in the military. The authority ranking model also applies to religious beliefs that involve a supreme deity who must be obeyed unquestioningly. In this context, suffering is seen as the will of

God, and people who are suffering misfortune tend to interpret it as punishment for their disobedience.

Equality Matching

Equality matching, as the name suggests, refers to relationships in which members have equal status and strive to maintain that equality. Unlike communal sharing relationships, the members of an equality matching relationship retain their individual identity and personal, as distinct from collective, responsibility. Tit-for-tat reciprocity and turn-taking lie at the heart of this model, with the receipt of a gift or benefit requiring that the favour be returned and members of the relationship being attentive to what the "score" is. Equally, offences against a person require "eye for an eye" vengeance. Decisions are made democratically. Members of an equality matching relationship are motivated by a principle of equality. This model is often applied to establish amicable relations among strangers, through equal exchange of goods and favours, or through synchrony of actions. Application of this model emerges in humans at about four years of age. In Western culture, friendship relations and the rules of competitive sports often involve an equality matching model.

Market Pricing

These relationships focus upon rates and proportions. Individuals receive benefits in direct proportion to their contribution or their needs. Decisions are made based on rational cost-benefit analyses and efficiency considerations. In the context of this model, objects and land are viewed in terms of their market value. Market pricing relationships are seen to be entered into voluntarily, and their central motivation is achievement. They are frequently exhibited in workplace relations. Humans begin to engage in market pricing relations from about age nine. As the most complex and cerebral of the social models, it is also has the least emotionality associated with it.

Asocial and Null Relationships

Fiske also notes that not all interactions among people are truly social. Asocial relationships occur where a person simply uses another as a means to an end without regard for the rules and standards implicit in any social model (cf. psychopathy). Null relationships involve people simply ignoring each other and apply to one's relationship with most other people most of the time.

Fiske (1991, 1992) argues that these four basic social models are universal to humans. However, there exist cultural and individual differences in the specific relationships to which each model is conventionally applied. For example, many cultures apply an authority ranking model to marital relationships, whereas modern Western culture is more likely to apply a communal sharing or equality matching model. There are also cultural differences in how widely used different models are.

For example, industrialised Western societies, in contrast to village communities, tend to show a general preference for market pricing models as professional and fair, and an antipathy towards authority ranking models as exploitative.

Where there is agreement among members of a relationship about the model to be applied, interactions can proceed in relative harmony. However, conflict can arise when different members of a relationship disagree about the model that applies, as the resulting behaviour that is appropriate to one model may be highly inappropriate to another model. Similarly, even if the members of the relationship agree about the model that applies, they may find themselves in conflict with their cultural milieu if they are seen to be applying a culturally inappropriate model. It is also common for the same relationship to conform to different models on different occasions or in different situations. For example, a parent may communally share food with children, but may adopt an authority ranking relationship with the same children in situations where the parent's greater knowledge or physical strength is relevant.

Social Models and Companion Animals

Fiske (1991, 1992) himself has little to say about how far his theory might generalise to the animal kingdom, but evidence exists that nonhuman animal species may be predisposed to engage in social behaviours that conform to particular social models. That is, at least some of the social models seem to extend to animal species beyond humans. For example, communal sharing behaviours are witnessed in many species, ranging from filial attachment in sheep (Val-Laillet, Meurisse, Tillet, & Nowak, 2009), rodents (Hennessy, Schiml-Webb, & Deak, 2009), and monkeys (Harlow & Zimmerman, 1959) to romantic partnerships in monogamous vole species (Young, Liu, & Wang, 2008). There is a burgeoning literature on commonalities in the neuroanatomical and neurochemical mechanisms associated with maternal love, romantic love and long-term attachment (Dunbar, 2010; Stein & Vythilingum, 2009) and the role of social touch and grooming in maintaining long-term relationships in primates (Dunbar, 2010). Authority ranking behaviours are observed in the dominance hierarchies of many bird and mammal species, where dominant individuals have better access to resources and greater responsibility for decision making. Interestingly, Fedurek and Dunbar (2009) observe a distinction between unidirectional grooming in chimpanzees, associated with inequalities of rank, and bidirectional grooming patterns, associated with enduring relationships with relatives and chimpanzees who live in close proximity. It is not entirely clear from the literature whether "bidirectional" or "equitable" grooming (Mitani, 2009) is consistent with a communal sharing model versus an equality matching model. The deciding factor would be the extent to which animals keep track of whose turn it is to groom whom. Of all the social models, the only one that appears to be exclusively human is market pricing.

This opens up several ways in which Fiske's social models could apply to human–animal relationships. First, humans could simply impose a social model on their relationship with a companion animal without the animal reciprocating.

This would be a case of anthropomorphism. A second possibility is that humans and their companion animals may mutually apply a particular social model to their relationship. This would require both parties to engage socially with the other and to converge upon a common social model. Third, both humans and animals might apply a social model to their relationship but not apply the same model; for example, one party might wish for a communal sharing relationship while the other expects an authority ranking relationship. In this situation, the relationship could be considered genuinely social, but the resulting human–animal interactions may not be harmonious. Finally, it is possible that humans and companion animals interact only asocially or in null relationships, essentially treating each other as a means to an end, or only as physical objects. This would be the most parsimonious default assumption.

Identifying Signs of Social Models in Human–Animal Relationships

According to Fiske (1992), it is possible to identify which of the models a person is applying to a relationship by examining the features of interactions that are salient to them, their intentions and expectations about it, the emotions they experience in relation to it, and their moral judgements about it. Empirically, researchers have not yet sought directly to investigate which social models (if any) humans apply to their relationships with their companion animals, or which aspects of human–animal relationships commonly conform to which model. Nevertheless, the existing data do provide some preliminary evidence for the relevance of some of the models.

It is worth noting that the communal sharing model is implicit in the word *companion* (from Latin *cum* meaning "with" or "together" and *panis* meaning "bread"—someone with whom one shares one's bread). To the extent that an animal shares food and shelter with a human, the chances of them engaging in a communal sharing relationship might be expected to increase. Similarly, actively seeking out physical contact with each other, distress at separation and joy at reunion would all be signs of a communal sharing relationship. A number of objective animal care behaviours that suggest a communal sharing model—free access to the house, sleeping inside, inclusion in family events, taking the animal on trips —are more frequent among owners with stronger pet attachment (Shore, Douglas, & Riley, 2010), although it should be noted that numerous other care behaviours that are not specific signs of communal sharing, such as walking the dog, also increase with reported attachment strength. It has also been reported that oxytocin, one of the neuropeptides believed to have a role in maternal and romantic partner bonding, increases significantly in female dog owners as a result of interacting with their dog after being separated from it, but not in male dog owners (Miller et al., 2009). This would be consistent with females being more likely than males to hold a communal sharing relationship with their dog, which would also link to their commonly reported stronger average attachment to their companion animal (Johnson et al., 1992) and greater average distress at the animal's death (Planchon & Templer, 1996).

Some of the qualitative responses from Davis et al. (2003) interviews with bereaved animal owners can also be interpreted as indicative of a communal sharing relationship. Objects associated with the animal took on a special significance. For example, one woman reported sitting on the cat's chair and crying herself to sleep for the first week after the cat died. Many reported that toys, food bowls and leashes of deceased animals were upsetting to them, that the house they had shared with the animal seemed "dead" without it. Loss of ritual activities with their animal was also a reported source of distress. Decisions about how to dispose of the animal's body also frequently revolved around communal sharing issues: either the desire to keep the animal's remains somewhere close or else to bury the animal in a place that was special to it while it lived. Idealising of the relationship as eternal was also relatively common: More than half of the sample believed that their animal had an afterlife, and a substantial minority still felt that they were in touch with the animal. When questioned on their beliefs about an afterlife, respondents frequently engaged communal sharing reasoning, either stating that animals fell into the same category as people, and therefore had an afterlife, or else that they fell into a different category and did not live on. Similarly, discussion of the issue of euthanasia sometimes elicited the response that owners chose euthanasia for their animal on the grounds that they would have done the same for themselves if they were in the animal's situation. Notwithstanding the signs of communal sharing evident in some pet owners, it should be noted that the human–animal partnership is far more arbitrary than the typical communal sharing relationship, which frequently represents a group that the individual is born into (Fiske, 1992). From this perspective, we would not expect it to be extremely common as the dominant model in human–animal relations, and we would expect people outside the relationship to question its legitimacy.

Authority ranking is also evident in human–animal relationships, most obviously where humans seek to control the behaviour of their animals through commands, rewards and punishments, where owners value obedience in their animal, where the animal is fed leftovers from the human's meal, where it has only restricted access to the house or yard, and where it is considered acceptable for the animal to be physically chastised by the human but not for the animal to hurt the human. Despite the clear relevance of authority ranking to pet ownership, research on the human–animal bond has tended to neglect this model as a meaningful relationship. Some comments around whether religion helped in coping with animal death tapped into an authority ranking model. Sometimes this was helpful: accepting that the animal belonged to God and that God took the animal when He was ready, but other times it was not: questioning why God would so cruelly take the animal from them (Davis et al., 2003).

There is less readily available evidence of people applying equality matching or market pricing models to their animals. One anecdotal example of an equality matching model comes from a young man who was driving around outback Australia with his dog. He described to the author how he had saved his dog's life once from floodwaters, and the dog had saved his life once when he found himself in a fight with a group of people at a remote tavern, so they were "even". An equality matching model may also apply when humans and animals engage in turn-taking play behaviours. It is possible that owners apply a market pricing model to working animals. Given, however, that even higher primates do not develop the necessary cognitive abilities to understand ratios and proportions, it seems unlikely that such a model would be mutual.

As well as evidence for social model use in human–animal relationships, it is likely that some owners engage in asocial or null relationships with their animals. For example, where a dog is primarily kept for home security purposes rather than companionship, this would represent an asocial relationship. Equally, where owners do not engage in interactions with their companion animal, either ignoring it completely or treating it as an object that requires some basic maintenance, this would be consistent with a null relationship. We might expect this to be more common among animals that are themselves less socially evolved and that do not provide their owners with social cues. It might also be more common among owners who do not choose to participate in pet-related surveys.

It bears reiterating that people do not consistently apply exactly the same social model to a human–human relationship in all situations and at all times, and we should not expect to find perfect consistency in human–animal relationships either. It is quite possible that any particular human–animal partnership is sometimes characterised by communal sharing principles, authority ranking at other times and a null relationship at others. Nevertheless, understanding which models are *ever* applied to the relationship and which models are *usually* applied to the relationship may help us to understand the variation in human responses when their companion animal dies, the issues that arise for them, and what is likely to help them through this transition if it is difficult.

Implications for Coping with Grief

In trying to understand the nature of a grief response, the social models could allow us to identify what exactly the grieving person has lost. If communal sharing was a person's dominant model of interaction with their companion animal, they would be at risk of emotional devastation by its loss. They would be likely to have identified strongly with the terminal suffering of their animal. The physical loss of contact with the animal would be distressing, as would be the loss of ritual interactions with it. They would have lost a source of intimacy, belonging and acceptance. They would have lost a recipient of their kindness. They may feel that that they have lost a part of themselves. It is likely that people who suffer an extreme grief response understand their relationship with their pet in communal sharing terms.

We might expect that human rituals and beliefs surrounding death would be helpful to a person who had a communal sharing relationship with their companion animal. They would likely see their relationship as ongoing, not something to forget about and move on, and if their belief system includes an eternal afterlife, it would likely apply to their animal. The animal's possessions would be likely to hold special significance and treating them with respect would be important to such an owner. We would also expect the grief process to take an extended period of time for such people, if their relationship with their animal was an important component of their own identity.

Less of a grief response would be expected from people in predominantly authority ranking relationships with their animal. They would be expected to identify with the animal less than the communal sharing owner. Nevertheless, the authority ranking relationship may still represent a significant loss to the owner. In particular, they may have lost a loyal follower who responded to their commands with obedience and implicit trust. They may have lost a source of status and authority. The needs of a bereaved authority ranking owner may be somewhat different from the communal sharing owner. It may be particularly important for them to feel that the death of their animal was not due to their failings as its protector and that their decision-making regarding the animal was sound.

Losing an equality matching relationship with an animal might equate to losing a nonintimate friend or playmate. Grief would probably not be extreme, but people may feel the loss of someone "like them." If their equality matching interactions took place in a play context, they may have lost an important source of fun. For the owner in an asocial or null relationship with their animal, grief is unlikely to be extreme. The benefits that the animal brought are likely to be easily replaced by a new animal.

One likely significant background factor is the number and type of other relationships the owner has either with humans or other animals. Regarding communal sharing, the data that show increased risk of extreme grief responses to animal death among childless people, and people who live alone (Field et al., 2009), suggest that a deficit of communal sharing relationships in one's life may make the loss of communal sharing relationship with an animal particularly difficult. The findings that females may be more prone to extreme grief than males may be due to them more readily entering into a mother–infant communal sharing relationship with an animal. Similarly, people who lack authority ranking relationships in their life, or whose social ranking is low in their existing relationships, might be expected to suffer more at the loss of an authority ranking relationship with their animal. Especially in Western societies where authority ranking relationships tend to be frowned upon, they may be deprived of the self-worth that comes from being a trusted leader.

Euthanasia also takes on different significance when viewed from a social model's perspective. While it is likely to be completely unproblematic when human–animal relationships are asocial or null, it raises several different issues within the social models. A person in an authority ranking relationship is likely to feel that he or she has the right to end the life of an animal in his or her care, but may feel that it is inconsistent with being a beneficent owner. In contrast, a person in a communal sharing relationship would be likely to have major difficulties with the issue and may well be torn between bringing about the death of a part of themselves and suffering along with the animal to the end of its natural life. Equality matching relationships may face a similar dilemma: If you have the animal euthanised, the act that would bring you back into equality is your own death. In each case, an owner's clear belief that it is (or is not) morally acceptable to end suffering including one's own would likely simplify the decision.

A social model approach makes sense of disenfranchised grief (Doka, 1989) that may be experienced by bereaved animal owners. Quite simply, if the feelings that a person experiences due to the demise of a relationship are consistent with the social model that they applied to that relationship, but that the application of that social model (or indeed *any* social model) to that relationship is not culturally acceptable or not legitimated by the people around him or her, disenfranchised grief is the likely outcome. From this perspective, belonging to a religion that teaches the oneness of all living things is likely to be protective of bereaved owners whose communal sharing relationship with their animal is consistent with this. Religions, such as those in the Judaeo-Christian tradition, that explicitly classify animals as distinct from humans may be problematic for a member who accepts the communal sharing teachings directed at humans, but extends them to a companion animal in a way that is not sanctioned by religious authorities, especially if religious group membership is an important part of the owner's self-concept. At a more local level, if friends and family members have an asocial or null orientation towards animals, they are unlikely to accept a bereaved owner's communal sharing response as legitimate.

Others who hold an authority ranking orientation towards animals may sympathise to some extent with a communal sharing grief response, as they would at least be ready to acknowledge that a socially meaningful relationship has been lost, rather than just an object. Nevertheless, it would be difficult to reconcile an authority ranking model with the extent of the communal sharing owner's distress. Authority ranking owners may be less likely to experience disenfranchised grief than communal sharing owners, as the distinction between an animal as an object and an animal as a lower-status partner in a social relationship is more subtle. Nevertheless, others who do not class animals as social beings may be inclined to ridicule a person who derives feelings of responsibility and authority from an animal.

Conclusions and Questions for Future Research

The foregoing discussion has endeavoured to interpret some of the existing literature on individual differences in grief response at the loss of a companion animal in terms of Fiske's (1992) theory of social models and to show how the theory might give a more comprehensive account of the range of human–animal relationships. While interpreting findings after the fact is a useful first step, further research is necessary to test a priori predictions of the theoretical framework. An important next step would be to design measurement instruments to assess the extent to which people apply the different social models to human–animal relationships. Several measures of human–companion animal attachment have been developed, such as The Companion Animal Bonding Scale (Poresky, Hendrix, Mosier, & Samuelson, 1987) and, more recently, the Lexington Attachment to Pets Scale (LAPS; Johnson et al., 1992). Viewed from a social model's perspective, the items on such measures tend to focus on communal sharing relations, or to be possible signs of more than one model. Some of the items on the LAPS, intended to quantify low levels of attachment, would be relevant to an asocial orientation. Interestingly, one of the three orthogonal factors to emerge from the LAPS items, labelled "animal rights/animal welfare," may be relevant to the authority ranking model. Nevertheless, while existing item pools might provide a starting point for an assessment of the application of social models to pet relationships, new items would certainly be needed to fully assess and disambiguate the models. Items might be adapted from Haslam and Fiske's (1999) questionnaire assessing human relationships.

Most obviously, an important research question would be whether the nature and extent of the owner's grief response to the loss of their companion animal is predictable from the social model that they applied to the relationship while the animal lived. The usefulness of the social model approach could be evaluated in terms of how well different avowed social models discriminated between grief responses and issues of concern. A more subtle issue to examine would be the range of models that applied to the human–animal relationship and whether the best predictor of distress is the *dominant* model, or the *mere presence* of a particular model in the range.

Future research may also seek to clarify whether specific gaps in one's human social model repertoire predict which model(s) an owner applies to his or her relationship with a companion animal and whether greater grief is associated with loss of a scarce model. This compensation model could be contrasted with a trait model, that certain individuals have a consistent preference for certain social model types over other types and tend to apply them broadly, putting some individuals at increased risk of extreme grief responses to deaths in general.

Another research question arising from the social model approach would be the extent to which humans and their companion animals *mutually* converge upon a model for interaction versus failing to agree on which model is appropriate, or only one party behaving as though any social model applies. This question would call for some ingenuity in measuring behaviours indicative of the animal's adherence to a particular social model, but it would pave the way to distinguishing between pathological grief arising from loss of a relationship based largely in wishful thinking and the extreme grief that is the natural response to the loss of a genuinely social, objectively observable relationship between human and companion animal.

References

Ainsworth, M., Blehar, M. C., Waters, E., & Wall, S. (1978). *Patterns of attachment: A psychological study of the strange situation*. Hillsdale, NJ: Erlbaum.

Archer, J., & Winchester, G. (1994). Bereavement following the death of a pet. *British Journal of Psychology, 85*(2), 259–271.

Bartholomew, K., & Horowitz, L. (1991). Attachment styles among young adults: A test of a four-category model. *Journal of Personality and Social Psychology, 61*(2), 226–244.

Beck, L., & Madresh, E. A. (2008). Romantic partners and four-legged friends: An extension of attachment theory to relationships with pets. *Anthrozoös, 21*(1), 43–56. doi: 10.2752/089279308X274056

Davis, H., Irwin, P., Richardson, M., & O'Brien-Malone, A. (2003). When a pet dies: Religious issues, euthanasia and strategies for coping with bereavement. *Anthrozoös, 16*(1), 57–74.

Diener, E., Suh, E. M., Lucas, R. E., & Smith, H. L. (1999). Subjective well-being: Three decades of progress. *Psychological Bulletin, 125*(2), 276–302.

Doka, K. J. (1989). Disenfranchised grief. In K. J. Doka (Ed.), *Disenfranchised grief: Recognising hidden sorrow* (pp. 3–11). Lexington, MA: Lexington.

Dunbar, R. I. M. (2010). The social role of touch in humans and primates: Behavioural function and neurobiological mechanisms. *Neuroscience and Biobehavioral Reviews, 34*, 260–268. doi: 10.1016/j.neubiorev.2008.07.001

Fedurek, P., & Dunbar, R. I. M. (2009). What does mutual grooming tell us about why chimpanzees groom? *Ethology, 115*(6), 566–575. doi: 10.1111/j.1439-0310.2009.01637.x

Field, N. P., Orsini, L., Gavish, R., & Packman, W. (2009). Role of attachment in response to pet loss. *Death Studies, 33*(4), 334–355. doi: 10.1080/07481180802705783

Fiske, A. P. (1991). *Structures of social life: The four elementary forms of human relations.* New York: Free Press.

Fiske, A. P. (1992). The four elementary forms of sociality: Framework for a unified theory of social relations. *Psychological Review, 99*(4), 689–723.

Forbes, A., & Roger, D. (1999). Stress, social support and fear of disclosure. *British Journal of Health Psychology, 4*(2), 165–179.

Gerwolls, M. K., & Labott, S. M. (1994). Adjustment to the death of a companion animal. *Anthrozoös, 7*(3), 172–187.

Gosse, G. H., & Barnes, M. J. (1994). Human grief resulting from the death of a pet. *Anthrozoös, 7*(2), 103–112.

Harlow, H. F., & Zimmerman, R. (1959). Affectional responses in the infant monkey. *Science, 130*(3373), 421–432.

Haslam, N., & Fiske, A. P. (1999). Relational models theory: A confirmatory factor analysis. *Personal Relationships, 6*(2), 241–250.

Hennessy, M. B., Schiml-Webb, P. A., & Deak, T. (2009). Separation, sickness, and depression: A new perspective on an old animal model. *Current Directions in Psychological Science, 18*(4), 227–231. doi: 10.1111/j.1467-8721.2009.01641.x

John, O. P., & Gross, J. J. (2007). Individual differences in emotion regulation. In J. J. Gross (Ed.), *Handbook of emotion regulation* (pp. 351–372). New York: Guildford.

Johnson, T. P., Garrity, T. F., & Stallones, L. (1992). Psychometric evaluation of the Lexington attachment to pets scale (LAPS). *Anthrozoös, 5*(3), 160–175.

Keddie, K. M. G. (1977). Pathological mourning after the death of a dog. *British Journal of Psychiatry, 131*, 21–25.

Kobak, R. (2009). Defining and measuring attachment bonds: Comment on Kurdek (2009). *Journal of Family Psychology, 23*, 447–449. doi: 10.1037/a0015213

Kübler-Ross, E. (1969). *On death and dying.* New York: Macmillan.

Kurdek, L. A. (2008). Pet dogs as attachment figures. *Journal of Social and Personal Relationships, 25*, 247–266. doi: 10.1177/0265407507087958

Kurdek, L. A. (2009). Pet dogs as attachment figures for adult owners. *Journal of Family Psychology, 23*, 439–446. doi: 10.1037/a0014979

Luiz Adrian, J. A., Deliramich, A. N., & Frueh, B. C. (2009). Complicated grief and posttraumatic stress disorder in humans' response to the death of pets/animals. *Bulletin of the Menninger Clinic, 73*(3), 176–187. doi: 10.1521/bumc.2009.73.3.176

McCutcheon, K. A., & Fleming, S. J. (2001). Grief resulting from euthanasia and natural death of companion animals. *Journal of Death and Dying, 44*(2), 169–188.

Mikulincer, M., & Shaver, P. R. (2003). Attachment theory and affect regulation: The dynamics, development, and cognitive consequences of attachment-related strategies. *Motivation and Emotion, 27*(2), 77–102. doi: 10.1023/A:1024515519160

Miller, S. C., Kennedy, C., DeVoe, D., Hickey, M., Nelson, T., & Kogan, L. (2009). An examination of changes in oxytocin levels in men and women before and after interaction with a bonded dog. *Anthrozoös, 22*(1), 31–42. doi: 10.2752/175303708X390455

Mitani, J. C. (2009). Male chimpanzees form enduring and equitable social bonds. *Animal Behaviour, 77*(3), 633–640. doi: 10.1016/j.anbehav.2008.11.021

Parkes, C. M. (1971). Psychosocial transitions: A field for study. *Social Science and Medicine, 5*(2), 101–115.

Planchon, L. A., & Templer, D. I. (1996). The correlates of grief after death of pet. *Anthrozoös, 9*(2–3), 107–113.

Planchon, L. A., Templer, D. I., Stokes, S., & Keller, J. (2002). Death of a companion cat or dog and human bereavement: Psychosocial variables. *Society and Animals, 10*(1), 93–105.

Poresky, R. H., Hendrix, C., Mosier, J. E., & Samuelson, M. L. (1987). The companion animal bonding scale: Internal reliability and construct validity. *Psychological Reports, 60*(1), 743–746.

Quackenbush, J., & Glickman, L. (1983). Social services for bereaved pet owners: A retrospective case study in a veterinary teaching hospital. In A. H. Katcher & A. M. Beck (Eds.), *New perspectives on our lives with companion animals* (pp. 377–389). Philadelphia: University of Pennsylvania.

Sanders, C. M. (1988). Risk factors in bereavement outcome. *Journal of Social Issues, 44*(3), 97–111.

Shore, E. R., Douglas, D. K., & Riley, M. L. (2010). What's in it for the companion animal? Pet attachment and college students' behaviors toward pets. *Journal of Applied Animal Welfare Science, 8*(1), 1–11. doi: 10.1207/s15327604jaws0801_1

Stallones, L. (1994). Pet loss and mental health. *Anthrozoös, 7*(1), 43–54.

Stein, D. J., & Vythilingum, B. (2009). Love and attachment: The psychobiology of social bonding. *CNS Spectrums, 14*, 239–242. Retrieved May 29, 2010, from http://www.cnsspectrums.com/aspx/articledetail.aspx?articleid=2074

Turner, W. G. (1997). Evaluation of a pet loss support line. *Anthrozoös, 10*(4), 225–229.

Val-Laillet, D., Meurisse, M., Tillet, Y., & Nowak, R. (2009). Behavioural and neurobiological effects of colostrum ingestion in the newborn lamb associated with filial bonding. *European Journal of Neuroscience, 30*(4), 639–650. doi: 10.1111/j.1460-9568.2009.06845.x

Weisman, A. D. (1990). Bereavement and companion animals. *Omega, 22*(4), 241–248.

Williams, S., & Mills, J. N. (2000). Understanding and responding to grief in companion animal practice. *Australian Veterinary Practitioner, 30*(2), 55–62.

Young, K. A., Liu, Y., & Wang, Z. X. (2008). The neurobiology of social attachment: A comparative approach to behavioral, neuroanatomical, and neurochemical studies. *Comparative Biochemistry and Physiology Part C: Toxicology and Pharmacology, 148*, 401–410.

Part IV
Animal Rights, Abuse, and Neglect

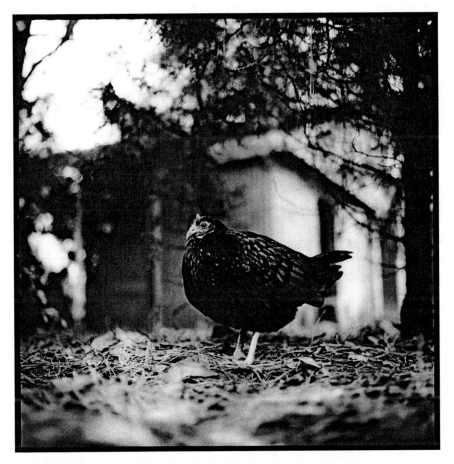

Kaola, Resident of United Poultry Concerns.
Kaola was rescued from a cockfighting operation and has lived at UPC for 11 years.

Chapter 14
A Triad of Family Violence: Examining Overlap in the Abuse of Children, Partners, and Pets

Sarah DeGue

Theoretical and Empirical Links Between the Abuse of Children, Partners, and Pets

The relationship between cruelty to animals and the abuse of women and children has been informally recognized throughout history (Ascione & Arkow, 1999). A folk proverb advised, "A woman, a horse, and a hickory tree; The more you beat 'em, the better they be" (cited in Adams, 1995). Similarly, George Cannon, leader of the Church of Latter Day Saints in the 1890s, warned, "Young ladies, never put yourself in the power or under the control of young men who treat their animals badly, for if you become their wives, they will abuse you" (cited in Quinlisk, 1999). More recently, popular belief in a link between animal- and human-directed violence has been codified in state legislation establishing cross-reporting systems that permit or require animal cruelty and child welfare investigators to refer families to parallel agencies for investigation (Long, Long, & Kulkarni, 2007). Such laws are based on the assumption that families experiencing one form of violence victimization will be at an increased risk for other forms of violence (DeGue & DiLillo, 2009). Additionally, several states have implemented laws permitting the inclusion of pets in protection orders for intimate partner violence (DeGue & DiLillo, 2009). Recognition of a link between the abuse of children, partners, and pets is also evident in the field. For instance, there has been increasing demand for the cross-training of veterinarians, animal and child welfare workers, and domestic violence shelter staff on issues of family violence or animal abuse in order to promote interagency communication and collaboration in the prevention of all forms of violence (Onyskiw, 2007). In addition, advocates have worked to increase the availability of animal housing for women seeking shelter from abusive partners who may be afraid to

The findings and conclusions in this report are those of the authors and do not necessarily represent the official position of the Centers for Disease Control and Prevention.

S. DeGue (✉)
Centers for Disease Control and Prevention, Atlanta, GA, USA
e-mail: sdegue@cdc.gov

C. Blazina et al. (eds.), *The Psychology of the Human–Animal Bond*,
DOI 10.1007/978-1-4419-9761-6_14, © Springer Science+Business Media, LLC 2011

leave their pet behind (American Humane Association, 2010; Kogan, McConnell, Schoenfeld-Tacher, & Jansen-Lock, 2004).

This progression from popular and anecdotal support for the link between animal abuse and family violence to tangible changes in policy and practice has been facilitated by a growing research base in this area over the past 30 years. Although still limited relative to the much larger scientific literature amassed during the same period on the predictors, correlates, and outcomes of child maltreatment and intimate partner violence (IPV), a compelling picture of the overlap in violence against children, partners and pets in the home is emerging. This chapter provides an overview of current knowledge regarding the extent and nature of this overlap, discusses possible explanations for the exposure of family members (human and nonhuman) to multiple types of violence victimization, and highlights potential implications for prevention and early intervention.

A Triad of Family Violence?

A substantial body of research suggests that child maltreatment and IPV[1] commonly co-occur within a family (e.g., Appel & Holden, 1998; Higgins & McCabe, 2000; Saunders, 2003; Slep & O'Leary, 2005). Although rates of overlap reported in the literature vary significantly by sample, methodology, and definitions of abuse, there is consistent evidence that the presence of one form of family violence in a home significantly increases the risk for other forms (Knickerbocker, Heyman, Slep, Jouriles, & McDonald, 2007). A smaller body of work, reviewed here, suggests that this pattern of co-occurring violence may extend to another set of vulnerable family members—pets. Indeed, citing evidence that the vast majority of pet owners view their animals as "members of the family," some authors have argued that the abuse of companion animals should be considered another form of family violence (Hutton, 1983; Lacroix, 1999).

Multiple mechanisms may account for the co-occurrence of animal cruelty and family violence in a home. For example, in some families, one perpetrator may be responsible for all of the violence experienced by family members. That is, a parent may engage in abuse of pets as well as aggression toward their partner or child. Alternatively, animal abuse may be perpetrated by a child or adult who is himself or herself a victim of family violence. For instance, a maltreated child may perpetrate animal abuse as a result of his or her own exposure to violence in the home through the development of emotional and behavioral difficulties or a process of

---

[1] The Centers for Disease Control and Prevention (CDC) defines *child maltreatment* as any act of commission or omission by a parent or other caregiver that result in harm, potential for harm, or threat of harm to a child, including child physical abuse, sexual abuse, psychological abuse, or neglect (Leeb, Paulozzi, Melanson, Simon, & Arias, 2007). *Intimate partner violence* (IPV) is defined by CDC as physical, sexual, or psychological harm, or threats of harm, by a current or former partner or spouse (Saltzman, Fanslow, McMahon, & Shelley, 2002). Definitions and measures of child maltreatment and IPV vary across the studies reviewed here. When possible, substantial deviations from these definitions are noted.

social learning. Finally, it is possible that animal abuse may occur within a dysfunctional and violent family context in which multiple family members engage in aggressive behavior toward each other, and animals become another intentional or unintentional victim. Of course, it is possible that different patterns of co-occurring animal and family violence exist in different families (e.g., with adult vs. child animal abusers) or that multiple mechanisms may be active within the same family. Each of these potential explanations and their application to the existing literature is discussed in depth below. First, I review current knowledge regarding the extent and nature of the overlap between violence toward children, partners, and pets in order to identify patterns of co-occurring violence and illuminate potential points for prevention or intervention.

Intimate partner violence and animal abuse. Much of the existing evidence regarding the co-occurrence of IPV and animal abuse is derived from surveys of women[2] seeking services from domestic violence shelters. For example, four studies using small samples of pet-owning women in shelters found that between 46.5 and 71% of respondents reported that their partner had threatened, harmed, or killed their pet (Ascione, 1998; Carlisle-Frank, Frank, & Nielsen, 2004; Faver & Strand, 2003; Flynn, 2000). Although the proportion of women in shelters who own pets or had a pet during the course of their current abusive relationship varies across studies, they represent a substantial portion of women seeking services for IPV (e.g., 40.2%, Flynn, 2000; 74%, Ascione, 1998). A somewhat lower rate of partner animal abuse was identified in a recent study of primarily Hispanic pet-owning women seeking services from two domestic violence programs in Texas near the US–Mexico border (Faver & Cavazos, 2007). In this study, with a larger sample, more than one out of three abused women (36%) indicated that their partner had threatened, injured, or killed an animal. Although these studies suggest that exposure to animal abuse may be common among women seeking shelter from an abusive partner, the lack of a nonabused comparison group makes it difficult to generalize and interpret these findings.

Using a much larger sample ($N = 1,283$) of women seeking services at an urban domestic violence shelter in Texas, Simmons and Lehmann (2007) found that only 25% of the sample reported that their partner had engaged in some type of pet abuse, including threats or harm to a companion animal. However, women who reported that their partners threatened or perpetrated animal cruelty were significantly more likely to report multiple forms of co-occurring partner violence, including sexual violence, emotional abuse, and stalking, compared to women who did not report pet

---

[2]Intimate partner violence (IPV) is perpetrated by and against both male and female partners. Indeed, there is evidence to suggest that a proportion of the partner violence that occurs is reciprocal (Kelly & Johnson, 2008). Also, IPV can and does occur in the context of same-sex relationships (Tjaden & Thoennes, 2000). However, due to the nature of the existing literature in this area, which focuses heavily on female victims of male perpetrators in domestic violence shelters, women are sometimes referred to in this chapter as the primary victims of violence within the home. Male victims of IPV may also be exposed to animal abuse perpetrated by their male or female partners. Additional research is needed to examine the experiences of male IPV victims.

abuse by their partner. Because almost all women in this study (>90%) had experienced physical partner violence, animal cruelty was not significantly related to the presence of this primary form of partner abuse. Furthermore, women in this study reported that male perpetrators who abused pets had used more forms of violence against their partners and engaged in more controlling behaviors than abusive men who did not abuse animals. Although this study was also limited by its lack of a comparison group, these findings suggest that animal cruelty in the context of IPV may be associated with a particularly high-risk relationship—at least among women in shelter settings.

Three recent studies provide additional information about the relative rate of exposure to animal cruelty for abused and nonabused women. Ascione et al. (2007) compared the reports of women in domestic violence shelters with a nonabused community sample and found that IPV victims seeking shelter were 11 times more likely to report that their partner had hurt or killed a pet (54% vs. 5%) and four times more likely to indicate that their partner had threatened a pet (52.5% vs. 12.5%) than the comparison group. In the same study, Ascione and colleagues found that scores on the Minor Physical Violence and Verbal Aggression subscales of the Conflict Tactics Scale (CTS; Straus, 1979) were the strongest predictors of *threats* toward pets, whereas the Severe Physical Violence subscale best predicted *actual harm or killing* of animals by a partner. These findings suggest that the severity of partner-perpetrated animal cruelty may increase as a function of the increasing the severity of IPV. A similar study compared Australian women seeking domestic violence services with a non-abused comparison group and found significantly higher rates of partner animal abuse (52.9% vs. 0%) or threats toward animals (46% vs. 5.8%) in the abused sample (Volant, Johnson, Gullone, & Coleman, 2008). Further, using the full sample, women who reported partner animal cruelty were five times more likely to be a victim of IPV than women who did not witness partner animal abuse.

Although the use of comparison samples in these recent studies provides important normative data that suggest abused women are at an increased risk for exposure to animal cruelty, women in shelters are not representative of the larger population of women or men in violent relationships (Kelly & Johnson, 2008). Kelly and Johnson (2008) highlight critical differences in IPV data originating from clinical samples (e.g., women's shelters, courts, police, or hospital sources) versus IPV data from community or national samples, pointing to evidence that the violence observed across these various settings and samples may have different patterns and etiologies. Importantly, these authors differentiate between two subtypes of IPV: *coercive controlling violence*, in which a pattern of emotional abuse, intimidation, coercion, and control accompanies physical violence by one partner (typically, the male partner) toward the other; and *situational couple violence*, which is not based in a pattern of coercive control and in which both partners engage in often less severe, bidirectional physical aggression. Johnson (2006) found that while IPV identified in a community sample consisted of 89% situational couple violence and 11% coercive controlling violence, the opposite pattern was identified in a shelter sample. Instead, in the shelter sample, 79% of the violence could be considered coercive controlling violence and only 19% constituted situational couple violence. Given evidence that these two forms of IPV vary significantly in their etiology, patterns, correlates, and consequences (Kelly & Johnson, 2008), it is reasonable to assume that the role of animal abuse in the context of these forms of IPV may vary as well.

Two studies have examined the link between animal abuse and IPV with nonshelter samples. In one large case-control study, researchers interviewed women from 11 US cities who had survived an attempted homicide by an intimate partner or the proxies of nonsurvivors (e.g., mother, sisters) and compared them with a randomly selected control group of community women in order to identify risk factors for severe IPV and IPV-related injury (Walton-Moss, Manganello, Frye, & Campbell, 2005). Multivariate analyses, including several sociodemographic and behavioral characteristics of the victim and perpetrator, identified the threat or actual abuse of a pet as one of five significant predictors of IPV perpetration. Other perpetrator-specific risk factors identified included not being a high school graduate, women's perception of the partner's mental health as fair or poor, and women's perception that the partner had an alcohol problem or a drug abuse problem. Of those risk factors identified, partner pet abuse had the largest effect on risk for IPV, with an adjusted odds ratio indicating that women who reported partner pet abuse were 7.59 times more likely to be victims of severe IPV than women whose partners did not abuse animals. Although this study did not use a shelter sample, the identification of cases from police and medical examiner records may have similar issues with respect to the representativeness of the sample. Like shelter samples, police, hospital, and court data may overrepresent cases of coercive controlling violence and underrepresent situational couple violence (Kelly & Johnson, 2008). However, this study may provide additional evidence, from a well-controlled study, of the role of animal abuse as a risk factor for severe partner violence marked by dynamics of power and control.

Finally, using retrospective reports of experiences with family violence and animal cruelty in a large, geographically diverse sample of US college students, DeGue and DiLillo (2009) found that 28.3% of respondents who witnessed parental violence while growing up were also exposed to animal abuse. When exposure was limited to severe parental violence, 33% of respondents reported some exposure to animal cruelty in their home. Further, in regression analyses, individuals who witnessed animal cruelty growing up were significantly more likely to have witnessed severe parental violence than those who did not. These findings suggest that IPV and animal cruelty also co-occur at relatively high rates in community samples. However, consistent with the studies reviewed above, animal cruelty may be more strongly associated with risk for more severe forms of IPV. It is notable that this study examined both witnessing and perpetration of animal cruelty by respondents. Thus, a portion of the overlap in IPV and animal cruelty exposure captured here can be accounted for by animal cruelty perpetrated by the respondent while growing up in a home marked by parental violence, rather than by an abusive adult. Perpetration of animal abuse by children exposed to family violence is discussed below.

Child maltreatment and animal abuse. Fewer studies have examined the overlap between animal cruelty and child maltreatment in a household, although existing studies provide initial evidence that these forms of family violence may also co-occur in many households. In one of the first studies in this area, DeViney, Dickert, and Lockwood (1983) examined 53 families involved in the child welfare system with substantiated cases of child maltreatment and found evidence of the concurrent abuse or neglect of a companion animal in 60% of these households. When the authors examined the type of maltreatment reported, they found that 88% of families with substantiated child physical abuse had existing records of companion animal abuse compared to 34% of families with either child sexual abuse or neglect. These findings suggest that the abuse of pets may be fairly common in families with substantiated reports of child maltreatment; however, animal cruelty may be more strongly linked to the presence of child physical abuse than other forms of maltreatment. Notably, studies examining the overlap of child maltreatment and animal cruelty have sometimes included any animal abuse perpetrated by a family member, including abuse by parents or children in the home. This is in contrast to much of the research described above in which IPV victims were asked specifically about animal abuse perpetrated by their partner. For example, in this study, although the majority of pet abuse reported was perpetrated by one or both parents, 14% of the animal cruelty involved a child perpetrator (DeViney et al., 1983).

A more recent study of Japanese children who were removed from their homes due to abuse or neglect indicated that these maltreated youth were significantly more likely to report witnessing animal abuse than a comparison group of elementary school children (44% vs. 23.8%; Yamazaki, 2010). The animal cruelty witnessed by maltreated children in this study was also significantly more severe, on average, than animal abuse witnessed by the comparison sample. However, like the studies of shelter and police samples described above, the inclusion of families involved in the child welfare system in this study and the previous one (DeViney et al., 1983) may have resulted in an oversampling of children and families with more severe or chronic histories of child maltreatment. Thus, these findings may not be representative of all families in which child abuse or neglect is present.

Miller and Knutson (1997) examined correlations between childhood exposure to animal abuse (witnessing or perpetrating) and retrospective reports of physical punishment and negative family home environment in two samples: inmates and college students. Results from both samples indicated significant correlations between animal cruelty exposure and being raised in a negative or physically punitive home environment; however, these correlations were small ($r = 0.12 - 0.28$). Because the measures used in this study captured indicators of family conflict and physical punishment, up to and including physical abuse but not including other forms of child maltreatment, the abusive experiences assessed in this study likely represent a lower level of severity, on average, than studies using official records of maltreatment (e.g., DeViney et al., 1983) or assessing the full range of maltreatment types using accepted definitions and thresholds (e.g., DeGue & DiLillo, 2009). The proportion of overlap between childhood exposure to animal abuse and child maltreatment was not provided in this study, but it is notable that general rates of animal cruelty exposure were high in both groups: 66% of inmates and 48.4% of college students reported witnessing and/or perpetrating animal abuse.

DeGue and DiLillo (2009) also asked a sample of college students to report retrospectively on their experiences with family violence and animal abuse in childhood. In this study, respondents with a history of childhood maltreatment (physical, sexual, or emotional abuse or neglect) were significantly more likely to report witnessing and/or perpetrating animal abuse than those who had no exposure to family violence (including child maltreatment or exposure to parental violence; 27.7% vs. 19.1%). Individuals with a history of childhood emotional abuse were 2.25 times more likely to have witnessed animal cruelty than their peers without a history of emotional abuse. However, other forms of child maltreatment, including physical abuse, sexual abuse, and neglect, were not significant predictors of witnessing animal abuse when other forms of family violence exposure (including parental violence) were controlled.

Together these findings suggest that animal cruelty is not uncommon among families with substantiated reports of abuse and child welfare involvement—indicators of severe maltreatment and lower overall family functioning. While there is also clear evidence of an overlap between animal- and child-directed violence in nonclinical samples, the rate of co-occurrence may be somewhat lower and proportional to the severity of abuse experienced. Thus, across samples, these findings suggest that when child maltreatment is more severe, co-occurring animal abuse may be more common. In some cases, the co-occurrence of child maltreatment and animal abuse in a home may be due to perpetration by children exposed to violence.

Animal cruelty by children exposed to family violence. Examining the perpetration of animal abuse by children exposed to IPV or child maltreatment widens the lens through which we view the overlap and etiological links between these forms of family violence. Research in this area has utilized multiple samples and methods to examine the overlap and potential links between family violence and child animal abuse. For instance, Duncan, Thomas, and Miller (2005) compared samples of conduct-disordered adolescent boys with and without a history of animal cruelty and found that the animal-abusing group was significantly more likely to report a history of physical and/or sexual abuse and exposure to domestic violence than the nonabusive group. Other studies have relied on maternal reports of family violence and child behavior, with child animal cruelty measured using an item on the Child Behavior Checklist (Achenbach, 1991). For instance, Currie (2005) found that mothers who reported that their children were exposed to IPV were almost three times more likely to report that their children had been cruel to animals than a matched sample of mothers who did not report IPV. Also, Ascione and colleagues found that a clinic-referred sample of children with a substantiated history of child sexual abuse were five times more likely to have a maternal report of animal cruelty than a comparison sample of nonabused children (Ascione, Friedrich, Heath, & Hayashi, 2003). However, it is notable that rates of animal cruelty in the sexually abused sample were similar to rates identified for a third sample of youth referred for psychiatric evaluation who had no history of sexual abuse, suggesting that the increased rate of animal cruelty observed in this study may be associated with the presence of emotional or behavioral disturbances rather than sexual abuse per se (Ascione et al., 2003).

Using a large, nonclinical sample of Italian youth (ages 9–17), Baldry (2003) found that individuals who engaged in animal cruelty were more likely to have witnessed animal cruelty perpetrated by their peers or parents, suggesting a link between witnessing and perpetrating animal cruelty. Youth exposed to parental violence were almost twice as likely as their nonexposed peers to report animal abuse perpetration and more than twice as likely to perpetrate animal abuse when the parental violence was severe. Exposure to animal abuse by peers and being male were the best predictors of animal cruelty in this study, followed by (in order of predictive value) maternal partner violence, maternal animal abuse, paternal partner violence, and being older. The use of a large, though nonrandom, sample of community adolescents and multivariate analyses in this study provides additional information about the strength of the relationship between animal abuse perpetration and IPV in the general population. Consistent with Baldry (2003), Thompson and Gullone (2006) reported that a history of witnessing animal abuse was associated with significantly higher levels of animal cruelty among adolescents, especially when the abuse was perpetrated by a family member or friend (vs. stranger) and when it was witnessed more frequently. These findings suggest that social learning may play a role in the abuse of animals by children, particularly when these behaviors are modeled by important figures in the child's life.

In a study of college students, DeGue and DiLillo (2009) found that 62.2% of those who retrospectively reported perpetrating childhood animal cruelty also reported exposure to at least one form of family violence (child maltreatment or IPV). Individuals who reported animal abuse were significantly more likely than nonperpetrators to report a history of sexual abuse, physical abuse, and neglect. Interestingly, no differences were identified for history of emotional abuse or exposure to IPV. It may be that these forms of abuse are more closely associated with witnessing animal abuse (perpetrated by another family member) than perpetration of animal abuse. Indeed, findings from the same study (as described above) suggest that emotional abuse and IPV were significantly associated with witnessing animal abuse as a child.

Finally, in contrast to other findings in this area, Dadds, Whiting, and Hawes (2006) examined a nonclinical sample of adolescent boys and found an association between animal cruelty and the presence of callous, unemotional personality traits, but did not identify a significant relationship between animal cruelty and a general measure of family conflict once these personality traits were accounted for. Similarly, Dadds, Whiting, Bunn, Fraser, and Charlson (2004) failed to find unique associations between measures of parenting behaviors (monitoring, positive parenting, inconsistent and extreme punishment) and childhood animal abuse, when controlling for other factors, using a large sample of Australian children. Null findings in these studies regarding the link between family violence and animal abuse may reflect differences in measurement; the family conflict and parenting measures utilized may capture less severe forms of aggression in the family than have been examined in other studies. If so, these findings would be consistent with other studies in which the presence of animal cruelty in a home was more strongly associated with severe forms of human-directed violence. Alternatively, the use of multifactorial models that account for child personality and behavior is unique to these studies and may suggest that the relationship between family violence and animal cruelty perpetration is mediated by other child-specific factors, such as the development of antisocial traits or conduct disorder.

Overall, these studies point to a significant relationship between childhood animal cruelty and exposure to family violence. However, the strength of this relationship may depend on the type and severity of violence experienced. In addition, although few studies have examined the role of potential mediators and moderators, it is possible that other factors such as the development of conduct disorder may account for this relationship. Nevertheless, the results of these investigations do suggest that when animal abuse at the hands of children is identified in a household, the likelihood that other forms of family violence are also present may increase.

Understanding the Overlap

There is substantial evidence to suggest that the co-occurrence of child maltreatment and IPV in a home is fairly common (Knickerbocker et al., 2007). For example, a recent study (Slep & O'Leary, 2005) using a representative sample of suburban families with at least one child found that 45% of respondents reported instances of both partner- and child-directed physical aggression in their household in the past year. Even when reports were limited to only severe physical aggression, one out of twenty families in this community sample reported experiencing severe violence towards both children and partners in the last 12 months. Studies of clinical samples, in which one form of serious violence was already identified, have also pointed to high rates of co-occurring family violence, with many studies identifying rates between 30 and 60% (Appel & Holden, 1998; Knickerbocker et al., 2007).

Several hypotheses have been proposed in the literature to account for the overlap between child maltreatment and IPV in some families (e.g., Appel & Holden, 1998; Knickerbocker et al., 2007). Given growing evidence that pet abuse may represent an additional form of co-occurring family violence, it is possible that one or more of these models may also explain the presence of animal cruelty in homes with concurrent child- and/or partner victimization. Thus, we briefly review several of these theories below, citing potential applications to co-occurring animal cruelty.

Shared risk factors. One hypothesis proposed to explain the overlap between child abuse and IPV in some homes surmises that these forms of violence perpetration may share common risk factors that increase the likelihood of either behavior (Knickerbocker et al., 2007; Slep & O'Leary, 2005). Such factors may include characteristics of the individual (e.g., personality traits, biological or psychological characteristics, historical risk factors), the environment or context (e.g., financial stress, low social support, child behavior problems), or dyadic factors (e.g., family role assignments, dysfunctional attributions for child and partner behavior; Knickerbocker et al., 2007). Although it is possible that shared environmental risk factors, for instance, might increase the risk of violence perpetration by multiple family members, this hypothesis is most commonly associated with the *single perpetrator* model, as described by Appel and Holden (1998), in which one family member (usually conceptualized as the male partner) is responsible for the abuse of other vulnerable family members, including female partners and children. This pattern of violence, involving only one aggressive partner, is also consistent with the coercive controlling violence subtype of IPV in which partner violence is unidirectional, often severe, and characterized by tactics of intimidation, coercion, and control (Kelly & Johnson, 2008).

One tactic that may be used to intimidate or control an intimate partner in the context of a coercive controlling relationship is harming or threatening to harm a companion animal. Indeed, as discussed above, female victims of coercive controlling violence, who represent the largest proportion of victims in shelter and police samples, report a very high prevalence of co-occurring animal cruelty. Abuse of pets is also listed as one possible tactic of intimidation on the Minnesota Power and Control Wheel, a conceptual model of IPV with limited empirical evidence but widespread clinical adoption among professionals and advocates working with victims and perpetrators in clinical settings (Dutton & Starzomski, 1997; Pence & Paymar, 1993). Further, some questionnaires and checklists designed to measure IPV have included items assessing animal abuse (e.g., Dutton, 1992; Renzetti, 1992; Straus, 1993).

Faver and Strand (2007) outline several ways in which an abuser may use threats or violence toward pets as a tactic to control and intimidate their partner. For example, they suggest that an abusive partner may injure or kill a pet to demonstrate power and convey to family members that no one is safe from the violence, perpetuating a context of terror. Animal abuse or the threat of animal abuse might also be used to incite fear in the partner to teach submission, prevent her from leaving, or to punish her after leaving. Killing a pet, who may represent a source of comfort or support to a victimized partner, may also serve to further isolate her from her network of support, maintaining exclusivity in the abusive relationship. The use of these tactics by perpetrators is also described by other authors and supported by both empirical evidence and anecdotal accounts (e.g., Onyskiw, 2007). Based on interviews with a large sample of abused women being evaluated at a community mental health center, Loring and colleagues found that some abusive partners may also threaten to harm or kill pets in order to coerce women into engaging in criminal behavior (Loring & Beaudoin, 2000; Loring & Bolden-Hines, 2004). Similar tactics or motives may explain the coexistence of animal abuse and child maltreatment in a single perpetrator context. For example, an abusive parent may threaten or harm a child's pets as a means of controlling their behavior, punishing them, or ensuring their silence about their own maltreatment (Adams, 1998; Davidson, 1998; Onyskiw, 2007). However, little work has been done to explore these hypotheses.

Shared risk factors for perpetration of IPV and child abuse have been well established (Knickerbocker et al., 2007), but we know less about whether these or other risk factors might also apply to co-occurring animal cruelty. McPhedran (2009) points to empathic deficits as one potential link between these behaviors, but cautions that there is not sufficient evidence to support empathy levels as a sole or primary driver of violent behavior. Instead, she argues that empathic traits likely interact with other experiences and characteristics (e.g., lack of prosocial parental behavior, childhood exposure to violence, antisocial traits) to produce a spectrum of aggressive behaviors, which may include both animal abuse and family violence. In another study, callousness was identified as a significant predictor of men's violence against both women and pets using a nonclinical, college sample (Gupta, 2008). In contrast, predictive models of IPV and animal abuse for female perpetrators identified unique, and not shared, predictors for each form of violence (Gupta, 2008). These findings suggest that while men's violence toward partners and pets may by rooted in underlying shared risk factors, these behaviors by women may have independent etiologies and be better explained by other models.

Overall, there is reason to believe that a model of shared risk factors, as proposed to explain coexisting IPV and child abuse, may also explain a portion of the overlap between animal abuse and other forms of family violence. Although shared risk factors may affect multiple members of a family, this hypothesis may be most consistent with co-occurring violence in the context of a single perpetrator model in which animal cruelty is used as a tactic of intimidation and control by an abusive adult. Thus, animal cruelty may most often manifest within a specific subset of family violence cases (e.g., coercive controlling violence) with a particular set of characteristics and risk factors. Indeed, the evidence suggests that prevalence estimates for animal abuse are highest in families with severe child and/or partner abuse (e.g., Ascione et al., 2007; DeGue & DiLillo, 2009; DeViney et al., 1983; Simmons & Lehmann, 2007; Walton-Moss et al., 2005). However, because animal abuse also co-occurs with child- or partner violence in homes that are not characterized by a single adult perpetrator or patterns of emotionally abusive intimidation and control, violence in other contexts may be better explained by additional hypotheses.

Violence begets violence. A second hypothesis posited to explain the overlap in IPV and child maltreatment suggests that the presence of one form of violence in the home may contribute directly to risk for the other (Knickerbocker et al., 2007). One common conceptualization of this hypothesis, referred to as the *spillover hypothesis* (Knickerbocker et al., 2007) or the *sequential perpetrator* model (Appel & Holden, 1998), is that male-to-female partner aggression results in female-to-child maltreatment. However, recent evidence provides little support for this theory, with regard to child and partner abuse, given that such households (with unidirectional partner violence and child abuse perpetrated by the victimized partner) constitute a very small proportion of those homes with co-occurring human-directed violence (Slep & O'Leary, 2005). However, it is not known whether this model might better explain animal abuse in a home. For instance, it is possible that victimized children or adults might act out their frustration or anger by abusing a pet. In the case of children, animal cruelty may be a learned behavior from their own exposure to violence and abuse in the home, including the witnessed abuse of pets (Ascione, 1998; DeGue & DiLillo, 2009). Further, it is possible that victimized adults in a household may not have the emotional or economic resources to provide the necessary care that their animals require (e.g., food, veterinary care, attention, training), resulting in neglect.

In addition to the possibility of victim-perpetrated animal abuse, the presence of one form of violence may also directly impact the perpetration of another form in other ways. With regard to child abuse and IPV, it has been suggested that child maltreatment by one parent may lead to partner conflict if the nonabusing parent disapproves; also, children may be injured unintentionally while caught in the middle or trying to intervene during parental conflicts (Knickerbocker et al., 2007). This pattern might also help explain the existence of animal abuse in a violent home. For instance, partners may argue about one partner's mistreatment of their animals, resulting in aggression or physical conflict. Pets may also be injured or killed during instances of physical aggression between partners, and children or pets may sustain injuries while caught in the crossfire or while trying to intervene on the other's behalf. Because the existing research has focused on single perpetrator contexts, little is known about whether these mechanisms might account for some portion of the overlapping violence between and among partners, children, and pets.

Multiple perpetrators. A third theory that has been proposed to explain the overlap between IPV and child abuse suggests that the co-occurrence of violence in a home may reflect a bidirectional or multidirectional pattern, in which both partners aggress against each other, one or both parents is aggressive toward the child or children, and the children engage in violence toward their parents. Appel and Holden (1998) describe the most severe model, in which both parents and children engage in reciprocal forms of violence, as one of *family dysfunction*. In this scenario, children's violence may be explained by one of several potential mechanisms (Appel & Holden, 1998). For instance, it may reflect involvement in a dysfunctional family system in which the parents and children all engage in behaviors that elicit conflict resulting in violence. It may also be explained by social cognitive theory, in which exposure to parental violence and the child's own abuse models and legitimizes their use of physical aggression. Alternatively, or in addition, this pattern of familial aggression may reflect a shared biological predisposition to violent behavior. It is possible that animal cruelty may also exist within this pattern of family dysfunction for some of the same reasons. For example, animals may represent just another potential victim in a home with multiple aggressive individuals and a pattern of violence against family members. The presence of several individuals with risk factors for violence perpetration in a home may increase the likelihood of a pet becoming an additional victim. Animals may also be abused directly by aggressive children in the home who have been exposed to multiple forms of violence, including parental violence, their own abuse, or parental violence toward the pets. These children may be re-creating abuse that they have witnessed or experienced, or violence toward pets may be a manifestation of externalizing behavior or callous unemotional tendencies resulting from their own maltreatment. In the same way that a child's externalizing behaviors may contribute to parental or parent–child conflict, it is also possible that pets, particularly dogs, in a dysfunctional home may become aggressive as a result of poor training, maltreatment, or intentional training to be aggressive. The pet's behavior may then elicit further violence from other family members in an attempt to control or punish them, creating a cycle of multidirectional family violence that extends to companion animals.

Conclusions. Unfortunately, the application of these theories of co-occurring family violence to the overlap with animal abuse has not yet received much attention from researchers. Thus, it is not possible to identify which theories may provide the best explanation for the apparently disproportionate rates of animal abuse in homes with child and partner violence, and vice versa. However, it is quite possible that each of these models, and possibly other models, may explain a portion of the overlap in violence within specific contexts. For example, a single perpetrator model in which animal abuse is used as a tactic of intimidation, control, and emotional abuse in the context of severe child or partner abuse may explain the high rates of overlap in clinical samples of, especially, women in shelters. In other families where animal cruelty is being perpetrated by a child, this violence may be best explained as a direct (e.g., social learning) or indirect (e.g., through development of antisocial traits) response to their own abuse or exposure to violence, or it may indicate a general pattern of child externalizing behavior and conduct problems that contribute to an overall pattern of conflict between family members in a dysfunctional home environment. Additional research is needed to differentiate between the various contexts in which animal abuse and family violence overlap and the mechanisms associated with co-occurrence in those contexts. Such information may have value for informing prevention and intervention efforts for violence against humans and animals.

Implications for Prevention and Early Intervention

Existing research, although limited in scope and methodology, provides preliminary evidence that animal cruelty and family violence co-occur in many households and that the presence of one form of violence may serve as a "red flag" for other forms of violence in a home. These findings have several implications for early intervention and the prevention of family violence. For instance, because many families exposed to animal cruelty may also be experiencing child and/or partner abuse, the use of cross-reporting legislation in which animal welfare investigators are permitted or required to report families with substantiated animal abuse to child or adult protection agencies for investigation may be useful; however, such policies should be evaluated to determine whether they are effective in identifying families at risk for violence and directing them toward prevention services (DeGue & DiLillo, 2009; Long et al., 2007). Recognition of a link between violence toward animals and humans may provide a useful means of identifying and intervening with families at highest risk for violence. These findings also suggest that educating health and social service providers about the potential relationship between these forms of violence may help in their identification of concomitant family violence when there is evidence of child animal cruelty, perhaps permitting early intervention and appropriate child protection efforts (Randour & Davidson, 2008). Further, given that child and adult victims of violence might view their pet as a source of comfort and emotional support in an otherwise traumatic or volatile home environment, witnessing or being forced to perpetrate abuse against their animal companion might have a profound negative emotional impact, especially for children without another source of social or emotional support (Flynn, 2000). Identifying individuals with exposure to multiple forms of violence, including pet abuse, might facilitate the provision of treatment to address these compound traumas.

Advocacy efforts in this area have often targeted female victims of IPV receiving services from domestic violence shelters. Data from several studies suggest that many women seeking shelter are concerned about the welfare of their pets and delay leaving their partner due to these fears (e.g., Ascione et al., 2007). Efforts to encourage screening for animal cruelty and concerns about pets may help service providers identify potential barriers to leaving and create safety plans that include pets. Many communities now offer programs that provide safe housing for pets when women seek shelter themselves from abusive partners (American Humane Association, 2010; Kogan et al., 2004). Although such interventions are most likely to reach those individuals who experience animal abuse in the context of severe IPV (e.g., coercive controlling violence) by a male perpetrator, as discussed above, this type of violence may account for many of the cases in which IPV and animal abuse co-occur. Because many women in these samples also report that their child has engaged in animal abuse, screening policies may also help identify children in need of services for behavioral or emotional problems.

From a prevention standpoint, several authors have suggested addressing the link between human- and animal-directed violence through the inclusion of universal humane education in elementary school curriculums (Faver, 2010). Humane education programs capitalize on children's interest in and identification with animals by incorporating animals or animal-related stories into lessons and activities that teach compassion, respect, and responsibility (Faver, 2010). Initial evidence from evaluations of these programs suggests that they may have positive effects on humane attitudes toward animals, human-directed empathy, attitudes toward aggression, and aggressive behavior (Arbour, Signal, & Taylor, 2009; Ascione & Weber, 1996; Sprinkle, 2008). Thus, although the humane treatment of animals is a core component of these programs, they may also have potential for preventing other forms of violence and aggression, including violence toward family members. However, more rigorous research is needed to understand the potential utility of these programs in preventing violence more generally, with particular attention to the effects on high-risk youth who have been exposed to violence in their home or community or who have already demonstrated emotional or behavioral difficulties.

Given the high prevalence and impact of child maltreatment and IPV on individuals and society, there is an urgent need for increased attention to the primary prevention of these forms of violence. A focus on the development and rigorous evaluation of prevention programs for these forms of violence has increased in recent years, but effective, innovative approaches are still needed in order reduce rates of perpetration and victimization at population level (Klevens & Whitaker, 2007; Murray & Graybeal, 2007). It is possible that further research attention to the relationship between animal cruelty and family violence, including the potential for a shared etiology, may shed light on promising approaches to addressing the prevention of all forms of violence in the home.

Need for Future Research

Given compelling evidence suggesting a meaningful overlap in the abuse of children, partners, and pets in the existing literature, prevention and intervention efforts, such as those described above, are currently being implemented, and national coalitions concerned with the welfare of human and animals victims of violence have begun to mobilize around this issue (National Link Coalition, 2008). However, relative to other areas of violence research, the literature in this area remains substantially limited in size, scope, and methodological rigor. For example, most of the research on overlapping IPV and animal abuse has been conducted with shelter samples of women. More research on rates and contexts of overlapping violence in nonclinical samples is indicated, including IPV involving female perpetrators and same-sex couples. The research on co-occurring child maltreatment and animal cruelty is similarly limited by the use of clinical samples as well as a failure to distinguish between children who witnessed and/or perpetrated animal abuse in some studies. Although a general assessment of exposure to animal cruelty is useful for establishing rates of overlap, the use of measures that distinguish between witnessing and perpetrating animal abuse and identify the perpetrator(s) will aid in the development and examination of etiological models to explain co-occurring forms of violence. The use of longitudinal or prospective designs in future research would also provide important evidence regarding the nature and etiology of the relationships between childhood maltreatment, exposure to violence, and the development of childhood animal cruelty. Finally, results from non-US samples (e.g., Baldry, 2003; Yamazaki, 2010) suggest that the relationships identified here may hold across cultures; however, additional cross-cultural research is needed.

An increased focus on the development and testing of etiological theories, including those suggested here, may help guide this nascent literature toward the next phase of development—beyond prevalence rates to an understanding of the contexts and mechanisms involved in producing these co-occurring forms of family violence. The work of the past three decades has increased awareness and provided some initial empirical support for a link between animal cruelty and family violence. Moving forward, attention to the ways in which these forms of violence interact and influence the development of other forms of violence will be critical for the translation of these findings into effective violence prevention and intervention strategies.

References

Achenbach, T. M. (1991). *Manual for the child behavior checklist/4-18 and 1991 profile.* Burlington, VT: University of Vermont, Department of Psychology.

Adams, C. J. (1995). Woman-battering and harm to animals. In C. J. Adams & J. Donovan (Eds.), *Animals & women: Feminist theoretical explorations* (pp. 55–74). Durham: Duke University Press.

Adams, C. J. (1998). Bringing peace home: A feminist philosophical perspective on the abuse of women, children and animals. In R. Lockwood & F. R. Ascione (Eds.), *Cruelty to animals and interpersonal violence: Readings in research and application* (pp. 318–340). West Lafayette, IN: Purdue University Press.

American Humane Association. (2010). *Pets and women's shelters (PAWS) program.* Retrieved August 15, 2010, from http://www.americanhumane.org/human-animal-bond/programs/pets-andwomens-shelters/

Appel, A. & Holden, G. (1998). The co-occurrence of spouse and physical child abuse: A review and appraisal. *Journal of Family Psychology, 12,* 578–599.

Arbour, R., Signal, T., & Taylor, N. (2009). Teaching kindness: The promise of humane education. *Society & Animals, 17,* 136–148.

Ascione, F. R. (1998). Battered women's reports of their partners' and their children's cruelty to animals. *Journal of Emotional Abuse, 1,* 119–133.

Ascione, F. R., & Arkow, P. (Eds.). (1999). *Child abuse, domestic violence, and animal abuse: Linking the circles of compassion for prevention and intervention.* West Lafayette, IN: Purdue University Press.

Ascione, F. R., Friedrich, W. N., Heath, J., & Hayashi, K. (2003). Cruelty to animals in normative, sexually abused, and outpatient psychiatric samples of 6- to 12-year-old children: Relations to maltreatment and exposure to domestic violence. *Anthrozoos, 16,* 195–211.

Ascione, F. R. & Weber, C. V. (1996). Children's attitudes about the humane treatment of animals and empathy: One-year follow up of a school-based intervention. *Anthrozoos, 9,* 188–195.

Ascione, F. R., Weber, C. V., Thompson, T. M., Heath, J., Maruyama, M., & Hayashi, K. (2007). Battered pets and domestic violence: Animal abuse reported by women experiencing intimate violence and by nonabused women. *Violence Against Women, 13,* 354–373.

Baldry, A. (2003). Animal abuse and exposure to interparental violence in Italian youth. *Journal of Interpersonal Violence,* 18, 258–281.

Carlisle-Frank, P., Frank, J. M. & Nielsen, L. (2004). Selective battering of the family pet. *Anthrozoos, 17,* 26–41.

Currie, C. L. (2005). Animal cruelty by exposed to domestic violence. *Child Abuse & Neglect, 30,* 425–435.

Dadds, M. R., Whiting, C., Bunn, P., Fraser, J., & Charlson, J. (2004). Measurement of cruelty in children: The Cruelty to Animals Inventory. *Journal of Abnormal Child Psychology, 32,* 321–334.

Dadds, M. R., Whiting, C., & Hawes, D. (2006). Associations among cruelty to animals, family conflict, and psychopathic traits in childhood. *Journal of Interpersonal Violence, 21,* 411–429.

Davidson, H. (1998). What lawyers and judges should know about the link between child abuse and animal cruelty. *American Bar Association Child Law Practice, 17,* 60–63.

DeGue, S. & DiLillo, D. (2009). Is animal cruelty a "red flag" for family violence? Investigating co-occurring violence toward children, partners, and pets. *Journal of Interpersonal Violence, 24,* 1036–1056.

DeViney, E., Dickert, J., & Lockwood, R. (1983). The care of pets within child abusing families. *International Journal for the Study of Animal Problems, 4,* 321–329.

Duncan, A., Thomas, J. C. & Miller, C. (2005). Significance of family risk factors in development of childhood animal cruelty in adolescent boys with conduct problems. *Journal of Family Violence, 20,* 235–239.

Dutton, M. A. (1992). *Empowering and healing the battered woman.* New York: Springer

Dutton, D. G., & Starzomski, A. J. (1997). Personality predictors of the Minnesota power and control wheel. *Journal of Interpersonal Violence, 12,* 70–82.

Faver, C. A. (2010). School-based humane education as a strategy to prevent violence: Review and recommendations. *Children and Youth Services Review, 32,* 365–370.

Faver, C. A., & Cavazos, A. M., Jr. (2007). Animal abuse and domestic violence: A view from the border. *Journal of Emotional Abuse, 7,* 59.

Faver, C. A. & Strand, E. B. (2003). To leave or to stay? Battered women's concern for vulnerable pets. *Journal of Interpersonal Violence, 18,* 1367–1377.

Faver, C. A. & Strand, E. B. (2007). Fear, guilt, and grief: Harm to pets and the emotional abuse of women. *Journal of Emotional Abuse, 7*, 51–70.

Flynn, C. P. (2000). Why family professionals can no longer ignore violence toward animals. *Family Relations, 49*, 87–95.

Gupta, M. (2008). Functional links between intimate partner violence and animal abuse: Personality features and representations of aggression. *Society and Animals, 16*, 223–242.

Higgins, D. J., & McCabe, M. P. (2000). Multi-type maltreatment and the long-term adjustment of adults. *Child Abuse Review, 9*, 6–18.

Hutton, J. S. (1983). Animal abuse as a diagnostic approach in social work: A pilot study. In A. H. Katcher & A. M. Beck (Eds.), *New perspectives on our lives with companion animals*. Philadelphia: University of Pennsylvania Press.

Johnson, M. P. (2006). Conflict and control: Gender symmetry and asymmetry in domestic violence. *Violence Against Women, 12*, 1003–1018.

Kelly, J. B., & Johnson, M. P. (2008). Differentiation among types of intimate partner violence: Research update and implications for intervention. *Family Court Review, 46*, 476–499.

Klevens, J., & Whitaker, D. J. (2007). Primary prevention of child physical abuse and neglect: Gaps and promising directions. *Child Maltreatment, 12*, 364–377

Knickerbocker, L., Heyman, R. E., Slep, A. M. S., Jouriles, E. N., & McDonald, R. (2007). Co-occurrence of child and partner maltreatment: Definitions, prevalence, theory, and implications for assessment. *European Psychologist, 12*, 36–44.

Kogan, L. R., McConnell, S., Schoenfeld-Tacher, R., & Jansen-Lock, P. (2004). Crosstrails: A unique foster program to provide safety for pets of women in safehouses. *Violence Against Women 10*, 418–434.

Lacroix, C. A. (1999). Another weapon for combating family violence: Prevention of animal abuse. In F. R. Ascione & P. Arkow (Eds.), *Child abuse, domestic violence, and animal abuse: Linking the circles of compassion for prevention and intervention* (pp. 62–80). West Lafayette, IN: Purdue University Press.

Leeb, R. T., Paulozzi, L., Melanson, C., Simon, T., & Arias, I. (2007). *Child maltreatment surveillance: Uniform definitions for public health and recommended data elements, Version 1.0*. Atlanta, GA: Centers for Disease Control and Prevention, National Center for Injury Prevention and Control. Available from: http://www.cdc.gov/ViolencePrevention/pub/CMP-Surveillance.html

Long, D. D., Long, J. H., & Kulkarni, S. J. (2007). Interpersonal violence and animals: Mandated cross-sector reporting. *Journal of Sociology & Social Welfare, 34*, 147–164.

Loring, M. T., & Beaudoin, P. (2000). Battered women as coerced victim-perpetrators. *Journal of Emotional Abuse, 2*, 3–14.

Loring, M. T., & Bolden-Hines, T. A. (2004). Pet abuse by batterers as a means of coercing battered women into committing illegal behavior. *Journal of Emotional Abuse, 4*, 27–37.

McPhedran, S. (2009). A review of the evidence for associations between empathy, violence, and animal cruelty. *Aggression and Violent Behavior, 14*, 1–4.

Miller, K. S. & Knutson, J. F. (1997). Reports of severe physical punishment and exposure to animal cruelty by inmates convicted of felonies and by university students. *Child Abuse & Neglect, 21*, 59–82.

Murray, C. E., & Graybeal, J. (2007). Methodological review of intimate partner violence prevention research. *Journal of Interpersonal Violence, 22*, 1250–1269.

National Link Coalition. (2008). *Strategizing the link*. Retrieved August 25, 2010, from http://www.nationallinkcoation.org

Onyskiw, J. E. (2007). The link between family violence and cruelty to family pets. *Journal of Emotional Abuse, 7*, 7–30.

Pence, E., & Paymar, M. (1993). *Education groups for men who batter: The Duluth model*. New York: Springer.

Quinlisk, J. A. (1999). Animal abuse and family violence. In F. R. Ascione & P. Arkow (Eds.), *Child abuse, domestic violence, and animal abuse* (pp. 168–175). West Layfayette, IN: Purdue University Press.

Randour, M. L., & Davidson, H. (2008). *A common bond: Maltreated children and animals in the home*. Washington, DC: American Humane Association.

Renzetti, C. M. (1992). *Violent betrayal: Partner abuse in lesbian relationships*. Newbury Park, CA: Sage.

Saltzman, L. E., Fanslow, J. L., McMahon, P. M., & Shelley, G. A. (2002). *Intimate partner violence surveillance: Uniform definitions and recommended data elements, version 1.0*. Atlanta, GA: Centers for Disease Control and Prevention, National Center for Injury Prevention and Control. Available from: http://www.cdc.gov/ncipc/pub-res/ipv_surveillance/intimate.htm

Saunders, B. J. (2003). Understanding children exposed to violence: Toward an integration of overlapping fields. *Journal of Interpersonal Violence, 18*, 356–376.

Simmons, C. A. & Lehmann, P. (2007). Exploring the link between pet abuse and controlling behaviors in violent relationships. *Journal of Interpersonal Violence, 22*, 1211–1222.

Slep, A. M. S., & O'Leary, S. G. (2005). Parent and partner violence in families with young children: Rates, patterns and connections. *Journal of Consulting and Clinical Psychology, 73*, 435–444.

Sprinkle, J. E. (2008). Animals, empathy, and violence: Can animals be used to convey principles of prosocial behavior to children? *Youth Violence and Juvenile Justice, 6*, 47–58.

Straus, M. A. (1979). Measuring intrafamily conflict and violence: The conflict tactics (ct) scales. *Journal of Marriage and the Family, 41*, 75–88.

Straus, M. A. (1993). Identifying offenders in criminal justice research on domestic assault. *American Behavioral Scientist, 36*, 587–600.

Thompson, K. L., & Gullone, E. (2006). An investigation into the association between the witnessing of animal abuse and adolescents' behavior toward animals. *Society & Animals, 14*, 221–243.

Tjaden, P., & Thoennes, N. (2000). *Extent, nature, and consequences of intimate partner violence: Findings from the National Violence Against Women Survey* (Publication No. NCJ181867). Washington, DC: US Department of Justice.

Volant, A. M., Johnson, J., Gullone, E., & Coleman, G. (2008). The relationship between domestic violence and animal abuse: An Australian study. *Journal of Interpersonal Violence, 23*, 1277–1295.

Walton-Moss, B. J., Manganello, J., Frye, V., Campbell, J. C. (2005). Risk factors for intimate partner violence and associated injury among urban women. *Journal of Community Health, 30*, 377–389.

Yamazaki, S. (2010). A comparison of maltreated children and non-maltreated children on their experiences with animals: A Japanese study. *Anthrozoos, 23*, 55–67.

Chapter 15
Urbanization and Animal Cruelty: What Role Does Utilitarianism Play?

Samara McPhedran

The majority of incarcerated offenders who report both violence toward humans and a history of animal cruelty also report growing up in urban or peri-urban settings. This may, in part, simply reflect the increased urbanization of Western society and a shift away from rural living and agricultural production. However, it has also been suggested that urban living and how that has affected the attitudes of humans towards animals may influence the development of animal cruelty behaviors by humans. In contrast, while the 'utilitarian' view of animals (where animals are seen in the context of their usefulness to humans) appears more prevalent in rural areas and has been linked by some with animal cruelty, it has been hypothesized – somewhat paradoxically – that utilitarian attitudes may also protect against the development of animal cruelty behaviors by humans. This theory, and what it means for understanding the relationships between humans and animals, is examined from the dual perspectives of philosophy and empirical study. Particular emphasis is placed on considering how the definition and measurement of animal cruelty has influenced existing theory and study in the field, and how that has shaped research into human–animal relationships.

Background

Potential relationships between animal cruelty and a range of interconnected dysfunctional behaviors, such as violence, substance abuse, theft, and arson, have received growing attention within psychological, criminological, and sociological discourse. There is increasing recognition that while animal cruelty may co-occur with other antisocial behaviors, it does not – as has sometimes been argued – 'cause' or 'lead to' those behaviors (see Patterson-Kane & Piper, 2009, for a thoughtful critique). Rather, that view has been replaced with the more nuanced perspective that in instances in which animal cruelty is found alongside other antisocial behaviors, this correlation is most probably due to the presence and influence of a shared set of underlying developmental and contextual factors.

S. McPhedran (✉)
e-mail: smcphedran@iprimus.com.au

C. Blazina et al. (eds.), *The Psychology of the Human–Animal Bond*,
DOI 10.1007/978-1-4419-9761-6_15, © Springer Science+Business Media, LLC 2011

Empirical research into the antecedents of co-occurring animal cruelty and other antisocial behaviors, however, remains limited to a relatively small number of now well-known and oft-cited studies (e.g., Arluke, Levin, Luke, & Ascione, 1999; Felthous & Kellert, 1986; Kellert & Felthous, 1985; Merz-Perez, Heide, & Silverman, 2001). Briefly, those studies provide some degree of evidence that among violent offenders who reported engaging in animal cruelty, many also reported early exposure to domestic violence, abuse as children, and/or parental alcohol/substance abuse.

However, these studies, while suggestive of common factors potentially associated with a spectrum of dysfunctional and antisocial behaviors, are constrained by a range of methodological limitations such as recall bias, over- or underreporting, and small/highly specific samples. In addition, there is a notable absence of longitudinal information following childhood animal cruelty perpetrators into adulthood, rendering it difficult to follow the developmental progression of those children or study their family functioning, for example. There have been few efforts to discern why some children who engage in cruelty to animals go on to exhibit dysfunctional behaviors in later life, whereas others do not, and what factors most strongly influence the trajectories of such children.

While there are considerable gaps in knowledge, one form of information that many available studies have provided is descriptive data about the socioeconomic and demographic characteristics of violent adult offenders who also report perpetrating animal cruelty. This has been augmented by a small number of studies into self-reported animal cruelty among broader populations (e.g., Baldry, 2003). Regarding the demographic characteristics of those who commit animal cruelty, the main characteristic that has been given attention is sex. The perpetrators of animal cruelty – whether children, adolescents, or adults – are generally male. For instance, in early clinical studies on youths (Rigdon & Tapia, 1977; Tapia, 1971) and in retrospective studies of criminals who reported abusing animals in childhood or adolescence (Felthous & Kellert, 1986; Kellert & Felthous, 1985), males were consistently overrepresented (however, the proportion of incarcerated males is substantially greater than that of incarcerated females, so this finding may simply reflect the demographics of the prison population as a whole).

The relationship that other characteristics such as education, race, employment status, and place of residence bear to animal cruelty is less well studied. It has been suggested, for example, that animal cruelty is associated with lower education levels (Hensley, Tallichet, & Singer, 2006). However, as this is a proposition arising largely from studies of incarcerated violent offenders (among whom relatively low levels of education is a common factor, irrespective of the presence or absence of a reported history of animal cruelty), its utility in relation to understanding animal cruelty is questionable. Indeed, this may simply offer further evidence of common characteristics across co-occurring violent and antisocial behaviors.

Interactions between place of residence during childhood, and subsequent animal cruelty have also been hinted at. Using a prison population, Hensley and Tallichet (2005) found an association between animal cruelty (which they defined as having 'hurt or killed' animals) and place of residence, with animal cruelty more common among inmates who were raised in urban areas. By way of explanation, the authors propose that a rural upbringing may engender heightened respect for animals, although this hypothesis was not tested.

A simple explanation for Hensley and Tallichet's (2005) finding that most offenders who also reported animal cruelty were raised in urban areas is that it may, in part, simply reflect the increasing urbanization of Western society and a demographic shift away from rural living and agricultural production (that is, a greater proportion of the population now live in urban areas). Indeed, connections between growing urbanization and the increasing occurrence of crime (particularly, juvenile crime) were noted as early as the eighteenth century in the United Kingdom (King, 1998). However, it is also possible that urban living, and how that has influenced the attitudes of humans toward animals and the nature of human–animal interactions, may relate to the development of animal cruelty behaviors by humans.

While it would appear, at face value, a relatively straightforward task to investigate relationships between cruelty and location (or other demographic variables), this is not the case. Rather, this seemingly innocuous question captures a complex set of theoretical and empirical issues that scholars in the field should be acutely aware of, ranging from philosophical perspectives about the nature of human–animal relationships, to how cruelty is defined and 'measured', and how philosophy and definitions can exert influence upon research methodologies and findings. The current chapter uses the example of animal cruelty and location to provide an introduction to these topics, with the aim of furthering critical inquiry in the field of human–animal interaction.

Philosophies of Human–Animal Interaction

For the purpose of this chapter, two broad, current views about the human–animal relationship require mention: utilitarianism and rights. Both of these perspectives have been written about at considerable length elsewhere, and it is beyond the scope of the present work to go into great detail. Briefly, though, utilitarianism refers to the view that it is acceptable for humans to 'use' animals (for example, for consumption or medical research). The utilitarian perspective accords to a considerable degree with what is commonly referred to as animal 'welfare,' which allows for the use of animals but holds that animals should, nonetheless, not be treated poorly. Within the utilitarian view, animals may be seen in the context of their usefulness to humans (for example, as a source of food or fibers).

The postmodern animal 'rights' position, however, rejects the concept that animal use may be justified under any circumstances and holds that it is morally wrong to use animals for human benefit. For instance, Regan (1983) contends that inherent value and moral consideration should be accorded independently of any being's potential or actual 'use' to others and independently of that creature being the object of anyone else's 'interests'. By invoking the concept of inherent value, the rights perspective rejects utilitarianism. Utilitarianism enables humans to view animals with reference to their usefulness to humans, whereas rights dictates the attribution of 'independent' value, that is, value that is not contingent on the role that an animal may play in the life of a human or the 'usefulness' of an animal to others.

It is important, at this juncture, to highlight that these two views about animal represent different philosophical (or, as some may argue, 'moral') perspectives about how humans 'should' see their relationship with animals. While different philosophies cannot be objectively evaluated with reference to data, or compared with one another using scientific methods to discern which is 'correct', these views can nonetheless influence the definition of cruelty and shape how the measures and methods used to conduct research into cruelty. This will be considered below.

The Difficulty of Definition

When evaluating research on animal cruelty, in addition to being aware of the contrast between utilitarianism and rights, it is vital to consider how cruelty is defined. Definitions of cruelty are often arbitrary and contested and frequently rely on operational definitions (that is, labeling specific behaviors as 'cruel'). However, as McPhedran (2010) notes, defining particular behaviors as 'cruel' without making reference to the *intent* of a behavior (thus, adopting a purely operational definition) reifies the concept of cruelty by assuming that a behavior has inherent properties of 'cruelty'. This is a flawed assumption which can lend itself to arbitrary assigning into the category of 'cruelty' those behaviors deemed by, for example, an interest group or researcher to be 'morally wrong'. A more meaningful approach to definition can be found in the concept that behavior does not have an inherent property of 'cruelty', but rather, is cruel if it is the result of an agent (i.e., the individual) acting with cruelty.

In an effort to overcome the reification of cruelty and move toward recognition of agency, there have been attempts to incorporate the concept of agency (i.e., intent) into definitions of cruelty. One of the more frequently encountered definitions of this nature is drawn from Ascione (1993), who defined cruelty as any "socially unacceptable behavior that intentionally causes unnecessary pain, suffering, or distress to, and/or death of, an animal" (p. 228). Under Ascione's (1993) definition, emotional or psychological pain (e.g., teasing, bestiality), as well as physical pain, could constitute cruelty. This definition excludes practices that are socially acceptable, such as the slaughter of farm animals or the use of animals in research. It also excludes unintentional acts (for example, unintentionally striking an animal while driving a vehicle).

Unfortunately, by invoking 'social unacceptability' as a condition for cruelty, this definition shifts emphasis away from the intent of a behavior onto a process through which certain behaviors come to be defined as 'unnecessary,' and thence 'cruel'. This reflects an uncomfortable effort to blend the fundamentally relativistic view that behaviors defined as 'cruel' are constantly shifting, with the view that 'cruelty' is a fixed construct – the specific intent of an agent. It implies that the intent of an agent to act with 'cruelty' can be inferred through their engaging in a behavior that has been socially constructed as 'cruel'. This is not a logically sustainable or empirically supported position.

Prior to Ascione (1993), Kellert and Felthous (1985) defined animal cruelty as "the wilful infliction of harm, injury, and intended pain on a non-human animal" (p. 1114). While such a definition accepts that behavior in itself does not constitute 'cruelty' and instead recognizes that cruelty is the action of an agent, it still fails to represent cruelty as an action undertaken by an agent for a particular reason. This shortcoming has been partially addressed by the definition of cruelty as "a pattern of socially and culturally unacceptable behavior in which an individual takes pleasure in, or shows indifference to, the deliberate, unnecessary pain, harm, or injury of another animate, vertebrate being" (Schiff, Louw, & Ascione, 1999, p. 26).

Although the latter definition retains the problematic criterion of social unacceptability, it also includes the concept that cruelty is the outcome of an agent acting with *intention*. By adopting the position that only very specific intentions for behavior should constitute 'cruelty,' this definition also sets forth exclusion criteria, whereby the *absence* of a specific intent precludes application of the label of cruelty. This allows for the utilitarian perspective of human–animal interaction, because it does not label human use of animals as cruelty.

However, the concept of 'unnecessary' remains open to interpretation and re-interpretation and lacks conceptual clarity. Illustrating this point, some consider animal cruelty to be any behavior that contributes to the pain or death of an animal or that otherwise threatens the welfare of an animal (Vermeulen & Odendaal, 1993) and that any behavior labeled 'unnecessary' should also be considered 'cruel'. This type of definition does not recognize any distinction between (for example) livestock production for the purpose of human consumption and deliberately torturing an animal until that animal dies. Nor does it allow for cruelty to be viewed with reference to intent or motivation. This understanding of cruelty relies heavily on the philosophical animal 'rights' perspective that any act that harms or kills an animal is 'unnecessary' and therefore inherently 'cruel.' Hence, definitions of cruelty can in some instances rest fundamentally on untestable belief systems, rather than setting out exclusion criteria for what does not constitute cruelty, or being open to scientific scrutiny and falsification. Examples of how this perspective can affect research in the field are considered below.

Assessment, Attitudes, and Cruelty

In many research settings, animal cruelty is assessed using a single question, such as 'have you ever been cruel to animals?' (This item is usually drawn from the Child Behavior Checklist, Aschenbach, 1991; see for example Currie, 2006.) There is, however, a selection of more detailed tools available. For example, Ascione's (1993) semi-structured 'Children and Animals (Cruelty to Animals) Assessment Instrument' (CAAI) considers nine different dimensions of behavior (e.g., the severity of an act, whether it was concealed, how frequently it occurred). The multidimensional approach of the CAAI recognizes the importance of considering different forms of human behavior toward animals and the context of those behaviors. However, this tool has not been well validated and – as it is a semi-structured tool – it is open to subjective interpretation and coding of responses (which is in turn open to be influenced by the way in which cruelty is defined).

One of the more comprehensive tools available is Boat's (1999) Inventory on Animal Related Experiences. This questionnaire covers a variety of different experiences regarding interaction with animals. Its dimensions range from pet ownership through to harming animals in different ways and for various reasons (such as controlling others, or out of fear of a particular animal). It differentiates between accidental and deliberate harm, considers 'why' an event took place, and includes rudimentary evaluation of how a respondent reacted to different animal experiences (a three-point scale of how bothered they were by a particular experience). However, the reliability and validity of this instrument have not been well established.

Due in part, perhaps, to the difficulties of defining cruelty and understanding 'cruel behavior', as well as the challenges of validating instruments designed to 'measure' cruelty, a small but increasing body of (mainly nonclinical) research has shifted emphasis onto the study of attitudes toward animals (e.g., Henry, 2004, 2009; Phillips & McCulloch, 2005; Preylo & Arikawa, 2008; Taylor & Signal, 2009). Inherent in the approach of many attitudinal studies, however, is the problematic assumption that attitudes reliably translate into behaviors, and that assessment of attitudes can provide meaningful information about behavior. This contrasts with more clinically oriented investigations into, for example, animal cruelty among children within the context of family violence, which tend to focus more on the use of behavioral indicators across a range of domains (rather than focusing only on interaction with animals). In addition, the assessment of attitudes is no less arbitrary than the definition of cruelty – with definitions of cruelty and philosophical views about human–animal interaction fundamentally shaping the methods and tools used to assess attitudes.

Arguably, the most commonly used tool in the study of attitudes toward animals is Herzog, Betchart, and Pittman's (1991) Animal Attitude Scale (AAS) (or a derivative of that scale, for example Knight, Vrij, Bard, & Brandon, 2009). This AAS uses questions such as 'much of the scientific research done with animals is cruel and unnecessary,' 'it is morally wrong to hunt wild animals for food,' and 'the use of animals in rodeos and circuses is cruel'. Agreement with such statements is scored such that higher agreement translates to higher levels of 'pro-animal' attitudes. From this, it is frequently inferred in studies using the AAS that lower pro-animal attitudes indicate a higher likelihood of engaging in animal cruelty (Henry, 2004; Vollum, Buffington-Vollum, & Langmire, 2004). However, studies using this scale are simply assessing levels of agreement with a philosophical perspective about the acceptability of animal use by humans.

The use of this measure will necessarily find that to disagree with particular ideological principles represents a 'negative attitude' toward animals, which is then interpreted as an indicator of potential animal cruelty. The scale does not allow for falsification of the premise that disagreement with the series of value statements it contains is indicative of a 'negative attitude'. Whether this assessment tool is able to provide meaningful data about anything other than levels of agreement with a particular belief system is questionable, casting doubt on the value of this measure within animal cruelty research.

Aside from philosophical preconceptions, this approach also demonstrates two leaps of faith common in existing literature – the assumption that attitudes necessarily translate to behaviors and conclusions about dysfunctional behaviors or behaviors of clinical significance can be validly drawn from the study of a 'normal' sample. The latter point, however, deserves scrutiny in itself. Sample selection within attitudinal studies is a notable shortcoming of such work. Typically, studies into attitudes toward animals utilize highly select samples (for example, persons who do not consume or otherwise use animal products; see Pallotta, 2008; Potts & Parry, 2010), or first-year psychology students (e.g., Furnham, McManus, & Scott, 2003). The latter cannot be considered a truly representative sample (Harton & Lyons, 2003). Hence, reliable normative data for attitudinal studies have not been well established, just as matched controls have seldom been utilized in studies of violent populations.

Utilitarianism and Rurality – Protection Against, or Risk for, Cruelty?

How, then, do the philosophy of human–animal interaction, the different definitions of cruelty, and the methods commonly used to assess 'cruelty,' relate to questions about location, cruelty, and violence toward humans, or to broader questions about human–animal interaction? The utilitarian and rights philosophies of human–animal interaction and the definitions of cruelty they inform create a paradox for understanding how location may relate to animal cruelty. On one hand, there is the suggestion that utilitarian attitudes toward animals may protect against the development of animal cruelty behaviors by humans. On the other hand, it is argued that utilitarian attitudes are associated with animal cruelty and that all animals – irrespective of their 'usefulness' to humans – should be accorded inherent value. The first proposal accords with the view that urbanization and animal cruelty are associated, while the second implies the opposite.

As discussed above, much of this apparent incongruity can be seen to relate to different definitions of cruelty, stemming from different philosophies of human–animal interaction. However, a different way to view these two seemingly contradictory perspectives may lie in Miller's (2001) suggestion that violent acts to 'socially valued' animals (such as pets) are more likely to be associated with interpersonal violence than abuses of 'less valued' animals (rodents are cited as one instance of a less-valued animal). Therefore, understanding the different ways in which animals are 'valued' bears particular relevance to the investigation of location and cruelty.

The manner in which 'value' is attached to animals has undergone considerable transformation in Western culture over the past centuries. Historically, the value of animals in society has been assigned within a utilitarian framework, with reference to their 'usefulness' to humans – for example, a dog valued as a hunting companion, a cat valued as a rat catcher, and a cow valued as a source of milk and meat (Driscoll, Macdonald, & O'Brien, 2009). While certainly not negating the possibility of emotional bonds between humans and those animals (rather, it highlights the presence of multiple, but concurrent, relationships between humans and animals and the complexity of the human–animal bond), this view – reminiscent of utilitarianism – nonetheless emphasizes the practical value of animals to humans (for example, as an economic/commercial resource), rather than assigning value in and of itself.

In the past two centuries, however, specific animals have increasingly had social value assigned to them not on the basis of their practical utility but on the basis of the symbolic role they play in humans' lives (especially, emotional lives) – for instance, they are valued as domestic 'pets' (or, more recently, 'companion animals'). It is this 'symbolic' value that Hensley and Tallichet (2005) suggest is most likely to make such animals the target of cruelty, and it is here that urban/rural differences may be drawn. In rural settings, animals continue to be accorded practical utility. Dogs, for example, as well as fulfilling a role as companions, are still used for farmwork, while other animals continue to represent an economic asset (for instance, cattle).

This contrasts with urban settings, where humans interact mainly with companion animals and where the 'value' of animals to humans is primarily emotionally based (McGreevy & Bennett, 2010). It is thus reasonable to suggest that value is accorded on the basis of emotional connections between humans and animals, rather than the 'usefulness' of that animal to a human.[1] While use is equated with value outside urban settings, value is not equated with use in urban settings. That is, 'usefulness' and 'value' have been separated in urban society, and certain animals (those most commonly found in domestic urban settings) have been accorded 'social value' without 'practical usefulness'.

In a dysfunctional setting (such as family violence), harming an animal can thus be a way of harming a human who has an emotional bond with that animal. Alternatively, acting with the intent of deliberate cruelty toward an animal could also be seen as indicative of an attitude that what happens to that animal has no bearing on humans, because in an urban setting that animal may be seen as not having *any* value or usefulness. Clearly, while neither of these situations is desirable, both can – theoretically – be linked to a shift away from the view of a particular animals having *practical* value to humans.

Oddly, urban living is also associated with a higher prevalence of anti-utilitarianism, with the majority of animal rights followers dwelling in urban areas (Jamison & Lunch, 1992). This may suggest that urban disconnection from utilitarianism increases the likelihood of finding one of two extremes: either viewing any animal use as cruel or not seeing animals as having any value and engaging in behaviors with the deliberate intention to be 'cruel'. This theory is consistent with the suggestion that rural living may engender heightened respect for animals; seeing animals from a 'utilitarian' perspective may also entail seeing animals as having

---

[1] There are, of course, exceptions to this principle; for example, animals are accorded practical utility in urban settings such as airports or in various police operations.

'value'. By accommodating the capacity for emotional bonds between humans and animals, but also enabling animals to be seen in light of their usefulness to humans, this perspective may reduce the likelihood of acting with the deliberate intent of 'cruelty.' While this may seem counterintuitive to some, it is consistent with observations from ecological and conservation study that people are more likely to protect that which they see as having practical value to them (Ando & Getzner, 2006; Beaumont, Austen, Mangi, & Townsend, 2008).

Clinical and Research Implications

To answer any of these questions, though, will require a rigorous approach that avoids the philosophical, definitional, and methodological pitfalls outlined in this chapter. A number of steps could be undertaken to advance this goal. For instance, it is necessary to undertake robust and multimodal research into whether attitudes do reliably translate to behaviors and to examine what motivations underlie different behaviors in different contexts. Also, if a specific interest is to understand how animal cruelty may relate to interpersonal violence, then careful investigation of which behaviors toward animals and – crucially – which corresponding motivations reliably co-occur with interpersonal violence (and those which do not) must be undertaken.

Should these studies find further support for Hensley and Tallichet's (2005) suggestions, as well as for Miller's (2001) views about cruelty toward 'socially valued' animals, then this may highlight a role for developing practical interventions in this area. Particularly, emphasis should be placed on means of addressing underlying issues that contribute to the mistreatment of animals. For instance, if a key link between animal cruelty and interpersonal violence is the direction of cruelty to animals to which a human has an emotional bond – which appears to be the case in family violence – then this highlights the need for intensive family interventions, strong responses to domestic violence, and social support programs, for instance.

While 'humane education,' where children are 'taught' to care about animals, has been proposed as a means of assisting at-risk children and youths and reducing animal cruelty, these interventions lack robust empirical support (McPhedran, 2009). Rather, the findings point to the importance of establishing positive relationships between young people and adults. There are ways in which practical interventions could be structured around this theme. For instance, concerning location, there is some support for the efficacy of programs that connect youths with rural or wilderness settings and enable those youths to build skills and self-esteem under adult supervision (for a review, see Hattie, Marsh, Neill, & Richards, 1997). This is an avenue for further consideration.

Summary

The purpose of this chapter has not been to answer questions about urbanization and animal cruelty, but rather, to demonstrate how seemingly straightforward questions about demography and animal cruelty are vastly complex. Nor was it the intent of this work to set out an empirical argument for particular relationships between location and cruelty; instead, it sought to introduce scholars to a range of theoretical possibilities arising from a very basic observation about urban living and animal cruelty among a prison population. The overall goal of this paper was to raise awareness of how philosophical preconceptions and their associated empirical limitations must be overcome, if such observations are to translate into robust research and meaningful clinical applications or interventions.

References

Ando, A. W., & Getzner, M. (2006). The roles of ownership, ecology, and economics in public wetland-conservation decisions. *Ecological Economics, 58,* 287–303.

Arluke, A., Levin, J., Luke, C., & Ascione, F. (1999). The relationship of animal abuse to violence and other forms of antisocial behavior. *Journal of Interpersonal Violence, 14,* 963–975.

Aschenbach, T. M. (1991). *Manual for the child behavior checklist/4-18 and 1991 profile.* Burlington, VT: University of Vermont Department of Psychiatry.

Ascione, F. R. (1993). Children who are cruel to animals: A review of research and implications for developmental psychology. *Anthrozoos, 6,* 226–247.

Baldry, A. C. (2003). Animal abuse and exposure to interparental violence in Italian youth. *Journal of Interpersonal Violence, 18,* 258–281.

Beaumont, N. J., Austen, M. C., Mangi, S. C., & Townsend, M. (2008). Economic valuation for the conservation of marine biodiversity. *Marine Pollution Bulletin, 56,* 386–396.

Boat, B. W. (1999). Abuse of children and abuse of animals: Using the links to inform child assessment and protection. In F. R. Ascione & P. Arkow (Eds.), *Child abuse, domestic violence, and animal abuse: Linking the circles of compassion for prevention and intervention* (pp. 83–100). West Lafayette, IN: Purdue University Press.

Currie, C. L. (2006). Animal cruelty by children exposed to domestic violence. *Child Abuse and Neglect, 30,* 425–435.

Driscoll, C. A., Macdonald, D. W., & O'Brien, S. J. (2009). From wild animals to domestic pets: An evolutionary view of domestication. *Proceedings of the National Academy of Sciences of the United States of America, 106,* 9971–9978.

Felthous, A. R., & Kellert, S. R. (1986). Violence against animals and people: Is aggression against living creatures generalized? *Bulletin of the American Academy of Psychiatry Law, 14,* 55–69.

Furnham, A., McManus, C., & Scott, D. (2003). Personality, empathy, and attitudes to animal welfare. *Anthrozoos, 16,* 135–146.

Harton, H. C., & Lyons, P. C. (2003). Gender, empathy, and the choice of psychology major. *Teaching of Psychology, 30,* 19–24.

Hattie, J., Marsh, H. W., Neill, J. T., & Richards, G. E. (1997). Adventure education and Outward Bound: Out-of-class experiences that make a lasting difference. *Review of Educational Research, 67,* 43–87.

Henry, B. C. (2004). The relationship between animal cruelty, delinquency, and attitudes toward the treatment of animals. *Society and Animals, 12,* 185–207.

Henry, B. C. (2009). Can attitudes about animal abuse be differentiated from attitudes about animal neglect? *Society and Animals, 17,* 21–37.

Hensley, C., & Tallichet, S. E. (2005). Animal cruelty motivations. Assessing demographic and situational influences. *Journal of Interpersonal Violence, 20,* 1429–1443.

Hensley, C., Tallichet, S. E., & Singer, S. D. (2006). Exploring the possible link between childhood and adolescent bestiality and interpersonal violence. *Journal of Interpersonal Violence, 21,* 910–923.

Herzog, H. A., Betchart, N. S., & Pittman, R. (1991). Gender, sex role identity, and attitudes toward animals. *Anthrozoos, 4,* 184–191.

Jamison, W. V., & Lunch, W. M. (1992). Rights of animals, perceptions of science, and political activism – profile of American animal rights activists. *Science Technology and Human Values, 17*, 438–458.

Kellert, S. R., & Felthous, A. R. (1985). Childhood cruelty toward animals among criminals and noncriminals. *Human Relations, 38*, 1113–1129.

King, P. (1998). The rise of juvenile delinquency in England 1780–1840: Changing patterns of perception and prosecution. *Past and Present, 160*, 116–166.

Knight, S., Vrij, A., Bard, K., & Brandon, D. (2009). Science versus human welfare? Understanding attitudes toward animal use. *Journal of Social Issues, 65*, 463–483.

McGreevy, P. D., & Bennett, P. C. (2010). Challenges and paradoxes in the companion-animal niche. *Animal Welfare, 19*, 11–16.

McPhedran, S. (2009). A review of the evidence for associations between empathy, violence, and animal cruelty. *Aggression and Violent Behavior, 14*, 1–4.

McPhedran, S. (2010). Misinterpretation, missing interpretation: Understanding animal cruelty and interpersonal violence. In A. M. Columbus (Ed.), *Advances in psychology research volume 65*. New York: Nova Publishers.

Merz-Perez, L., Heide, K. M., & Silverman, I. J. (2001). Childhood cruelty to animals and subsequent violence against humans. *International Journal of Offender Therapy and Comparative Criminology, 45*, 556–573.

Miller, C. (2001). Childhood animal cruelty and interpersonal violence. *Clinical Psychology Review, 21*, 735–749.

Pallotta, N. R. (2008). Origins of adult animal rights lifestyle in childhood responsiveness to animal suffering. *Society and Animals, 16*, 149–170.

Patterson-Kane, E. G., & Piper, H. (2009). Animal abuse as a sentinel for human violence: A critique. *Journal of Social Issues, 65*, 589–614.

Phillips, C. J. C., & McCulloch, S. (2005). Student attitudes on animal sentience and use of animals in society. *Journal of Biological Education, 40*, 17–24.

Potts, A., & Parry, J. (2010). Vegan sexuality: Challenging heteronormative masculinity through meat-free sex. *Feminism and Psychology, 20*, 53–72.

Preylo, B. D., & Arikawa, H. (2008). Comparison of vegetarians and non-vegetarians on pet attitude and empathy. *Anthrozoos, 21*, 387–395.

Regan, T. (1983). *The case for animal rights*. Berkeley, CA: University of California Press.

Rigdon, J. D., & Tapia, F. (1977). Children who are cruel to animals: A follow-up study. *Journal of Operational Psychiatry, 8*, 27–36.

Schiff, K.-G., Louw, D. A., & Ascione, F. R. (1999). The link between cruelty to animals and later violent behavior against humans: A theoretical foundation. *Acta Criminologica, 12*, 25–33.

Tapia, F. (1971). Children who are cruel to animals. *Clinical Psychiatry and Human Development, 2*, 70–71.

Taylor, N., & Signal, T. (2009). Pet, pest, profit: Isolating differences in attitudes towards the treatment of animals. *Anthrozoos, 22*, 129–135.

Vermeulen, H., & Odendaal, J. (1993). Proposed typology of companion animal abuse. *Anthrozoos, 6*, 248–257.

Vollum, S., Buffington-Vollum, J., & Langmire, D. R. (2004). Moral disengagement and attitudes about violence towards animals. *Society and Animals, 12*, 209–235.

Chapter 16
Broken Bonds: Understanding the Experience of Pet Relinquishment

Bruce S. Sharkin and Lisa A. Ruff

Broken Bonds: Understanding the Experience of Pet Relinquishment

Every year in the United States, thousands of pets (namely dogs and cats) are relinquished to animal shelters. Although there are a multitude of reasons why people relinquish their pets, the recent economic downturn and rising number of home foreclosures are likely to result in greater numbers of pets being relinquished than ever before (One million pets, 2009; Schultz & Verdon, 2008). Some pet owners simply find themselves incapable of properly caring for their pets and may have no choice but to relinquish them. Thus, there are cases in which pet relinquishment is unfortunate but perhaps unavoidable. However, there still appear to be many cases in which pets are relinquished rather casually as if they were disposable objects.

The relinquishment of pets can be devastating to both pets and people alike. For pets, the experience of being relinquished can be traumatic, places them at risk of being left with no permanent home, and, as a result, leaves them vulnerable to being euthanized if not adopted within a reasonable time period. For many people, the act of relinquishing a pet can be similarly traumatic and compromise their well-being. Pet owners who relinquish pets may struggle with feelings of doubt, guilt, regret, and other difficult emotions. In essence, the emotional toll for both animals and people as a result of pet relinquishment can be significant.

Because pet relinquishment is such a vital aspect of animal and human welfare and is so prevalent in the United States, it needs to be thoroughly examined and well understood in order to find ways to prevent or at least minimize it from occurring. Hence, the purpose of this chapter is to examine the experience of pet relinquishment from several vantage points. First, research on the reasons why people relinquish their pets and factors that might place pets at risk for relinquishment to shelters will be reviewed. Second, the question of what may or may not constitute a valid reason for relinquishing a pet will be explored. Third, recommendations for reducing cases of pet relinquishment will be offered. Finally, a discussion of

B.S. Sharkin (✉)
Department of Counseling and Psychological Services, Kutztown University, Kutztown, PA, USA
e-mail: sharkin@kutztown.edu

C. Blazina et al. (eds.), *The Psychology of the Human–Animal Bond*,
DOI 10.1007/978-1-4419-9761-6_16, © Springer Science+Business Media, LLC 2011

directions for future research and implications for mental health practitioners will be presented. This chapter will address the relinquishment of dogs and cats, given that they represent the most common household pets, and as such, the most frequently relinquished pets in the United States.

Definition of Terms

Before proceeding, it is important to first define and clarify a few terms that tend to be used frequently and sometimes interchangeably in the pet relinquishment literature. The term *relinquishment* will be used throughout this chapter, for it is the term that seems to best represent the experience being addressed here: when pet owners voluntarily give up their pets to a shelter, sometimes for reasons unforeseeable or not within their control (e.g., illness, loss of home). Pets that are given to family members or friends when owners can no longer keep or care for them can also be considered a form of relinquishment, though the pet is essentially transferred directly to a new owner. Perhaps "transferred" is a more appropriate way to characterize such situations. As will be discussed later, this process of transferring pets to specific people and not to a shelter is often problematic, even though the intention is for continued and proper care of the pets.

Another term that is often used in a similar vein as relinquishment is *surrender*. Although these terms may be conceptualized as quite similar in meaning, the term surrender implies an element of involuntariness. Therefore, pet surrender is perhaps best reserved for those situations where owners are made to give up their pets, for example, for reasons of abuse or neglect.

Finally, the term *abandonment* is similarly used to describe the experience of people giving up their pets. However, the term abandonment connotes an element of deliberate abuse. Vermeulen and Odendaal (1993) proposed that abandonment be defined as a specific form of companion animal abuse: "When an animal is temporarily or permanently left without adequate care or intention of resuming care again" (p. 255). Indeed, in some states, abandonment of a companion animal is a criminal offense. Although giving up a pet, whether to another home or shelter, may be perceived by some as a form of abandonment, it can be differentiated from abandonment because people are ensuring that the pets are properly cared for as opposed to intentionally leaving them behind or not transferring them to new owners.

Despite overlapping associations and continued use as interchangeable terms, the terms *relinquishment, surrender,* and *abandonment* can clearly be conceptualized as having different and distinct meanings. The material discussed in this chapter is most appropriately defined by the term *relinquishment*.

Why Do People Relinquish Their Pets?

Over the past several years, researchers have examined the reasons why people relinquish their pets to shelters in order to identify risk factors for relinquishment. Most of the research is based on surveys of shelters or owners who relinquished their pets.

In some studies, interviews rather than questionnaires were used to elicit information about the reasons people relinquished their pets. The findings of these studies will be divided into five subsections representing different domains of data obtained about why pets are relinquished: owner demographics, how pets are acquired, pet characteristics, pet behavior problems, and personal circumstances or problems of owners.

Owner Demographics

Data regarding demographics of people who relinquish their pets are available, albeit somewhat limited in scope. Researchers have reported that those more likely to relinquish pets are male (Kidd, Kidd, & George, 1992; New et al., 2000), younger than 35 (New et al., 2000), married (Miller, Staats, Partlo, & Rada, 1996), and parents (Kidd et al., 1992). First-time pet owners were found to be more likely to relinquish pets in one study (Kidd et al., 1992), though another study found that previous owners were less tolerant of behavior problems when acquiring a new pet (Mondelli et al., 2004). When moving was given as a primary reason for relinquishment, the relinquisher was more likely to be female, white, in the 25–39-year-old age group, educated beyond high school (New et al., 1999), and of lower income (Shore, Petersen, & Douglas, 2003).

How Pets Are Acquired

The way pets are acquired represents another potential contributing factor in why pets are relinquished. For example, several studies on relinquishment found that a significant number of the relinquished pets were obtained from friends, relatives, or neighbors (Arkow & Dow, 1984; Miller et al., 1996; Salman et al., 1998), including pets that were relinquished because of owners needing to move (New et al., 1999). DiGiacomo, Arluke, and Patronek (1998) referred to pet owners who inherited pets from friends or relatives as "unintentional owners" who may consider these pets as temporary rather than permanent. They also used the term *nonconsensual ownership* to refer to people who are reluctantly talked into getting pets because of the wishes of others such as children convincing parents or one spouse convincing the other spouse to get a pet. It has also been found that in many cases pets that have been relinquished were originally obtained at little or no cost (New et al., 2000; Patronek, Glickman, Beck, McCabe, & Ecker, 1996a), including pets that were relinquished due to moving (Shore et al., 2003).

Oftentimes, people who relinquish their pets may have limited knowledge, may have unrealistic expectations, or are otherwise ill-prepared to care for pets. For example, many reported animal behavior problems that are given as reasons for relinquishment are actually normal and to-be-expected behaviors (Miller et al., 1996). When owners report that the care of a pet was more work and responsibility than expected (Patronek et al., 1996a) or when people return pets within a week of adoption (Mondelli et al., 2004), this tends to suggest that people were not ready for the responsibility of pet care. In contrast, problems such as unprovoked aggressive behavior toward people and other pets represent "real" behavior problems that may justify relinquishment.

Pet Characteristics

There have been some significant findings regarding the characteristics and status of pets that have been relinquished. This includes age, with younger pets more likely to be relinquished (Miller et al., 1996; New et al., 1999, 2000), size, with smaller pets less likely to be relinquished (Posage, Bartlett, & Thomas, 1998), and breed, with toy, terrier, hound, and nonsporting dogs less likely to be relinquished (Posage et al., 1998). Being sexually intact has been identified as a risk factor for relinquishment for both dogs (Patronek et al., 1996a) and cats (Patronek, Glickman, Beck, McCabe, & Ecker, 1996b). When owners relinquish their pets because they move, the pets are more likely to be dogs than cats (Shore et al., 2003), and are generally young and have not been in the household for long (New et al., 1999; Shore et al., 2003).

Researchers have looked at the relationship between how much time pets spend inside versus outside and their risk for relinquishment. Mondelli et al. (2004) found that having a yard or outdoor space for dogs has a positive influence on the length of adoption, whereas Patronek et al. (1996a) reported that dogs that spent most of the day in a yard appear to be more at risk for relinquishment. Posage et al. (1998) found that a history of indoor residence among dogs was associated with successful adoption, though this was primarily for specific, smaller breeds. Also, dogs that spend a lot of time in a crate may be more at risk for relinquishment (Patronek et al., 1996a). Unlike dogs, cats can remain indoors all of the time, and, in fact, cats that are allowed outdoors are more at risk for relinquishment (Patronek et al., 1996b; Posage et al., 1998).

Pet Behavior Problems

The behavior problems of pets may play a key role for many in the decision to relinquish them. In some surveys, owners report pet behavior problems as the primary reason for relinquishment (Arkow & Dow, 1984; Miller et al., 1996; Mondelli et al., 2004). Although behavior problems are risk factors for relinquishment of both dogs (Patronek et al., 1996a) and cats (Patronek et al., 1996b), it appears to be more of a risk factor with dogs (Miller et al., 1996; New et al., 2000). Examples of commonly reported behavior problems for dogs are excessive or unwanted barking, unwanted chewing, disobedience, biting, unprovoked aggression toward people or other pets, and inappropriate elimination (Mondelli et al., 2004; Salman et al., 1998). For cats, the most common behavior problem reported by relinquishing owners is inappropriate elimination and house soiling (Patronek et al., 1996b; Salman et al., 1998).

An interesting aspect of behavior problems as a reason for relinquishment is that some of the reported problems appear to be within the normal range of the pet's behavior, suggesting that in some cases expected behaviors of pets are simply not tolerated well by owners (Miller et al., 1996). In one study (New et al., 2000) some owners characterized the behavior problem of their relinquished dogs as "being overly active," which may have been more indicative of a mismatch between owner and pet rather than a true behavior problem. For example, if a person who is relatively inactive chooses a particular breed because of its appearance without realizing that it is a highly energetic breed, this is likely to result in the "perception" of a behavior problem.

In the case when some type of intervention is appropriate to resolve actual behavior problems, some owners report that they do not have the time or finances for such intervention (DiGiacomo et al., 1998). When interventions are made, they sometimes fail to resolve the behavior problems because owners are poorly informed about either the nature of the problems or how to properly correct them (DiGiacomo et al., 1998; New et al., 2000). Not surprisingly, when proper intervention is made such as the use of obedience training for dogs, the risk of relinquishment is lessened (Patronek et al., 1996a).

Personal Circumstances or Problems of Owner

People may choose to relinquish a pet due to specific circumstances or problems experienced in their lives. Indeed, some of the most common reasons people give for pet relinquishment fall in the domain of personal circumstances or problems (Arkow & Dow, 1984; Miller et al., 1996; Mondelli et al., 2004; New et al., 1999; Salman et al., 1998; Scarlett, Salman, New, & Kass, 1999). Some of the more common scenarios reported by owners are pregnancy or birth of baby, divorce, illness, unemployment, and need to move. When health issues are identified as a reason, it is often allergy-related problems, which are especially common as a reason for the relinquishment of cats (Miller et al., 1996; Salman et al., 1998; Scarlett et al., 1999). Owners have also claimed that they needed to relinquish pets because of having a small home or not enough room, having too many pets, and not being able to afford the cost of pet maintenance and veterinary care. Not having enough time for the pet is especially prevalent as a reason for relinquishing dogs (Miller et al., 1996; Mondelli et al., 2004; Salman et al., 1998; Scarlett et al., 1999). In some instances, pets are relinquished due to the death of the owner (Scarlett et al., 1999).

Because moving is commonly given by owners as a primary reason for relinquishment, researchers have further examined cases of relinquishment due to moving and discovered that such cases often involve landlord restrictions for people renting homes (Miller et al., 1996; Salman et al., 1998; Shore et al., 2003). Even in cases when moving is given as the primary reason for relinquishment, New et al. (1999) found that other reasons such as personal problems often played a role in the decision to relinquish the pet.

What Constitutes a Valid Reason for Pet Relinquishment?

As the review of research on pet relinquishment demonstrates, there are numerous and varied reasons why people relinquish their pets. Unfortunately, the literature has thus far not adequately addressed the question of what would constitute a valid reason for pet relinquishment. Can we consider all of the reasons identified to be valid ones? Are some of these reasons more or less justified than others? These are difficult questions to answer because how we respond may depend largely on our values, biases, and specific experiences with pets. In other words, what one person views as a valid reason for relinquishment may be viewed as questionable by another person.

Beliefs about the role of pets in people's lives will undoubtedly influence how they assess the validity of any reason for relinquishment. For example, for those people who form strong bonds with pets and consider them as family members will likely judge most reasons for relinquishment as unacceptable except under extenuating circumstances. In contrast, people who do not get as attached to their pets and see them more as possessions may not object to most of the reasons given for relinquishment. As the authors of this chapter, we believe it is important to inform the reader of our own position. We are both of the perspective that the human–animal bond is as significant or important as any human–human bond. As such, we view many cases of pet relinquishment as unnecessary and difficult to comprehend. With that in mind, the following discussion will attempt to provide some insight into how to objectively assess the reasons given for relinquishment.

One way to assess the validity of reasons given for relinquishment is to consider the circumstance of how owners obtain their pets and how well prepared they are for the responsibilities of pet ownership. According to Miller et al. (1996), there is evidence to suggest that owners are sometimes ill-informed about what is involved in caring for a pet. This may be because (a) people fail to do the needed research before taking on the responsibility of pet ownership, (b) breeders or shelters neglect to provide enough information to ensure that owners are well informed, or (c) people end up with pets accidentally or suddenly, for example, when they are given pets by others who can no longer care for them. In most instances, being ill-informed should not be an excuse for relinquishing a pet. People need to be proactive in informing themselves when they plan to purchase or adopt a pet and should not necessarily rely on others to inform them. As Miller et al. state, "Owners need to know what to expect is normal pet behavior and how to care for and manage their pet" (p. 741). However, if people do not intend to have a pet but acquire one as a result of unusual circumstances (e.g., following the death of a family member), then it may be understandable in such instances that people will be less prepared and perhaps poorly equipped for pet ownership, which could in turn result in relinquishment.

When people relinquish their pets due to pet behavior problems, the following questions can be used to determine the validity of the decision to relinquish: First, how much was known about the behavior problem(s) at the time the pet was acquired? If the behavior problem already existed but was not disclosed or otherwise known to the new owner, then it would be difficult to hold the person responsible for needing to relinquish the pet. Second, how severe or troublesome was the behavior problem? Whether the problem behavior is known from the outset or emerges after the pet is acquired, the degree of difficulty or distress it causes can justify relinquishment. For example, unprovoked aggressive behavior toward people or other animals, if unable to be corrected, would certainly be cause for concern and would seem to be a valid reason for relinquishment. On the other hand, something such as mild destruction of furniture from chewing or scratching could be considered less severe and perhaps more easily correctable. It can be challenging to fairly assess the degree of severity in some cases because people vary significantly in how much they can tolerate different types of pet behavior problems. The problem of house soiling, for instance, may be something that some pet owners will simply not tolerate under any circumstances, even if due to a health problem.

Third, what types of efforts were made to address and remedy the problem behavior? How much time and energy people can or are willing to spend to deal with pet problem behavior will vary considerably. As previously noted, some owners will simply not be able or willing to devote the necessary time and resources for proper intervention such as obedience training (DiGiacomo et al., 1998). If one knows about the problem behavior from the beginning and agrees to assume responsibility for the pet, then it could reasonably be expected that the owner would make every effort to try to properly deal with the matter until resolved unless the behavior is incorrigible. For instance, dogs that suffer from separation anxiety may be prone to behaviors such as chewing and barking. Separation anxiety is treatable with medication and other measures such as doggy day care, but owners need to take these additional steps to remedy the problem.

Perhaps the most difficult domain to assess fairly is personal circumstances or problems of the owner. Certainly if people experience serious hardship such as prolonged illness, loss of employment, or other circumstances that make it challenging or impossible to continue providing proper care to their pets, then relinquishment may be the only choice. When people have severe allergy reactions, which in one study was the most common personal reason given for the relinquishment of cats (Scarlett et al., 1999), this may be an understandable reason as well. But how do we judge other personal or life circumstances that result in pet relinquishment such as divorce, pregnancy, or the birth of a baby? Why would people need to relinquish their pets because of such events? Unfortunately, most of the survey data on reasons for relinquishment give only the reasons without any deeper understanding of that particular reason. For example, relinquishing a pet because of pregnancy or the birth of a child may not fully explain the circumstances. Is it because there will not be enough time for the pet? Are there concerns about how the pet will behave around an infant? It is interesting to note that in one study (Scarlett et al., 1999) about 1/3 of the pets relinquished because of the birth of a new baby were acquired during the previous 9 months. This suggests that in many cases the relinquished pet was obtained when the pregnancy was known. If so, this may be another example of poor planning or poor timing for assuming ownership of a pet. In the case of a divorce where property is divided, it is unclear why a pet would not be retained by one spouse (especially if one is more attached to the pet than the other) or a joint custody arrangement made. Children are not relinquished when people divorce, so why are pets?

The need to move is another type of personal circumstance that has been frequently reported as a reason for relinquishment (Arkow and Dow, 1984; Miller et al., 1996; New et al., 1999; Salman et al., 1998). Like circumstances such as divorce or the birth of a baby, relinquishment of a pet due to moving appears to be valid in some situations but not in others. If someone has to move into an apartment or dwelling that does not allow pets, and there are no other options, then relinquishment may be justified. Landlord restrictions are an often-cited factor in relinquishment due to moving (Shore et al., 2003). A key question is whether the pet was obtained with the knowledge that a move was going to happen. Shore et al., for example, suggest that renters (as opposed to homeowners) be advised to adopt cats or small dogs, given that larger dogs are more commonly relinquished than cats and smaller dogs when people move. Another key question is how much the pet is considered in the decision or need to move. In other words, were all options explored in an effort to avoid relinquishment or was the decision to move made without consideration of what would be best for the pet? In some instances, such as when people move out of the country, they may opt to relinquish rather than try to arrange transport for the pet. Perhaps relinquishment is justified if the pet is older and will have trouble with long-distance travel and the adjustment. Otherwise, why would someone not keep their pet (assuming no pet restrictions in housing) regardless of where they move?

Some pet owners have reported not having enough room, too many pets, or not enough time for their pets as reasons for relinquishment (Miller et al., 1996; Mondelli et al., 2004; Salman et al., 1998; Scarlett et al., 1999). All of these reasons beg the question, "Why were pets acquired in the first place?" Unless circumstances changed after the pet was acquired, these do not appear to represent valid reasons for relinquishment. If, for example, pet owners allow pets to have litters and as a result relinquish pets because they have too many, then that would be a case of poor planning or decision making on their part. Not having enough room may result from failure to consider the adult size of a dog obtained as a puppy. Not having enough time may result from being ill-prepared or having unrealistic expectations regarding the responsibilities of pet ownership.

For some people, especially those involved in pet rescue work, there may be a perception that many owners relinquish their pets in an almost callous or thoughtless manner, as if they are mere objects that can be disposed of easily. This perception has been challenged by the findings of a qualitative study in which people who relinquished their pets to a private shelter were interviewed about their experience. DiGiacomo et al. (1998) discovered that cases of relinquishment may be more complex than previously assumed. They found that the majority of people truly struggled with the decision for long periods of time, experienced guilt and sometimes regret, and resorted to relinquishment to the shelter only as a last resort. It was reported that many of the relinquishing owners tolerated their situations for as long as possible and some made attempts to find proper homes themselves for their pets before finally relinquishing them to the shelter. This finding was supported in a subsequent study by Shore et al. (2003), who similarly found that the experience of relinquishment was very difficult for people who had to do so because of landlord restrictions when they moved. Shore et al. also found that many of the people in their study reported being quite attached to the pets they relinquished.

In sum, it is difficult to say what percentage of cases of relinquishment is for valid reasons and what percentage is for reasons that might be considered questionable. Clearly, there is a need for more research to understand not just the reasons given for relinquishment but the underlying issues or concerns that influence the decision to relinquish a pet. In the meantime, however, the existing research does have implications for how pet relinquishment can be minimized. Five recommendations to help lessen the frequency of pet relinquishment will be offered in the following section.

Recommendations for Reducing Cases of Pet Relinquishment

People Need to Be Well Informed Before Acquiring a Pet

Several researchers made note of how important it is for people to be prepared for pet ownership, analogous to how prospective parents prepare for the birth or adoption of a child. For example, Miller et al. (1996) observed that "pet owners commonly lack knowledge and awareness of the responsibilities of pet ownership" (p. 742). This may be especially true when it comes to pet behavior problems, as attempts to resolve such problems are oftentimes unsuccessful because pet owners are ill-informed about the problems and how to correct them (DiGiacomo et al., 1998; New et al., 2000). Thus, it is incumbent upon prospective pet owners to do the necessary research before purchasing or adopting a pet. This includes finding an appropriate match between owner and pet based on one's circumstances and lifestyle (New et al., 2000; Scarlett, Salman, New, & Kass, 2002). Indeed, Shore (2005) found that many individuals who relinquished a pet said that they would make a different choice (e.g., regarding the size or breed of pet) if they were to adopt again.

People Need to Plan Ahead as Much as Possible Before Acquiring a Pet

A major theme that emerged in the study by Shore (2005) was that people needed to devote more thought and planning both to the consideration of adoption and the process of adoption. Based on many of the reasons given for relinquishment, it seems reasonable to expect people to try to anticipate foreseeable events in their lives such as the need to move or the birth of a child if such events might subsequently make the experience of pet ownership too challenging or burdensome. Another circumstance that warrants consideration is who would assume care for the pet in the event of an owner having to go into a nursing home or dying. This requires planning and consultation with potential caretakers to ensure that proper care will be anticipated and carried out successfully. Granted, there will always be circumstances either unforeseeable or unanticipated, but as the research suggests, there are clearly cases in which more forethought may prevent unnecessary relinquishment of pets. For example, the amount of time that one will have to devote to a pet should be given considerable consideration before acquiring a pet, particularly if considering a dog.

People Should Be Discouraged from Transferring Pets to Relatives, Friends, or Neighbors Without the Assistance of a Shelter

There is strong support for this recommendation from studies that show a significant number of relinquished pets that result from being transferred without the involvement of shelters (Arkow and Dow, 1984; Miller et al., 1996; New et al., 1999, 2000; Salman et al., 1998). Although there may be many cases in which such transfers work out well, there is a significant risk for pets that are given to other people without the benefit of more thorough screening to ensure that it will be a good home for them. Shelters and animal rescues typically take the time to find matches between the interests and circumstances of people seeking a pet and the needs of the pet. If someone needs to relinquish a pet and there is someone in mind such as a friend, then it would be best if that person could consult with and enlist the assistance of a local shelter.

Obedience Training Should Be Required for People Who Adopt or Purchase Dogs

Obedience training may reduce the risk of relinquishment as a result of reducing the emergence of behavior problems (Patronek et al., 1996a; Salman et al., 1998). Obedience training also represents an ideal way for people to bond with their dogs, especially for individuals obtaining a dog for the first time. Also, obedience training reinforces the owner as leader within the hierarchy of the pack order. For these reasons, many animal rescues make obedience training a requirement of adoption.

Veterinary Practitioners Should Play an Important Role in Reducing Relinquishments

In addition to the fact that regular veterinary care may reduce the risk of relinquishment (Salman et al., 1998), veterinary practitioners can help in the overall effort to reduce relinquishments in a number of ways (Scarlett et al., 2002). First, they can provide appropriate guidance for people who are interested in acquiring a pet or additional pets. This can be in the form of giving vital information about the responsibility of pet ownership including type and frequency of routine health care required. Second, veterinary practitioners can help people choose the right pet (based on breed, age, size, gender, etc.), given their circumstances and lifestyle. Third, veterinary practitioners can be especially helpful when it comes to educating about and properly intervening with pet behavior problems.

Directions for Future Research

Our understanding of the experience of pet relinquishment can be further enhanced with additional research. As noted earlier, most of the research to date on pet relinquishment has examined only the specific reasons for relinquishment. The process of how people come to the decision to relinquish a pet may be much more complex than the research thus far demonstrates. For example, there may be interactions of various factors (e.g., owner losing employment plus pet behavior problems) that ultimately contribute to relinquishment. Surveys of pet owners need to delve deeper into not only the reasons for relinquishment but also their thoughts and feelings involved in the experience. In other words, how much thought is devoted to the matter and how much do one's emotions play a role?

It would also be helpful if research could be done to further explore the question examined earlier in this chapter: What constitutes a valid versus invalid reason for relinquishment? What influences people to perceive a reason as valid or not? How do the perceptions of pet owners who have relinquished pets compare with pet owners who have never relinquished a pet? What are the perceptions about relinquishment held by pet rescue and shelter workers who deal with cases of relinquishment on a daily basis? How much anger versus acceptance do they experience in response to people relinquishing their pets? Despite the obvious biases they may have because of the work they do, do they differentiate between valid and invalid reasons for relinquishment? If so, how does this influence them when conducting interviews or home visits with people applying for adoption?

Implications for Mental Health Practitioners

The material reviewed and discussed in this chapter has important implications for mental health practitioners who work with clients who consider relinquishing a pet or have already done so. For clients who are trying to make a decision regarding relinquishment, clinicians can be helpful in the process by exploring and weighing various options, exploring a client's thoughts and feelings associated with the decision, and providing support through the process. With clients who have already made the decision to relinquish a pet, clinicians can be instrumental in working with them in terms of the range of feelings they may experience, such as grief and sadness, anger, guilt, and regret. This process would be similar to how clinicians can provide assistance for people going through the grief process after a pet dies (Sharkin & Knox, 2003).

Of course, in contrast with most cases of pet death (at least ones that result from illness or natural causes), the experience of relinquishing a pet may involve complicated grief reactions, given the voluntary nature of the vast majority of relinquishment cases. Clinicians need to be careful not to miss or inadvertently dismiss any conflicted feelings or sense of regret expressed by a client, for such feelings would often be expected to emerge. A related issue has to do with clinicians' own feelings about pets and their views on people relinquishing pets. As with almost everything that is explored in therapy, the subject of pet relinquishment can evoke countertransference reactions. Because the goal of therapy is focused on helping clients to achieve a sense of resolve and peace about their decisions, it behooves clinicians to manage their own feelings and potential biases so that they do not pass judgment or confront their clients when they choose or have chosen to relinquish a pet. However, if in the process of helping clients to make the decision, it does seem appropriate to at least raise thoughtful questions for clients to ponder as they make such an important decision that can have ramifications for themselves and their pets.

Summary and Conclusion

This chapter was devoted to an examination of the experience of pet relinquishment in this country, which has negative consequences for both animals and people. Based on a review of the research on relinquishment, people give a number of reasons for relinquishing their pets, including pet behavior problems and personal problems experienced by owners. An attempt was made to objectively assess the validity of the identified reasons given for relinquishment. Although some reasons may be understandable, we have raised questions about the necessity to relinquish pets under many of the circumstances described by those who have relinquished pets. In an effort to help reduce cases of pet relinquishment, recommendations based on the research review were offered. Suggestions for future research and implications for mental health professionals were also provided. It is our hope that this chapter will help promote more awareness about the devastating effects of pet relinquishment and the need for prospective and current pet owners to make every effort to avoid ever having to relinquish a pet.

References

Arkow, P. S., & Dow, S. (1984). The ties that do not bind: A study of the human–animal bonds that fail. In R. K. Anderson, B. L. Hart, & L. A. Hart (Eds.), *The pet connection: Its influence on our health and quality of life* (pp. 348–354). Minneapolis, MN: University of Minnesota.

DiGiacomo, N., Arluke, A., & Patronek, G. (1998). Surrendering pets to shelters: The relinquisher's perspective. *Anthrozoos, 11*, 41–51.

Kidd, A. H., Kidd, R. M., & George, C. C. (1992). Successful and unsuccessful pet adoptions. *Psychological Reports, 70*, 547–561.

Miller, D. D., Staats, S. R., Partlo, C., & Rada, K. (1996). Factors associated with the decision to surrender a pet to an animal shelter. *Journal of the American Veterinary Medical Association, 209*, 738–742.

Mondelli, F., Previde, E., Verga, M., Levi, D., Magistrelli, S., & Valsecchi, P. (2004). The bond that never developed: Adoption and relinquishment of dogs in a rescue shelter. *Journal of Applied Animal Welfare Science, 7*, 253–266.

New, J. C., Salman, M. D., King, M., Scarlett, J. M., Kass, P. H., & Hutchinson, J. M. (2000). Characteristics of shelter-relinquished animals and their owners compared with animals and their owners in U.S. pet-owning households. *Journal of Applied Animal Welfare Science, 3*, 179–201.

New, J. C., Salman, M. D., Scarlett, J. M., Kass, P. H., Vaughn, J. A., Scherr, S., et al. (1999). Moving: Characteristics of dogs and cats and those relinquishing them to 12 U.S. animal shelters. *Journal of Applied Animal Welfare Science, 2*, 83–96.

One million pets believed at risk during economic downturn. (2009, March). *DVM: The Newsmagazine of Veterinary Medicine, 40*, 14.

Patronek, G. J., Glickman, L. T., Beck, A. M., McCabe, G. P., & Ecker, C. (1996a). Risk factors for relinquishment of dogs to an animal shelter. *Journal of the American Veterinary Medical Association, 209*, 572–581.

Patronek, G. J., Glickman, L. T., Beck, A. M., McCabe, G. P., & Ecker, C. (1996b). Risk factors for relinquishment of cats to an animal shelter. *Journal of the American Veterinary Medical Association, 209*, 582–588.

Posage, J. M., Bartlett, P. C., & Thomas, D. K. (1998). Determining factors for successful adoption of dogs from an animal shelter. *Journal of the American Veterinary Medical Association, 213*, 478–482.

Salman, M. D., New, J. G., Scarlett, J. M., Kass, P. H., Ruch-Gallie, R., & Hetts, S. (1998). Human and animal factors related to the relinquishment of dogs and cats in 12 selected animal shelters in the United States. *Journal of Applied Animal Welfare Science, 1*, 207–226.

Scarlett, J. M., Salman, M. D., New, J. G., & Kass, P. H. (1999). Reasons for relinquishment of companion animals in U.S. animal shelters: Selected health and personal issues. *Journal of Applied Animal Welfare Science, 2*, 41–57.

Scarlett, J. M., Salman, M. D., New, J. G., & Kass, P. H. (2002). The role of veterinary practitioners in reducing dog and cat relinquishments and euthanasias. *Journal of the American Veterinary Medical Association, 220*, 306–311.

Schultz, K., & Verdon, D. (2008, April). Animal relinquishments climb with housing foreclosures. *DVM: The Newsmagazine of Veterinary Medicine, 39*, 28.

Sharkin, B. S., & Knox, D. (2003). Pet loss: Issues and implications for the psychologist. *Professional Psychology: Research and Practice, 34*, 414–421.

Shore, E. R. (2005). Returning a recently adopted companion animal: Adopters' reasons for and reactions to the failed adoption experience. *Journal of Applied Animal Welfare Science, 8*, 187–198.

Shore, E. R., Petersen, C. L., & Douglas, D. K. (2003). Moving as a reason for pet relinquishment: A closer look. *Journal of Applied Animal Welfare Science, 6*, 39–52.

Vermeulen, H., & Odendaal, J. (1993). Proposed typology of companion animal abuse. *Anthrozoos, 6*, 248–257.

Chapter 17
Children and Adolescents
Who Are Kind to Animals

Camilla Pagani

Children's and adolescents' positive attitudes and behaviors toward animals are analyzed in the general context of their attitudes to and interactions with animals, and within a theoretical framework that places great emphasis on the significance of humans' relationship with diversity. Here I will adopt a broad definition of diversity, whereby diversity is all that is not the self or, more precisely, all that is not the present self. The sense of diversity is a fundamental aspect of human experience, and its development is achieved through extremely complex cognitive and emotional processes. The role of empathy, the effect of a caring and affectionate attitude toward animals on the child's cognitive and emotional development, the relationship between attachment to animals and interest in their welfare on one hand and positive interhuman relations on the other hand, the relationship between attachment to animals and experience of and attitude toward nature, and the role of cultures are discussed. Children's and adolescents' benevolent attitudes and behaviors toward animals are juxtaposed with the competitive life pattern that is now prevailing in our societies. The role of adults in affecting children's and adolescents' interactions with animals is also considered, especially with reference to social contexts like the family and school and to social institutions like zoos and circuses where animals are used. In order to illustrate these points data are also drawn on some studies we conducted on Italian children's and adolescents' attitudes and behaviors toward animals.

Children and Adolescents Who Are Kind to Animals

In this chapter, I will analyze children's and adolescents' positive attitudes and behaviors toward animals[1] in a more general context, which includes the following:

---

[1] In this chapter I will refer to nonhuman animals as "animals".

C. Pagani (✉)
Institute of Cognitive Sciences and Technologies, National Research Council, Rome, Italy
e-mail: camilla.pagani@istc.cnr.it

C. Blazina et al. (eds.), *The Psychology of the Human–Animal Bond*,
DOI 10.1007/978-1-4419-9761-6_17, © Springer Science+Business Media, LLC 2011

1. The significance of humans' relationship with diversity
2. Youth's attitudes to and interactions with animals
3. Some of the distinguishing features of the relation between youth and animals
4. The relationship between positive attitudes and behaviors toward animals on one hand and attitudes toward and experience of the larger natural world on the other
5. The relationship between positive attitudes and behaviors toward animals and interhuman relations
6. The roles of cultures and education in affecting youth's attitudes and behaviors toward animals

The Significance of Humans' Relationship with Diversity

It is undisputable that the child–animal relationship is an extremely useful cognitive and emotional situation in which the child can be led on to attain that difficult and particularly significant task in her/his socialization path, which is constituted by the understanding of diversity (Pagani & Robustelli, 2005; Pagani, Robustelli, & Ascione, 2008; Robustelli, 2000; Robustelli & Pagani, 1994). In this chapter, I will adopt a broad definition of diversity (Pagani & Robustelli, 2005; Robustelli, 2000) whereby diversity is all that is not the self or, more precisely, all that is not the present self. It is a fact that the relationship with diversity is a basic and continuous aspect of human experience. At any moment of their lives humans are unavoidably and in various ways affected by the sense of diversity. This occurs in their relations with the environment, both natural and nonnatural, namely in their relations with the other people, the other species, the rest of the natural world, and the built environment as well as in their relations with themselves. Indeed, we should bear in mind that a single human being in different periods of her/his life (e.g., ten years ago, a month ago, yesterday, one hour ago) is also diverse from herself/himself. The concrete *self* is the present *self*, the *self* now (Robustelli, 2000). Human identity is the continuously evolving outcome of our relationship with diversity. As also Myers and Saunders (2002) point out, "from the beginning the self is constituted through its *relations* with others who are distinct from the self" (p. 159). I will analyze this point in more detail by referring to the child's relationship with animals and to humans' relationship with themselves.

There are at least two reasons why an animal can provide a child with an excellent opportunity for developing and improving the understanding of diversity. First of all, compared with, for example, a peer, an animal is very different from the child and sooner or later the child is able to acknowledge this diversity. In fact, though at the beginning children are not aware of animals' diversity and often tend to anthropomorphize them, subsequently, often with adults' help, they can learn to understand diversity. At the same time, and in many cases always with adults' help, children also learn that, compared with, for example, stones or trees, animals (and especially higher animals) share many characteristics with humans, like, for instance, the capacity for suffering and for feeling pleasure. Indeed, it is possible "that a great diversity, like the diversity between children and animals, can, as it were, shake children's *self*, strengthen their process of cognitive and affective decentering, and mobilize their empathic abilities" (Pagani, Robustelli, & Ascione, 2008, p. 247). Identifying similarities in what is diverse can be particularly stimulating, like "understanding pieces of a mystery" (Pagani, Robustelli, & Ascione, 2008, p. 247). These two processes – acknowledging diversity and acknowledging similarity – can constitute the first significant steps toward child's development of empathy and, in case, also of sympathy and caring attitudes and behavior. At the beginning the target of the child's empathy, sympathy and care can be limited to an animal, but later, as we will see, the target can expand so as to include the other animals and the other human beings.

As regards humans' relationship with themselves, I would like to quote a few lines from J. D. Salinger's *The Catcher in the Rye*. During his desperate search of someone willing to spend a few hours with him and, possibly, share his unhappiness, after having flunked out of college, the young Holden Caulfield walks all the way through Central Park over the Museum of Natural History. He had been there several times when he was a kid at school. There are two beautiful pages in the book where he describes "the whole museum routine", which he knew "like a book", when he visited the museum with his teacher and classmates. The most striking characteristic of these visits was that everything in the museum was immutable. Below is the ending part of this description of immutability, unexpectedly followed by an acute analysis of a concomitant sense of diversity, this time relating to the self, to the perception of one's identity.

> The best thing, though, in that museum was that everything always stayed right where it was. Nobody'd move. You could go there a hundred thousand times, and that Eskimo would still be just finished catching those two fish, the birds would still be on their way south, the deers would still be drinking out of that water hole, with their pretty antlers and their pretty, skinny legs, and that squaw with the naked bosom would still be weaving that same blanket. Nobody'd be different. The only thing that would be different would be *you*. Not that you'd be so much older or anything. It wouldn't be that exactly. You'd just be different, that's all. You'd have an overcoat on this time. Or the kid that was your partner in line the last time had got scarlet fever and you'd have a new partner. Or you'd have a substitute taking the class, instead of Miss Aigletinger. Or you'd heard your mother and father having a terrific fight in the bathroom. Or you'd just passed by one of those puddles in the street with gasoline rainbows in them. I mean you'd be *dif*ferent in some way [...] (Salinger, 1969, pp. 121–122).

One can easily realize how Holden's cognitive and emotional capabilities of acknowledging the diversity of his self and of penetrating into it are extremely sophisticated. Interestingly, Holden seems to possess similar capabilities, mainly empathic capabilities, also as far as individuals from a nonhuman species are concerned. On a number of occasions in the course of the story his mind almost obsessionally goes to the ducks in the lagoon in Central Park, as he is concerned about what happens to them and where they go "when it gets all frozen over." In spite of the great diversity of these animals, Holden also feels the presence of some commonalities with the ducks so as to almost identify with them, and above all with their being there in the cold, probably neglected or even completely abandoned by humans.

Contrary to what people usually think, the relationship with diversity does not inevitably involve fear and rejection. Indeed, it can involve, instead, such feelings and attitudes as interest, identification, empathy, and sympathy (Pagani, Robustelli, & Martinelli, 2010). In fact, though some authors (e.g., Kottak, 2002) maintain that intergroup negative biases and, thus, fear of diversity have some innate evolutionary origin, given their self-serving protective function, "secure attachment" helps individuals "to feel safe and confident enough to explore the unknown" (Magid, 2008, p. 353), so that interest and curiosity toward the unfamiliar outweigh fear and perception of threat.

Youth's Attitudes to and Interactions with Animals

Here, my considerations will especially draw on some of the data we obtained from a research study we conducted with 800 participants (9–18 years) on Italian youth's attitudes and behaviors toward animals (Pagani, Robustelli, & Ascione, 2007) with the use of an anonymous questionnaire. Our sample was constituted by 217 pupils aged 9–10 (108 F + 109 M), 221 pupils aged 11–12 (114 F + 107 M), and 362 pupils aged 13–18 (181 F + 181 M). This wide-ranging study aimed to investigate different aspects of child–animal relationships in current Italian culture, such as pet ownership (currently and in the past), pet loss, worries about pet, reasons for never having had a pet, possible desire to have a pet, animal abuse experiences (as witness), animal abuse experiences (as perpetrator), fear of animals, being comforted by an animal in difficult times, empathic attitudes toward animals (feelings toward road kill, opinions about hunting, zoos, the use of animals in circuses, and the use of furs and leather clothes). Twelve schools participated in the study: three primary schools, five middle schools, and four high schools. All the schools were located in central Italy: ten in Rome, one in a small town in the province of Rome, and one in a small town in the province of Florence. All the pupils in the involved classes took part in the research. We developed a six-page, self-administered questionnaire based on the "Children and Animals Assessment Instrument" (CAAI) (Ascione, Thompson, & Black, 1997) and the "Boat Inventory on Animal-Related Experiences" (BIARE) (Boat, 1999) in three versions, one for each age group: 9–10, 11–12, and 13–18.[2] The questionnaire includes multiple-choice questions and open-ended questions. Participants had only to indicate their gender. No other demographic information was requested, as the questionnaire was anonymous. However, we were able to infer pupils' age from the grades they were attending, since the questionnaires were collected separately from each class. Pupils aged 11–18 years were given two hours to complete their questionnaire, while pupils aged 9–10 years were given one and a half hours.

---

[2]The questionnaire in its three versions, as well as its English translation, can be viewed at the following Web address: http://www.istc.cnr.it/createhtml.php?nbr=53 (go to the "Reports, Magazines, etc." section). A sample of the questionnaire can also be found in Pagani, Robustelli, and Ascione (2008).

The data I will discuss here will especially refer to the following aspects of youth's relations with animals: (a) worries about pet; (b) pet loss; (c) being comforted by an animal in difficult times; (d) opinions about zoos, hunting, the use of animals in circuses, and the use of furs and leather clothes. I will only focus on those points that are especially relevant to the topic of children's and adolescents' kindness toward animals.

The experience of being worried about a pet is quite common among Italian youth. More than two thirds of our participants stated they were or had been worried about their pets. Though one participant, a boy of 10, wrote that he had "all kinds of fears" for his pet, pupils' worries often relate to different and more specific kinds of fears. I will now mention the most notable of these fears followed by a few extracts, exemplifying different kinds of fears, from our participants' most significant open-ended answers to the item regarding the nature of their worries (participants' answers referred to their experiences during their lifetime):

(1) Fear of pet being killed:
    "That someone might kill her/him." (a number of participants, both girls and boys, of different ages, between 9 and 18 years)
    "That she/he might be poisoned." (a number of participants, both girls and boys, of different ages, between 9 and 18 years)
(2) Fears regarding pet's physical welfare:
    "That my rabbit might choke with an iron wire attached to its bowl." (girl, 13 years)
    "That he might hurt himself when at home alone." (girl, 11 years)
(3) Fears regarding pet's psychological well-being:
    "My concern for my dog was about his solitude." (boy, 17 years)
    "I was worried when he was at home alone. I thought he might need something or some help." (girl, 16 years)
    "That he [her pet] might believe I did not love him." (girl, 15 years)
(4) Fears regarding participants' capabilities of taking proper care of pet:
    "That I might fail to understand when my pet was sick." (boy, 14 years)
    "That we might overfeed our fish." (girl, 9 years)
(5) Fears regarding pet loss:
    "That I must separate from them [her pets]." (girl, 14 years)
    "That I might wake up and find my dog dead." (boy, 14 years)
    "I feared I might lose my dog." (her mother had given away participant's cat, when she was a little child) (girl, 16 years)
    "I used to wake up at night and go and see whether he was still there." (boy, 11 years)
    "That I would not see him any longer." (girl, 11 years)
    "That she might die while giving birth." (boy, 9 years)
    "The only worry was death." (boy, 18 years)

These examples indicate that children's attachment to their pets is usually deep, durable, and not devoid of anxious concern. On the other hand, it is noteworthy that, as our research findings also indicate, adults often tend to ignore or underestimate this fact. The extremely negative consequences for children's and adults' psychological well-being as well as for animals' welfare of what we can define as a dearth or lack of understanding of children on the part of adults can be easily grasped. Suffice it to consider that among our participants who lost their pet, 22% lost it because their pet had been given away – a very high percentage indeed. In fact, not infrequently, in some Italian families a pet can be taken without thoroughly considering all the consequences of this decision both for the pet and for one or more members of the family, especially the children. A girl of 16 wrote that when her pet – a hound puppy – was given away, her suffering had been "unbelievable."

Another example of some adults' "careless" attitude and behavior can be inferred from some, especially younger, participants' answers, when they seem to implicitly express their regret as to the fact that their mothers or both parents threw their dead fish or another kind of small pet into the toilet bowl or into the garbage can.

In general, as also our research findings suggest, adults often ignore, underestimate or are not aware of children's deep experiences with animals. In our study on youth's attitudes and behaviors toward animals (Pagani, Robustelli, & Ascione, 2007), 55% of respondents who were cruel to animals spoke to someone about their behavior. Of these only 38% spoke to one or both parents (to mothers almost three times more frequently than to fathers), 8% to other adult relatives, and 1% to teachers (the remaining percentage spoke to peers). Besides, 55% of those who witnessed animal abuse spoke to someone about their experience. Of these, 49% spoke to one or both parents (almost four times more frequently to the mother than to the father), 10% to other adult relatives, and 6% to teachers and police officers (also in this case the remaining percentage spoke to peers). But communication between youth and adults is often poor or absent also when youth's deepest experiences, emotions and thoughts regarding other basic aspects of reality are involved. For example, Whitney and Smith (1993) and Fonzi (1997) demonstrated that only 50% of children who are victims of bullying speak about their problem to teachers, parents, or friends and this percentage diminishes with increasing age (Menesini & Fonzi, 2003). Moreover, the absence, scarcity, and poor quality of communication between children and adults are frequently present in those situations when children are confronted with the problem of death (e.g., Pagani, 1992).

The majority of our participants (63%) stated that at least once in their life, in difficult times, they had been comforted by an animal. When describing the situations when this happened, some pupils explicitly referred to a more or less specific cause of their troubles, like in the examples below:

"When my parents scold me." (girl, 14 years)
"When my grandma died." (girl, 10 years)
"When I was alone." (boy, 15 years)

Others refer to a more or less generic feeling of distress without mentioning its causes:

"When I feel sadder." (boy, 17 years)
"I felt comforted by my cat when I hated the whole world." (boy, 15 years)

All these examples naturally conjure up the idea of "trust". The concept of trust is certainly a fundamental epistemological tool in order to understand positive, both interhuman and – in many cases – human–animal, relations. In this chapter I will not address the issue of the death of a companion animal, as in this book there are some chapters specially dedicated to this subject.

Some participants' answers clearly present specific situations where pupils displayed particularly benevolent behaviors toward animals: participants in various ways defended or rescued animals that were being maltreated, buried their pets or other small animals they were taking care of, fed stray animals, played with their pets and with other animals, kept them company, or rescued small birds fallen from their nests.

The majority of our participants were against hunting (83%), the use of furs and leather clothes (91%), the use of animals in circuses (77%), and zoos (58%). The lower percentage of participants against zoos probably relates to children's frequent belief that zoos have an educational role and are useful for the conservation of some animal species (Pagani, Robustelli, & Ascione, 2007; Robustelli & Pagani, 1994; Wells & Hepper, 1995). I will briefly comment on the issue of zoos and of the use of animals in circuses later in this chapter. On the whole, these high percentages further support the idea that most children and adolescents are aware of the psychological and physical needs of animals and feel empathetic toward them.

However, the data we obtained (from both this and other research studies we conducted) that most directly and unequivocally testify that many youth are deeply knowledgeable, thoughtful, and compassionate as far as their relations with animals are concerned, relate to their broad, refined, and complex concept of animal cruelty (Pagani, Robustelli, & Ascione, 2007, 2008; Pagani, Robustelli, & Ascione, 2010). This concept includes socially unacceptable and acceptable, direct and indirect, and intentional and unintentional behaviors, resulting in injury or harm to an animal (Ascione, 1993; Beirne, 1999). Suffice it to mention the question that one of our participants involved in another study[3] asked us: "If you do not rescue a fish lying almost dead on the shore, is it hurting it?" (boy, 10 years) (Pagani, Robustelli, & Ascione, 2010). Unfortunately, our data suggest that, again, adults often do not acknowledge children's cognitive and emotional maturity also as regards their attitudes and behavior toward animals (Pagani, 2003a).

Some of the Distinguishing Features of a Positive Relation Between Youth and Animals

I will now present a few considerations on some of the distinguishing features of a positive relation between youth and animals. I will analyze these features as compared with some of those features that mostly characterize interhuman relations

---

[3]The main aim of this study, which involved 137 pupils aged 9–16 (70 F and 67 M) in three Italian schools, was to field-test and validate the Italian version of the child self-report form of the CAI (The Children and Animals Inventory, Dadds et al., 2004).

and with some of those features that mostly characterize human–robotic animal interactions.

Though interhuman relations and human–animal relations (and in particular humans' relations with higher animals) share a notable number of elements, it is undisputable that many animals, as compared with humans, establish deep affective bonds with humans only on the basis of the actual (as opposed to pretended), inner (as opposed to exterior), and primary (as opposed to secondary) characteristics of their relationship (Pagani, 2003b). In this context the adjectives "actual", "inner", and "primary", though not synonymous, concretely strengthen each other and all together contribute to creating a comprehensive idea of the basic elements of this relationship. The adjectives in opposition to them, namely "pretended", "exterior", and "secondary", should further clarify the meaning of this idea. In brief, the final idea that the first three adjectives and their opposites should conjure up has very much to do with such concepts as trust, honesty, freedom, respect, and affection. We all know that an animal, for example, a dog, primarily understands, and is interested in, those aspects of the relationship with a human being that belong to the core or the essence of this relationship. This means that, from animals' point of view, their relationship with humans is absolutely untouched by sociocultural conditionings, that is by considerations relating to those aspects (i.e., social status) of human beings' lives and histories that do not specifically pertain to the core or the essence of the relationship itself, in sum by those elements that make interhuman relations particularly complex and, in most cases, problematic. These elements in various ways have to do with "pretending", "appearing", and "being unessential" and are the basic ingredients of the competitive life pattern that is prevailing the world over and has set up hierarchies of individuals on the basis of the amount of power each individual has over others (e.g., Pagani, 2000; Pagani & Robustelli, in press; Robustelli & Pagani, 1994, 1996).

The special features characterizing animals' bond with humans can easily affect humans' attitudes toward them, but can easily affect humans' personality in general and, hence, also their interpersonal relations. Since the pressure of sociocultural conditionings is very often heavy both for children and adults, the effect of a positive relationship with an animal can only be liberating. Besides, given that in our society animals usually occupy the lowest rungs in the social ladder, when a child or an adolescent establishes a deep and affectionate bond with an animal, she/he establishes a deep and affectionate bond with a somewhat weak and vulnerable individual, thus implicitly subverting this specific life pattern, which assumes that weak and vulnerable individuals can easily become the target of abuse on the part of the more powerful ones. In sum, a positive relationship between an animal and a child or an adolescent can be very beneficial also from an educational point of view.

Within this context a few words should also be spent on human–robotic animal interactions. In the last few years there has been an enormous technological progress in virtual reality and interactive computing, which has resulted in the creation of more and more sophisticated emulations of the natural world. Robotic pets, which are technological emulations of companion animals, are one of the outcomes of this trend (Melson, Kahn, Beck, Friedman, Roberts, Garret, & Gill, 2009). Thus, it is important to identify the basic specific characteristics of children–robotic pets interactions as compared to children–animal interactions and to analyze the differences between these characteristics and the possible different ways in which these differences can affect children's psychological well-being. In their excellent paper, which has recently appeared in the *Journal of Social Issues*, Melson, Kahn, Beck, and Friedman (2009) put forward two important points, which are supported by their research findings. They maintain that, with respect to a living dog, children tend to consider a robotic dog, like AIBO, "as a much more restricted interactive partner" (p. 556). They also state that "Over time, and with greater sophistication and capabilities on the side of the robotic technology, it is possible that children will develop deeper attachments to robotic dogs and the distinctions between their responses about living and robotic dogs may narrow" (p. 556). Three considerations may be useful here. First of all, it is proven that, as Serpell also points out, some animals possess an extremely refined sensitivity to unconscious human signals "that so far exceeds the blunted sensibilities of *Homo sapiens* that it can appear magical [...]"(Serpell, 2009, p. 638). It is the refined sensibilities that our human and animal fellows sometimes display (compared with those shown by robots) that make our interactions with them so complex, unique and fascinating. It is difficult to foresee whether, in the future, human–robotic animal interactions and humans' interactions with human-like robots will present these characteristics in the same degree. Second, in some cases the choice to own a robotic animal versus a living animal as a companion may be the product of some fears commonly associated with the interactions with a living being. For example, a fourth-grade girl who participated in one of the studies conducted by Melson and her collaborators (Melson, Kahn, Beck, & Friedman, 2009) declared: "The robotic dog would never die, and so I would never be sad" (p. 556). Couldn't owning a robotic animal versus a living animal lead children to avoid some important, complex, and unavoidable tasks, like coping with someone's death or tackling the problems that any interaction either with humans or animals involves? Third, my personal view, which is basically dictated by moral considerations, is that it would be preferable for children to interact with and take care of living animals instead of interacting with and taking care of robotic animals, given the enormous number of animals in the world that already exist and that may need our help, especially when they live in poor or desperate conditions.

Youth's Relationship with Animals and the Larger Natural World

Some authors (e.g., Myers & Saunders, 2002; Pagani, 2003b) maintain that a positive relationship with an animal can foster people to develop attitudes of interest in and concern for the larger natural world. A part of the rationale supporting this assumption is the idea that if an individual, a child or an adolescent in our case, shows a deep understanding of and affection for an animal, she/he will necessarily be more conscious of those environmental characteristics that are most suitable for the physical and psychological well-being of the animal. Thus, the child or the adolescent will learn that these environmental conditions must be preserved and that she/he has to do her/his best so that this happens. Moreover, as regards people's relationship with other animals, research findings (e.g., Ascione, 2005; Henry, 2004; Knight, Vrij, Cherryman, & Nunkoosing, 2004; Melson, 1998, 2001; Pagani, Robustelli, & Ascione, 2007; Paul, 2000; Podberscek, 1997; Robertson, Gallivan, & MacIntyre, 2004; Taylor & Signal, 2005; Taylor, Williams, & Gray, 2004) indicate that pet ownership or, more frequently, pet attachment is associated with empathic attitudes toward animals in general.

In the study mentioned above on Italian youth's attitudes and behaviors toward animals we found a significant relationship between deep attachment to pets and empathic attitudes toward animals in general (Pagani, Robustelli, & Ascione, 2007). For example, those participants who were "very fond" of their pets were more frequently "very sorry" when they saw roadkill and were more frequently against hunting, the use of furs and leather clothes, the use of animals in circuses, and zoos. The results regarding attitudes toward zoos and the use of animals in circuses are particularly significant, as children very often like visiting zoos as well as watching animals performing in circuses. Knight et al. (2004) justly point out that the theoretical justification for the association between positive experience of animals and attitudes toward animals may relate to the "contact hypothesis" (e.g., Allport, 1954), whereby positive contact with one or more members of an outgroup (which in this case is constituted by animals) can reduce prejudice toward that group and foster a mutual understanding between the two groups.

But there is a problem that many children who are attached to their pets sooner or later come across. Since a generalization process easily leads them on to feel interest in and affection for other animals, they can realize, for example, that some of these animals are often served to them as food. In many cases this discovery can be quite shocking. My 8-year-old nephew, who has had a pet – a tomcat – for one year and is very fond of him and who likes meat very much, said to me one day: "I am not yet mature for becoming a vegetarian." It seems that this young boy is actually aware of the contradiction between loving his cat (and, certainly, other animals, and, presumably, also animals in general) and eating animals at the same time. He also realizes that he is not yet ready for a radical change in his life – becoming vegetarian – also considering that his parents are not vegetarian. In other cases children may find out that the pet for whom they feel deep affection likes catching birds and eating them or that the food they give their pet has been obtained through the slaughtering of another animal. Indeed, this awareness violently pushes the child into the heart of those particularly conflictual attitudes toward animals that characterize our societies. But also – and this new kind of awareness may be even harder to sustain – the child realizes that nature is no Eden and that violence plays a major role there also, not only in human societies.

The Relationship Between Positive Attitudes and Behaviors Toward Animals and Interhuman Relations

Some research findings also indicate that pet ownership status or, more frequently, pet attachment and affection and respect for animals are associated with human-directed empathic concern and positive interhuman relations (e.g., Ascione & Weber, 1996; Melson, 1989; Poresky, 1990; Robertson, Gallivan, & MacIntyre, 2004; Taylor & Signal, 2005; Vidović, Štetić, & Bratko, 1999). As I said above, taking care of an animal or being interested and involved in animals' well-being in most cases also means being involved with an individual or group of individuals usually weaker and more vulnerable with respect to humans' greater cognitive capabilities. Given that the relationship with an animal, as compared with another human being, is usually easier, the process of identification with and sympathy toward the animal's weakness and vulnerability is also easier. When a child or an adolescent is capable of acknowledging the inevitable weaknesses and vulnerabilities of her/his self, she/he can also become more capable of acknowledging the weaknesses and vulnerabilities of others, and of feeling concern for them (Pagani, 2003b).

The themes of weakness, kindness, and power in both humans and animals and the process of mutual identification are extremely frequent in many folk fairy tales in different cultures. In these stories, where the motif of grateful or helpful animals is usually present (Sax, 2009), there is often a dynamic and dialectic play of different and interchangeable forces: the skill and kindness of the human main character (the hero), the weakness of the animal, the weakness of the human main character, and the skill and kindness of the animal. The pattern is quite simple: the animal is in a critical situation, the hero helps the animal to get out of it, later the hero in his turn is in a dangerous or difficult situation, and the animal rescues him. Here also the hierarchical and competitive life pattern is almost miraculously subverted. When the hero helps the animal, a creature that is usually considered inferior and despicable, not only the hero's behavior is not criticized or mocked but, contrary to what is usually the case in the real world, he is also rewarded with the best of the prizes (his life, the hand of the princess, etc.). This fantasy is clearly the expression of wish fulfilment, a process that is mostly elaborated by the common people, and especially by the poor and the weak. But it is also the expression of the great trust that humans often put in animals' kindness and affection toward human beings. In order to better clarify these points, I will refer to Grimm's fairy tale "The White Snake" (1856/1987). The structure and the formal style of the tale are not only perfect and precise but its meaning is also notable. Interestingly, in this story the pattern I have outlined above is repeated three times. The hero, a poor and honest servant, rescues three gasping fish caught in the reeds of a pond, and the three fish promise him they will remember his good act and will reward him. Later, he meets an ant who is complaining about people's horses as they tread heavily on ants and kill them. The servant, who is riding on horseback, makes a detour so that his horse does not crush the ants with its hooves. The ant tells him they will remember what he did for them and will reward him. Then the hero saves three little ravens, whose parents had cruelly and prematurely thrown them out of the nest, and the little ravens promise him they will remember his good action and will reward him. When, later on, the hero is set three almost impossible tasks – fishing a golden ring out of the bottom of the sea, picking all the millet seeds that had been contained in three sacks and had been scattered in the grass, and finding a golden apple that grows in the end of the world – in order to marry the princess, the animals he has been kind to bring him help. The three fish get him the golden ring, the ants pick the millet seeds, and the three ravens bring him the golden apple.

The Roles of Cultures and Education

In the last decade some authors have underlined the role of cultures in human–animal relationships in general (e.g., Flynn, 2001; Pagani, 2000; Podberscek, 2009; Serpell, 2009) and also, more specifically, in child–animal relationships (Flynn, 2008; Pagani, Robustelli, & Ascione, 2007, 2008; Pagani, Robustelli, & Ascione, 2010). Surprisingly, in the past the interest in the role of cultures had been very low or nonexistent among scholars in this research area. It is a fact that psychological phenomena are sometimes deeply influenced by culture (Robustelli & Pagani, 2005). Kardiner (1939), for example, elaborated the concept of *basic personality*, according to which a specific cultural context tends to foster the development of a specific type of personality, though the relation between culture and personality is not always straightforward. Indeed, culture produces tendencies, and individuals may sometimes respond in different ways to the same cultural influences. Therefore, the theoretical principle whereby all human psychological phenomena develop in and, hence, are affected by sociocultural conditions (Brislin, 1994) is to be applied also to the study of child–animal relations. Even among western cultures differences as regards people's attitudes toward animals and the larger natural world do occur. For example, with respect to English-speaking countries, Italy has been traditionally characterized by a weaker interest in nature, including animals. In some countries, like Cambodia, China, Thailand, and Vietnam, the practice of consuming dogs and cats is still alive (Podberscek, 2009). Also, regarding conceptualizations of animal abuse, there are notable cultural differences from one country to another, and even within a single country (e.g., Agnew, 1998; Merz-Perez, Heide, & Silverman, 2001; Pagani, Robustelli, & Ascione, 2007, 2008; Pagani, Robustelli, & Ascione, 2010; Piper, Johnson, Myers, & Pritchard, 2003; Podberscek, 2009). Besides, it is important to point out that a cultural context is characterized by temporal aspects as well, and not only by geographical and social features (Pagani, Robustelli, & Ascione, 2008). For instance, in Italy, acts of animal abuse perpetrated by children at the present time are to be interpreted and judged according to criteria that should differ, at least in part, from the criteria we might use in the interpretation and judgment of similar acts perpetrated by Italian children 50 years ago. At that time, children were not yet familiar with issues such as the preservation of the environment, respect for animals, ethological research, animal behavior, and animal mind. As a rule, all these topics were not debated at school, in the family, and in the media and, thus, were not an integral part of the Italian culture. It thus follows that, in general, from an educational point of view, animal maltreatment perpetrated half a century ago might in some cases be considered as a less serious problem compared to current animal maltreatment (Pagani, Robustelli, & Ascione, 2008; Pagani, Robustelli, & Ascione, 2010). Also Flynn (2001) underlined the strength of the link between culture and animal abuse when he stated that the high level of socially acceptable violence toward animals contributes to producing socially unacceptable violence toward them.

The research findings we obtained from our studies have been mostly analysed, discussed, and interpreted on the basis of the cultural contexts that produced them. Moreover, it is important to point out that, as I said above when I commented on the broad definition of animal cruelty given by many young participants in our research studies, youth are often able to also challenge traditional sociocultural views and perspectives as far as our relations with animals are concerned. And the significance of this challenge could not be completely grasped if cultural context should not be taken into due consideration. Hence, in psychological research the role of cultures should always be taken into account.

In any discussion of the child–animal relationship a reference to educational issues is obligatory. Earlier in this chapter I happened to make a few short comments on some parents' poor educational role as regards their children's relationship with their pets and with animals. Here, I will only touch on two points: the use of animals in circuses and the role of zoos. In an earlier paper (Robustelli & Pagani, 1994), I focused on the dangerous habit of taking children to places like circuses or zoos, where violence against animals is exhibited as "a normal, legitimate, even educational fact." (p. 14)

At the present time most children know that wild animals should live in their natural environment and that, anyway, both wild and domestic animals are not happy when they live in cages and are forced, for example, to learn useless, complex, grotesque, and unnatural behaviors, which humiliate their dignity and their intelligence. Nowadays Italian schools, and especially elementary schools, play a greater role, as compared with the past, in promoting children's knowledge of and compassion for animals. This fact seems to be related to the tendency, indicated by our research findings (Pagani, Robustelli, & Ascione, 2007), in children between 9 and 10 years, with respect to older participants, to feel more empathetic toward animals, especially as regards their attitudes toward zoos, the use of animals in circuses, the use of furs and leather clothes, and to be less frequently afraid of animals.

The animals that children watch at the circus are not animals freely displaying their specific natural characteristics, but often only animals that have been reduced to artificial and caricatural creatures. At a deep psychological level children experience these exhibitions as a message of abuse perpetrated by humans against weaker individuals.

Both zoos and the shows with animals in circuses can provide a social learning model that can be very dangerous as it inevitably affects children's relationships with both animals and human beings. Children can be led to the conclusion that abusing the weaker ones on the part of the more powerful ones is acceptable and, hence, they are allowed to imitate this behavior. Zoos and shows with animals in circuses can also contribute to strengthening that phenomenon which has been especially studied by social psychologists and which has been called "desensitization to violence" (e.g., Ascione, 1992, 1993; Donnerstein, Slaby, & Eron, 1994). Another psychological consequence for children's development may relate to the fact that children, who easily may identify with the animals they see in circuses or in zoos, learn that some adults are mean, violent, and abusing. Consequently their confidence in adults can deteriorate, which can negatively affect children's socialization process.

It is of no use trying to propose new life patterns based on justice and solidarity if we continue to consider the human species as "the ruler" of the earth. The idea that human beings can exercise their power over our planet and the idea that some human beings can exercise their power over other human beings are strictly connected. It is generally believed that zoological gardens play a positive educational role, thus forgetting that nothing can provide a better educational teaching than the view of freedom of others and of respect for them.

Conclusions

In this chapter, I analyzed children's and adolescents' positive attitudes and behaviors toward animals, mainly focusing on such themes as humans' relationship with diversity, the identification of the distinguishing features of the relation between youth and animals, the association between a caring attitude toward animals and a respectful attitude toward the larger natural world, the association between positive children–animal relations and children's interpersonal relations, and the roles of cultures and of education. Through the analysis of these issues I tried to underline and explain the deep significance of youth's positive attitudes and behaviors toward animals, a significance that society at large should take into greater consideration. Within this context, research can certainly provide a useful contribution. In particular, I would suggest some future directions for research in this area. For example, the study of the role of trust in children–animal interactions could be extremely important and could complement and shed light on the meaning of trust in interpersonal relations. Also the study of youth's fear of animals should deserve more attention on the part of researchers (Pagani, Robustelli, & Ascione, 2010), as fear can be an obstacle to the development of a positive relation between a child and an animal and, in some cases, can even lead to animal cruelty (Pagani, Robustelli, & Ascione, 2007).

I would like to conclude my chapter with the words of children themselves. In 1997, an article (Sartori, 1997) in an Italian newspaper told the story of a fallow deer wandering in the meadows to the north of the Garda Lake in northern Italy. The deer was killed by three hunters, who had been authorized to do so by the municipal council, as the animal was considered dangerous for the traffic. But the article especially addressed the theme of the rage and sadness of some children who had established an affectionate bond with the deer and reported their comments.

These are Daniel's (11 years) words:

> "I wrote him a poem. [...] It was on that occasion that I met him for the first time. [...] It all started about a month ago. One morning, I go out of the house to take a walk and the deer is there, standing still, staring at me. [...] I called my brother Matthew [...]. We started going near the deer, up to about 5 meters. Since then, almost every morning, while going to school, I used to leave him a small dried sandwich on the ground. On the way back from school, I used to check: the sandwich was never there. Sometimes I would see him: I would look at him without hiding and he would look back at me.
>
> Again, on Sunday I left him a sandwich. In the evening I went checking but the sandwich was still there. 'How strange', I thought. Later I found out that the deer had been killed."

This is Massimo's (14 years) story:

> "One Friday morning, at 7.00, I was going to school and he was there grazing the grass on my front lawn. Peaceful and happy. Wonderful. He did not lose his composure. [...] They killed him right here, at the field border. On Sunday, around 4 pm, I heard some shooting, at first quite far but then really near. I was even afraid of moving. So I saw him, at the end, lying on the ground, bleeding. Poor him. My dad got really mad at the hunters because they shot near our home. I was really mad for the deer."

And this is Katiuscha's (12 years) comment:

> "I would have never thought that somebody could kill him. On Sunday I got scared, but not for me, for him, for the deer. I thought about his fear, the escape, the shots that he must have felt coming on him."

References

Agnew, R. (1998) The causes of animal abuse: A social-psychological analysis. *Theoretical Criminology, 2*, 177–209.

Allport, G. W. (1954). *The nature of prejudice*. Cambridge, MA: Addison-Wesley.

Ascione, F. R. (1992) Enhancing children's attitudes about the humane treatment of animals: Generalization to human-directed empathy. *Anthrozoös, 5*, 176–191.

Ascione, F. R. (1993) Children who are cruel to animals: A review of research and implications for developmental psychopathology. *Anthrozoös, 6*, 226–247.

Ascione, F. R. (2005). *Children and animals: Exploring the roots of kindness and cruelty*. West Lafayette, IN: Purdue University Press.

Ascione, F. R., Thompson, T. M., & Black, T. (1997) Childhood cruelty to animals: Assessing cruelty dimensions and motivations. *Anthrozoös, 10*, 170–177.

Ascione, F. R., & Weber, C. V. (1996) Children's attitudes about the humane treatment of animals and empathy: One-year follow up of a school-based intervention. *Anthrozoös, 9*, 188–195.

Beirne, P. (1999) For a nonspeciesist criminology: Animal abuse as an object of study. *Criminology, 37*, 117–147.

Boat, B. W. (1999). Abuse of Children and Abuse of Animals. In F. R. Ascione & P. Arkow (Eds.), *Child abuse, domestic violence and animal abuse: Linking the circles of compassion for prevention and intervention* (pp. 83–100). West Lafayette, IN: Purdue University Press.

Brislin, R. W. (1994). Cross-cultural psychology. In R. J. Corsini (Ed.), *Encyclopedia of psychology* (Vol. 1, 2nd ed., pp. 352–361). New York: John Wiley & Sons.

Dadds, M. R., Whiting, C., Bunn, P., Fraser, J. A., Charlson, J. H., & Pirola-Merlo, A. (2004) Measurement of cruelty in children: The cruelty to animals inventory. *Journal of Abnormal Child Psychology, 32*, 321–334.

Donnerstein, E., Slaby, R. G., & Eron, L. D. (1994). The mass media and youth aggression. In L. D. Eron (Ed.), *Reason to hope* (pp. 219–250). Washington, DC: American Psychological Association.

Flynn, C. P. (2001) Acknowledging the "zoological connection": A sociological analysis of animal cruelty. *Society & Animals, 9*, 71–87.

Flynn, C. P. (2008). A sociological analysis of animal abuse. In F. R. Ascione (Ed.), *The international handbook of animal abuse and cruelty: Theory, research, and application* (pp. 155–174). West Lafayette, IN: Purdue University Press.

Fonzi, A. (1997). *Il Bullismo in Italia. Il Fenomeno delle Prepotenze a Scuola dal Piemonte alla Sicilia.* Firenze: Giunti.

Grimm, J., & Grimm, W. (1856/1987). *The complete fairy tales of the Brothers Grimm.* (J. Zipes, trans.). New York: Bantam Books.

Henry, B. C. (2004) Exposure to animal abuse and group context: Two factors affecting participation in animal abuse. *Anthrozoös, 17*, 290–305.

Kardiner, A. (1939). *The individual and his society.* New York: Columbia University Press.

Knight, S., Vrij, A., Cherryman, J., & Nunkoosing, K. (2004) Attitudes towards animal use and belief in animal mind. *Anthrozoös, 17*, 43–62.

Kottak, C. P. (2002). *Anthropology: The exploration of human diversity.* New York: McGraw Hill.

Magid, K. (2008). Attachment and Animal Abuse. In F. R. Ascione (Ed.), *The international handbook of animal abuse and cruelty: Theory, research, and application* (pp. 335–373). West Lafayette, IN: Purdue University Press.

Melson, G. F. (1989) Availability of and involvement with pets by children: Determinants and correlates. *Anthrozoös, 2*, 45–52.

Melson, G. F. (1998). The role of companion animals in human development. In C. C. Wilson & D. C. Turner (Eds.), *Companion animals in human health* (pp. 219–236). Thousand Oaks, CA: Sage.

Melson, G. F. (2001). *Why the wild things are: Animals in the lives of children.* Cambridge, MA: Harvard University Press.

Melson, G. F., Kahn, P. H., Jr., Beck, A., & Friedman, B. (2009). Robotic pets in human lives: Implications for the human–animal bond and for human relationships with personified technologies. *Journal of Social Issues, 65*(3), 545–567.

Melson, G. F., Kahn, P. H., Jr., Beck, A., Friedman, B., Roberts, T., Garret, E., & Gill, B. T. (2009) Children's behavior toward and understanding of robotic and living dogs. *Journal of Applied Developmental Psychology, 30*, 92–102.

Menesini, E., & Fonzi, A. (2003) La definizione del bullismo: alunni e insegnanti a confronto. *Età Evolutiva, 74*, 68–75.

Merz-Perez, L., Heide, K. M., & Silverman, I. J. (2001) Childhood cruelty to animals and subsequent violence against humans. *International Journal of Offender Therapy and Comparative Criminology, 45*, 556–573.

Myers, O. E., Jr., & Saunders, C. D. (2002). Animals as links toward developing caring relationships with the natural world. In P. H. Kahn, Jr. & S. R. Kellert (Eds.), *Children and nature* (pp. 153–178). Cambridge, MA: The MIT Press.

Pagani, C. (1992) L'oro dei bambini. Analisi della comunicazione tra il bambino e l'adulto e tra gli adulti in genere sul problema della morte e della malattia. *Bambini, 10*, 24–35.

Pagani, C. (2000) Perception of a common fate in human–animal relations and its relevance to our concern for animals. *Anthrozoös, 13*, 66–73.

Pagani, C. (2003a) Il bambino e il dolore. *A, 287*, 18–24.

Pagani, C. (2003b). Il bambino e l'animale: significati formativi della relazione con l'animale d'affezione. In *Atti del Convegno "Pet-therapy: il valore della relazione con l'animale", Reggio Emilia, 18–19 ottobre 2003* (pp. 33–40). Reggio Emilia: Provincia di Reggio Emilia.

Pagani, C., & Robustelli, F. (2005). *Marek a scuola. Gli insegnanti e l'inserimento degli alunni stranieri nella scuola italiana.* Milano: Franco Angeli.

Pagani, C., & Robustelli, F. (in press). Youths, multiculturalism, and educational interventions for the development of empathy. *International Social Sciences Journal.*

Pagani, C., Robustelli, F., & Ascione, F. R. (2007) Italian youths' attitudes toward, and concern for, animals. *Anthrozoös, 20,* 275–293.

Pagani, C., Robustelli, F., & Ascione, F. R. (2008). Animal abuse experiences described by Italian school-aged children. In F. R. Ascione (Ed.), *The international handbook of animal abuse and cruelty: Theory, research, and application* (pp. 247–268). West Lafayette, IN: Purdue University Press.

Pagani, C., Robustelli, F., & Ascione, F. R. (2010) Investigating animal abuse: Some theoretical and methodological issues. *Anthrozoös, 23,* 259–278.

Pagani, C., Robustelli, F., & Martinelli, C. (2010). *School, cultural diversity and multiculturalism.* Manuscript submitted for publication.

Paul, E. S. (2000). Love of pets and love of people. In A. L. Podberscek, E. S. Paul, & J. A. Serpell (Eds.), *Companion animals and us* (pp. 168–186). Cambridge: Cambridge University Press.

Piper, H., Johnson, M., Myers, S., & Pritchard, J. (2003) Children and young people harming animals: Intervention through PSHE?. *Research Papers in Education, 18,* 197–213.

Podberscek, A. L. (1997) Illuminating issues of companion animal welfare through research into human–animal interactions. *Animal Welfare, 6,* 365–372.

Podberscek, A. L. (2009). Good to pet and eat: The keeping and consuming of dogs and cats in South Korea. *Journal of Social Issues, 65*(3), 615–631.

Poresky, R. (1990). The young children's empathy measure: Reliability, validity, and effects of companion animal bonding. *Psychological Reports, 66,* 931–936.

Robertson, J. C., Gallivan, J., & MacIntyre, P. D. (2004) Sex differences in the antecedents of animal use attitudes. *Anthrozoös, 17,* 306–317.

Robustelli, F. (2000). Psicologia della diversità. In B. M. Pirani (Ed.), *L'abbaglio dell'occidente* (pp. 189–198). Roma: Bulzoni.

Robustelli, F., & Pagani, C. (1994) Bambini e animali. *Bambini, 5,* 10–17.

Robustelli, F., & Pagani, C. (1996) L'educazione contro la violenza. *Psicologia contemporanea, 136,* 4–10.

Robustelli, F., & Pagani, C. (2005) Le variabili della violenza umana. *Psicologia contemporanea, 187,* 60–63.

Salinger, J. D. (1969). *The catcher in the rye.* New York: Bentam Books.

Sartori, M. (1997, March 19). Le poesie tristi e la rabbia degli amici di Bambi. *L'Unità.*

Sax, B. (2009) The magic of animals: English witch trials in the perspective of folklore. *Antrozoös, 22,* 317–332.

Serpell, J. A. (2009). Having our dogs and eating them too: Why animals are a social issue. *Journal of Social Issues, 65*(3), 633–644.

Taylor, H., Williams, P., & Gray, D. (2004) Homelessness and dog ownership: An investigation into animal empathy, attachment, crime, drug use, health and public opinion. *Anthrozoös, 17,* 353–368.

Taylor, N., & Signal, T. D. (2005) Empathy and attitudes to animals. *Anthrozoös, 18,* 18–27.

Vidović, V. V., Štetić, V. V., & Bratko, D. (1999) Pet ownership, type of pet and socio-emotional development of school children. *Anthrozoös, 12,* 211–217.

Wells, D. L., & Hepper, P. G. (1995) Attitudes to animal use in children. *Anthrozoös, 8,* 159–170.

Whitney, I., & Smith, P. K. (1993) A survey of the nature and extent of bullying in junior/middle and secondary schools. *Educational Research, 35,* 3–25.

Chapter 18
Rational Emotions: Animal Rights Theory, Feminist Critiques and Activist Insight

Carol L. Glasser

Most animal rights theories forward rational and objective criteria as justification for granting nonhuman animals rights and often reject emotional connection with nonhuman animals as an adequate justification for granting rights. In this chapter, I use the terms "animal rights" and the "animal rights movement" broadly. I discuss philosophies, theories, and activism that are concerned with the moral consideration given to nonhuman animals as well as the question of whether animals should have rights. "Moral consideration" is not the same as "animal rights," since the concept of rights is theoretical and has specific political implications. Though I do think that these distinctions are important and meaningful, they are beyond the scope of this chapter. The varied beliefs regarding why human animals should not exploit or use nonhuman animals are colloquially discussed in a broad fashion as "animal rights" or the "animal rights movement," as such I will use also these terms broadly in this chapter. I focus on the animal rights movement in the United States and research conducted in the United States. Though many of the theories and philosophies discussed are important in other national, social, and cultural contexts, I am only considering the animal rights movement as it functions presently in the United States. Feminist philosophies critique these theories and argue that emotions and an ethic of care need to be incorporated into philosophies of animal rights. I argue that rational and emotional ontologies are not mutually exclusive; theories that combine feminist ethics of caring and emotion with rational arguments for animal rights are the most useful since activists and veg'ns understand via complex emotional, relational, and rational processes that nonhuman animals should not exist for food, clothing, entertainment, or human experiments. I also contend that there needs to be a more dynamic philosophy of animal rights. The homogeneous nature of the people involved in the animal rights movement suggests that animal rights theories do not adequately address the concept of oppression. I stress the need for a more robust and dynamic theory of animal rights that accounts for interlocking systems of oppression and draws simultaneously on emotion and reason.

C.L. Glasser (✉)
Department of Sociology, University of California, Irvine, CA, USA
e-mail: cglasser@gmail.com

C. Blazina et al. (eds.), *The Psychology of the Human–Animal Bond*,
DOI 10.1007/978-1-4419-9761-6_18, © Springer Science+Business Media, LLC 2011

Praxis: Theory Guiding Action, Activists Guiding Theory

While social movement participation often springs from personal experiences of oppression, the animal rights movement is rooted in philosophy, based on theory, and propelled in important ways by academics (Jasper and Nelkin, 1992). However, the driving force of the animal rights movement, and what makes it a formidable social movement rather than an ideological bent of academia, is that activists maintain it. As such, the efficacy and validity of animal rights theories should be reflected by, have practical implications for, and applications in the animal rights movement. The founding theories of the current wave of animal rights in the United States are in need of development and refinement. To do this we should look beyond academics and to activists. This dialectical route to theory building is of particular interest to the social scientist, as it grounds theory in practice.

Animal rights theories can be refined and improved by asking a few key questions: What are the arguments and experiences that compel activists? How do activists conceptualize and describe their reasons for recognizing and preserving the rights of animals? If the goal is to develop a theory that can end the suffering of nonhuman animals at the hands of humans, then we should learn from the processes that those who became animal rights activists went through in coming to the conclusion that nonhuman animals do not exist for human consumption and use.

The majority of animal rights activists and veg'ns made a conscientious choice in adolescence or adulthood to reject using animals in ways that most consider 'normal' or 'common,' and so the process of their shifting attitudes toward nonhuman animals is available for examination. As such, this is a unique point in the movement in which the experiences and motivations of activists can be utilized to develop and refine theories of animal rights. When we observe those who reject the exploitation of animals, understand the impetus for their attitudes toward animals and what it is that propels their commitment to behaving in a manner consistent to these attitudes, we can better understand *how* people decide that animals have rights, thereby allowing for the development of more robust and comprehensive theories of animal rights.

Rationalism in Animal Rights Theory

The theoretical underpinnings of the current wave of the animal rights movement in the United States are most closely associated with Peter Singer and Tom Regan. In *Animal Liberation* (1975), Singer uses the logic of utilitarianism to argue that nonhuman animals deserve moral consideration. According to Singer, nonhuman animals are sentient, meaning they have the ability to feel pain and to suffer; this ability is the prerequisite for having interests, and having interests is a basis for deserving equal consideration. As such, the fact that nonhuman animals have an interest in staying alive and avoiding pain means that they have a right not to be exploited or abused by humans.

Regan approaches animal rights from a natural rights philosophy, extending a Kantian framework to incorporate nonhuman animals. In *The Defense for Animal Rights* (1983), he argues that nonhuman animals deserve rights based on their mental capacities and subjective consciousness. Because they have active mental lives, nonhuman animals are "subjects of a life," and being subjects of a life makes nonhuman animals deserving of rights.

Rationalism is an epistemology that makes appeals to reason without reliance on personal experiences. A justice-based ethical framework advocates fairness and impartiality; justice-based ethics attempt to develop guidelines for decision making in which moral decisions can be made impartially without considering specific individual circumstances. In placing reason above emotion and valuing objective rules to subjective experiences as a basis of knowledge, both Regan and Singer explicitly reject personal experiences and relationships with nonhuman animals as relevant to their theories.

The Feminist Critique

Regan and Singer are often referred to as the "fathers of animal rights" (Donovan, 1990), and while their works are necessary, powerful, and compelling, they are not without fault. Addressing inadequacies with these philosophies allows for future theory to grow from their foundations in fruitful directions. In their attempts to establish their claims as rational, both Singer and Regan disassociate themselves from sentimentality and a 'love' for animals. They intentionally move away from 'emotion' and frame their arguments as 'reasonable' and thus 'rational.' Feminist critiques of these theories argue it is necessary to reject rationalist philosophy, as it reflects and bolsters a patriarchal (and thereby oppressive) ontology. These critiques argue "[r]ationalism is the key to the connected oppressions of women and nature in the West" (Plumwood, 1991, p. 3): the solution is for philosophy to embrace relational, empathetic, emotional, and caring ways of knowing (see Tong and Williams, 2009).

Feminists have also broadly critiqued traditional ethics for bolstering masculine traits and discounting feminine ones:

> Traditional ethics overrates culturally masculine traits like "independence, autonomy, intellect, will, wariness, hierarchy, domination, culture, transcendence, product, asceticism, war, and death," while it underrates culturally feminine traits like "interdependence, community, connection, sharing, emotion, body, trust, absence of hierarchy, nature, immanence, process, joy, peace, and life" (Tong and Williams, 2009).

Feminist critiques specific to Regan's and Singer's philosophies also address their rejection of emotional and interpersonal connections to nonhuman animals, arguing they embrace the very system of domination that is responsible for the oppression of nonhuman animals:

> In accepting as two primary texts, Singer's *Animal Liberation* and Regan's *The Case for Animal Rights*—texts that valorize rationality—the animal defense movement reiterates a

patriarchal disavowal of emotions as having a legitimate role in theory making. The problem is that while on the one hand it articulates positions against animal suffering, on the other hand, animal rights theory dispenses with the idea that caring about and emotionally responding to this suffering can be appropriate sources of knowledge (Adams, 2007 [2006], p. 201).

Looking to activists it is apparent that feminist contributions are necessary for animal rights philosophy, if only for the fact that most animal rights activists and veg'ns in the United States are women (Lowe and Ginsberg, 2002; Plous, 1991). Harold Herzog (2007) conducted a meta-analysis of research addressing gender differences in human–animal interactions and concluded that gender imbalances are notable: somewhere between 67 and 80% of animal rights activists in the United States are women, men are more likely than women to hunt recreationally and to have abused animals in both childhood and adulthood, and women are more likely to be involved in grassroots animal rights activism.

Though women predominate in the animal rights movement, they do not necessarily take on leading roles. Gender politics among activists can reproduce and reflect notions of the emotional/rational dichotomy. Julian McAllister Groves (2001) examined the animal rights movement at the grassroots level via in-depth interviews with activists and participant observation of a grassroots organization. She found that women are in a difficult position due to the gendering and devaluation of emotions:

> Women face a double bind when it comes to emotional expression: If they dismiss their compassion, they may be dismissed as trivial; if they express their anger, they may be dismissed as hysterical (p. 228).

Groves found this was reflected in gendered organizational structures such that, while the majority of movement participants are women, men held positions of power and served as public figureheads because movement members (men and women) believed them to be more rational and less emotional.

Care-focused feminists have critiqued traditional theories of animal rights for discounting relationships and caring as a basis of knowing. The care-based tradition (see Gilligan, 1982) makes a distinction between justice-based ethics and care-based ethics. The justice framework, in which Regan and Singer sit, is interested in the applicability of generalized rules of conduct and in resolving claims of conflict and interest (Luke, 2007 [1992]). Justice-based theories of ethics suggest that justice precedes care, whereas care-based theories argue caring is necessary before justice can occur. Caring places an emphasis on connections, the specific, and the satisfaction of individual needs (Tong and Williams, 2009).

It is the case that animal rights activists are focused on caring. Kenneth Shapiro (2007 [1994]) examined the autobiographies of 14 movement leaders as well as surveys from 21 activists and found animal rights activists share a number of key traits, and salient among these is a focus on caring. For most animal rights activists, their first remembered moment of caring for a nonhuman animal occurred at a young age, somewhere between five and ten years old. As Shapiro also highlights, the importance of caring is clear even in Regan's work; though Regan philosophically treats emotion as antithetical to reason, he describes the death of his dog as the catalyst for his animal rights work.

For vegetarian ecofeminists the oppression of women, nature, and animals are interlocking systems of oppression. Any theory of animals and nature must acknowledge that the structure of domination is also oppressive to women. Likewise, any theory explaining women's oppression must also recognize how their oppression is tied to the oppression of animals and nature. In *The Sexual Politics of Meat* (1990), Carol J. Adams makes the argument that the oppression of animals is directly linked to and reinforces the oppression of women. She introduces the concept of the "texts of meat," explaining that meat is itself an encoded form of patriarchy:

> [T]he coherence [meat] achieves as a meaningful item of food arises from patriarchal attitudes including the idea that the end justifies the means, that the objectification of other beings is a necessary part of life, and that violence can and should be masked (p. 24).

Though Regan and Singer do not explicitly suggest that the "end justifies the means," both engage in reproducing patriarchal value hierarchies by creating rules that establish some groups as inherently more important than others. Rather than dealing with the particular, as feminists in the care tradition encourage, they attempt to develop a set of 'rules' that can make their theories universally and objectively applicable in all situations in which animal rights may be called into question. To push the limits of their philosophies and show their broad applicability, they react to constructed "what-if" situations:

> Tom Regan requests, for example, that we imagine a man and a dog adrift in a lifeboat while Peter Singer explains why the life of one's child ought to be preferred to that of the family dog in the event of a house fire. I argue that such scenarios are not the usefully abstract analytic tools they purport to be... (Bailey, 2007 [2005], p. 129).

These situations are problematic for multiple reasons. First, they are unlikely to occur. Second, when they do, the child and the dog and their circumstances will never be the same twice, so one set of rules will not suffice. Rather, they reaffirm the notion that a set of rules can be established to place definitive boundaries around different groups and that these groups should then be valued differently. Ecofeminism highlights the ways this type of logic reasserts the same systems of domination that the animal rights movement is trying to deconstruct.

One important fault in the work of Regan and Singer is their reliance on the rational/emotional dichotomy. Raia Prokhovnik (2002) argues against a dichotomous way of knowing in favor of a relational way of knowing (i.e. learning through subjective experiences and interpersonal relationships) and identifies the characteristics of dichotomies, including an opposition between two identities, a hierarchical ordering of the pair and the assumption that the pair, when taken together, sums up and defines the whole. This dichotomous way of thinking is a definitional part of patriarchy. Ecofeminism recognizes oppression as "an ideology whose fundamental self/other distinction is based on a sense of self that is separate/atomistic" (Gaard, 1993, p. 2). Embracing a definition of oppression as something rooted in dichotomous constructs makes it a more viable theoretical framework for animal rights.

A dichotomy presumes only two opposite ways of being (Prokhovnik, 2002), and anything that is not on the valued end of the dichotomy is, by default, devalued. Under patriarchy, anything that is not male, white, or masculine assumes lower status on the hierarchy. Adams (1994) refers to this rank ordering as a value hierarchy. Dichotomous thinking not only reinforces a gender hierarchy through the man/woman dichotomy that devalues women and feminine traits (e.g. emotion as opposed to reason) but also reinforces a species hierarchy through the man/nature dichotomy. The problem with the theories for animal rights forwarded by Regan and Singer is that while they reject the latter dichotomy (man/nature), they embrace and perpetuate the former (man/woman). The ecofeminist critique asserts that to dismantle oppression it is necessary to deconstruct and reject philosophies that perpetuate dichotomous, value-ordered thinking in any way.

This argument also highlights the need to find a philosophy of animal rights that does not establish rationality and emotion as opposite and antithetical to one another. Feminist theories that establish themselves purely in opposition to rationalism risk reproducing the same dichotomous and rule-oriented perspective forwarded by theories that rely on rationality. For, if patriarchy is established in part by dichotomous ways of knowing, then establishing a care-based or emotion-based theory in *opposition* to a rationally based theory reproduces this problem in that it doesn't argue against a value hierarchy, it just argues for reconceptualizing what ideas should be on the valued end of the hierarchy.

While some feminist philosophers urge complete rejection of rationalism (e.g. Plumwood, 1991), most theorists and philosophers who advance feminist ethics do not deny all ties to rationality or rationalism, rather they seek to emphasize care-based and relational ontologies. A more fruitful approach is to develop philosophy that explicitly forwards a worldview in which emotion and rationality are not mutually exclusive. It is not irrational to be emotional or to care, nor is it impossible to be rational when acting on or reacting to emotional stimuli. As will be discussed in the following section, both emotions and rationality are at the forefront of humans' understandings of nonhuman animals' rights. People are simultaneously emotional and rational and so, if we are to root theory in practice, animal rights theory should as well.

Though much feminist work on caring and emotion does not reject any notion of rationalism, very little work attempts to address and incorporate *both* rationalism and emotionality. Philosophers have long questioned and investigated the linkages between emotion and reason; this question was discussed as early as the 300s B.C. by Aristotle and is still discussed by philosophers today (e.g. Elster, 1999). However, there are few attempts to apply these philosophical traditions to academic research in other fields, though there are some examples such as in the field of nursing (e.g. Botes, 2000).

Little work, however, has focused on animal rights philosophy. Though Herzog (1993) explicitly studies how both reason and emotion are important in developing animal rights activists' commitment to activism and veg'nism, his work is empirical and does not seek to advance a theory for animal rights that merges rational and relational epistemologies. Thomas G. Kelch (2007 [1999]) has made the only attempt of which I am aware that explicitly attempts to theoretically incorporate both, though his work is limited to advancing animal rights within the framework of legal theory. What is needed is a justification for animal rights based in appeals to experiences gained through emotions such as sympathy and caring (emotion and care-based philosophy) that are explained and justified as rational and reasonable experiences (rationalism). Such a theory is desperately needed, since both emotional and rational experiences are integral to activists' decisions to be veg'n and/or become activists.

Gaining Insight from Activists

There is a dearth of literature that examines the demographic composition or attitudes of animal rights activists and/or veg'ns. The research that does exist highlights that this is a homogeneous group demographically but that, individually, they experience a varied and complex interplay of emotions, the human–animal bond, compassion, and rationality in developing their attitudes toward nonhuman animals. Many activists and veg'ns note particular emotive experiences in changing their ways of thinking about nonhuman animals, but emotional impetus is not the only cue to which they react. Herzog (1993, p. 107) interviewed 23 activists in order to study the cognitive and emotional effects of the animal rights movement on its participants and he concluded that "the stereotype that activists are highly emotional clearly did not apply" across all of the activists he interviewed; while some claimed that emotional experience triggered their animal activism, many also worked to "buttress their initial emotional responses with logic in order to adequately discuss their positions on animal issues with others" (p. 108).

Shapiro (2007 [1994], p. 164) concluded that while caring is the "foundation of the animal rights movement," it is not the only aspect that influences activists: "[T]he caring of animal rights activists is informed by a sophisticated understanding of animals, both their suffering and the institutional and ideological origins of that suffering." The ability to empathize with and recognize the suffering of nonhuman animals was a relevant factor for the activists that Shapiro studied; however, these activists also worked to become more informed and enact change. Thus, emotional experiences became the impetus that encouraged activism, which is a pragmatic and rational way to try to change the plight of nonhuman animals.

What is also clear is that the ways in which emotions and rationality intermingle and inform each other are complex. Harold Herzog and Lauren L. Golden (2009) used survey measures to gauge peoples' attitudes toward animals as well as their sensitivity to disgust. They found that animal rights activists are more sensitive to visceral disgust than veg'ns who are not activists. This suggests a complex interplay of emotion and action in which varying degrees of activism, which is a rational way to try to combat animal cruelty, are paired with varying degrees of emotional connection to animals' suffering.

There are varied possibilities regarding how the interplay of reason and emotion functions: (1) emotional response to animals' suffering triggers a reasoned response to try to ease that suffering (i.e. becoming an activist), (2) being an activist and understanding why the torture and abuse of nonhuman animals is irrational or immoral creates a willingness to experience emotional connections with the animals they try to protect, and/or (3) a certain type of person simultaneously experiences reason and emotion when deciding to stop exploiting animals in conjunction with trying to convince others to do so as well.

It is likely that all three scenarios are occurring, and the interplay of emotion and reason are different for each activist as each individual activist's biography, psychology, and the circumstances that informed their activism (or veg'nism) are specific. In the earlier-mentioned study by Herzog (1993), activists described their emotional attachment to animals in varied ways—some were directed by reason, some by emotion, but most simultaneously by emotion and reason. Shapiro (2007 [1994]) found that once a concern for animals became pervasive in activists' lives, they handled it in different ways. Some embraced an ethic of care and sought out veg'n activist communities, some suppressed the care by distancing themselves from direct contact with the suffering they sought to reduce, and still others lost touch with caring—all are rational and sometimes calculated responses to the pain and frustration that can come with caring, particularly when there is often little these activists can do to help those for whom they care.

Since activists have such varied experiences drawing upon and melding emotional and rational reasons for embracing animal rights, an adequate theory should as well. A major problem with rationalism is that it attempts to determine rules that can objectively and fairly be applied to all situations. However, since activists have such varied ways of coming to recognize that nonhuman animals should not be exploited by humans, a single theory based in rationalist thought may not adequately forward the idea that nonhuman animals deserve the same moral consideration as do humans. As care-focused ethics highlight, concentrating on the specific and particular is important. This is especially the case if animal rights are the topic of concern.

One of the constructs that allows for nonhuman animals' oppression is that they are not viewed as individuals. Rather, individual animals are conceived of as an undifferentiated part of a species. This identification of individual animals with animal groups is what Adams (2007 [2006], p. 23) refers to as using "false mass terms:"

> Mass terms refer to things like water or colors; no matter how much of it there is or what type of container it is in, water is still water... Objects referred to by mass terms have no individuality, no uniqueness, no specificity, no particularity.

Theories that attempt to establish rules that group together 'types' of animals or 'sets' of circumstances in order to assign rights or value reproduce the very structures that allow for the oppression of animals.

Moving forward, philosophers and theorists should avoid the urge to develop a macro-level theory that seeks to develop a singular 'objective' set of logic and rules for giving nonhuman animals moral consideration. Philosophers can learn from social scientists, who are more concerned with praxis and often engage in meso-level theory building rather than macro-level theory building. Meso-level theories attempt to explain phenomena within the bounds of particular social and cultural settings; philosophies of animal rights could attempt to seek truth within the contexts of specific cultural constraints and in light of the particular traits and needs of the specific nonhuman animals living within those contexts.

Another issue with the dominant animal rights theories is that they do not adequately explain oppression. This is evidenced by the fact that adherents to an animal rights philosophy are not diverse, with most participants in positions of economic and ethnic and racial privilege. This suggests that current arguments for animal rights are not compelling to ethnic minorities or the economically disadvantaged. Animal rights activists and veg'ns are a very homogeneous group: mostly women (Herzog, 2007; Lowe and Ginsberg, 2002; Plous, 1991), well educated (Herzog, 2007; except see Jerolmack, 2003), white (Jamison and Lunch, 1992), and middle class or affluent (Herzog, 2007; Lowe and Ginsberg, 2002; except see Jerolmack, 2003). Future research should investigate why people choose not to embrace animal rights philosophy and focus on how this relates to issues of race and class. In doing so, insight can be gained as to how to develop a more robust theory of animal rights that will speak more cogently to oppression.

Thus, traditional theories and feminist theories of oppression and animal rights should also be evaluated in light of their ability to address varied oppressions. For example, the dichotomous thinking that perpetuates the oppression of women and nonhuman animals also perpetuates racial inequality. Yen Lee Espiritu explains the consistent oppression of Asian Americans and Asians in the United States as resulting from being defined by dominant culture as "not-American," which relegates them as a group to being "forever foreigners" (2001; see also 2000). This is just one example of how a dichotomous construct is used to forward racist ideology. An inclusive animal rights theory needs to be able to address oppression more coherently and broadly so that the characteristics of domination, which simultaneously oppress multiple groups, can be more clearly recognized.

This is a difficult task, as a versatile and robust explanation of oppression needs to explain that all oppression is equally important but that no two groups experience oppression in the same way. While all oppression must be valued equally and all oppression is rooted in the dominant group's desire to maintain power, the way that different groups experience oppression and their histories of domination are varied, and these histories must be understood as theory moves forward. For example, a parallel that is sometimes drawn in the animal rights community is between factory farming and chattel slavery. For an animal rights activist who truly rejects speciesism and racism, this may be a very clear parallel—the oppressor class systematically enslaves, tortures, extracts labor from, and murders individuals for profit. However, this parallel has often been rejected and viewed as racist. One such example is the negative response to a campaign by People for the Ethical Treatment of Animals that featured pictures of black men hanging by nooses next to pictures of cows hanging in slaughterhouses. Scott X. Esdaile, the president of the Connecticut chapter of the NAACP in 2005, responded: "Once again, black people are being pimped. You used us. You have used us enough. Take it down immediately" (Hall, 2005).

Knowledge of and sensitivity to the ways that racial oppression in the United States functions makes clear why some might feel that this comparison is racist. First, it is usually coming from someone in the privileged racial class, since most animal rights activists and veg'ns are white. Second, black Americans and other racial minorities have historically and are currently degraded by having their bodies paralleled to animal bodies. Examples of the use of animal parallels to degrade non-white ethnic and racial minorities in the United States abound. For example, in the late nineteenth century, racist sentiment toward Chinese immigrants was apparent in advertisements that depicted Chinese men as rats. Current racist sentiment, such as the statement that Latinas "breed like dogs" (see Hondagneu-Sotelo & Avila, 2007), also attempts to degrade racial and ethnic minorities by equating them with nonhuman animals.

From the perspective of someone who is discriminated against because of such parallels, embracing them in any way can reproduce racial inequality. Further, these comparisons do not take the necessary step to empower nonhuman animals by forwarding the idea that they are inherently deserving of rights; rather, even if unintentionally, it suggests that it is only because they are like humans that they deserve rights. As Adams (2007 [2006], p. 212) explains:

> It is not for us to compare suffering. We should *acknowledge* suffering, but not compare it. Acknowledging grants the *integrity* of the suffering, while comparing assumes the *reducibility*, the objectification of suffering... [A]nimal suffering is ignored unless appropriated to human suffering to make it expressible... Instead of saying, "animal's suffering is like humans"... why not say animal suffering in their bodies is *theirs*?

A more fruitful way to develop the idea that ethnic and species oppression are both important and intertwined is to highlight the ways that oppression of nonhuman animals and human minorities are used to mutually reinforce each other's oppression. For example, meat eating simultaneously reflects multiple oppressions in US society. There are arguments to reject meat eating from feminist, class-based, antiracist, and animal rights perspectives. Veg'ns reject eating meat out of concern for nonhuman animals that are slaughtered to produce it, but there are human-focused reasons to reject meat as well. As previously discussed, feminists may reject meat because it is a vestige of patriarchy. There are reasons to reject eating meat from the perspectives of race and class struggle as well.

Just as meat encodes patriarchy, it encodes colonialism. For example, though meat is now viewed as a staple in the Latino diet, it was not until colonization that regular meat consumption was introduced (Serrato, 2010). Meat also reflects a system of classism and labor exploitation. Government subsidies to agribusiness and the meat industries encourage mass production in such a way that it exploits and endangers nonhuman animals as well as human workers (see Eisnitz, 2003; Marcus, 2005). The conditions in factory farms and the pace of slaughterhouse kill-lines cause immeasurable suffering and egregious deaths for nonhuman animals as well as unhealthy dangerous conditions for human laborers (Eisnitz, 1997; Schlosser, 2001). Importantly, laborers in these industries are often poor and non-white. The exploitation of workers in slaughterhouses is so egregious that in 2004 Human Rights Watch issued a statement identifying meatpacking plants as the most dangerous factory job in the United States (Human Rights Watch, 2004):

> But meatpacking and poultry workers face more than hard work in tough settings. They perform the most dangerous factory jobs in the country. U.S. meat and poultry employers put workers at predictable risk of serious physical injury even though the means to avoid such injury are known and feasible (Compa and Fellner, 2005).

Further, these subsidies create a situation in which fast food, which is simultaneously an unhealthy by-product of and catalyst for the mass production of meat, becomes one of the most affordable means of eating for the economically disadvantaged. This leads to increased rates of disease such as obesity, heart disease, and diabetes in poor communities (Schlosser, 2001). Though some animal rights theory links systems of capital to oppression across nonhuman and human animals (e.g. Nibert, 2002; Torres, 2007), dominant philosophies of animal rights embrace some of the same logic as capitalism by accepting value hierarchies (i.e. emotion/reason); this might account for the lack of working-class and poor participants in the animal rights movement.

A comprehensive theory of why animals deserve moral consideration should be able to speak to the economically disadvantaged and the working class, since exploitation of nonhuman animals, the poor, and workers are integrally tied in a system of capital that benefits only those who hold positions of economic power.

Conclusion

Activists and veg'ns are varied in the way they approach animal rights; most draw upon emotions, such as compassion and caring, as well as reason and rationality in embracing animal rights. This suggests a need for dynamic philosophies of animal rights. Currently, theory that acknowledges both the rational and emotive ways of understanding nonhuman animals is the best. Additionally, the fact that movement participants are demographically homogenous signals the need for current animal rights theories to be more robust.

Feminist insights into rationalist animal rights philosophy highlight important ways in which theories of animal rights can be developed. Part of making these theories more robust is to root them in practice. In understanding motivations for becoming and remaining committed to activism and/or veg'nism it is clear that both emotional experiences and rational arguments have a role and the two are not mutually exclusive. Further, there is a lack of racial and ethnic minorities as well as middle- and working-class veg'ns and activists. As such, a dynamic and robust theory of animal rights must address rational and emotional justifications for animal rights and seek to forward a more comprehensive explanation that broadly addresses oppression as well as specifically arguing against human exploitation of nonhuman animals.

The paradigm shift that is necessary for animal rights to be embraced by a majority is for the oppression of nonhuman animals to be recognized as equally important as the oppression of disadvantaged human groups. Current feminist theories addressing animal rights encourage this in a couple key ways. First, they define ways in which the underlying structure of oppression is common to all domination; namely through value hierarchies, dichotomies, and patriarchy. Second, they develop and address important linkages between the oppression of human women and nonhuman animals. Animal rights theory needs to go further in defining oppression in such a way that linkages can be made between nonhuman animals and oppressed human groups. This theory must also argue why the species barrier is no less important than barriers of race, class, gender, nationality, or sexuality. In this chapter I have argued that the best way to do this is for academics to leave the library and hit the streets; their focus should be on praxis by using motivations for becoming activists and veg'n to develop theory. The end goal is an animal rights theory that addresses interlocking systems of oppression and simultaneously forwards emotional, relational, reasoned, and rational justifications for granting animals rights.

References

Adams, C. J. (1994). Bringing peace home: A feminist philosophical perspective on the abuse of women, children, and pet animals. *Hypatia, 9*, 63–84.

Adams, C. J. (1990). *The sexual politics of meat: A feminist-vegetarian critical theory*. New York: Continuum.

Adams, C. J. (2007 [2006]). The war on compassion. In J. Donovan & C. J. Adams (Eds.), *The feminist care tradition in animal ethics* (pp. 21–36). New York: Columbia University Press.

Bailey, C. (2007 [2005]). On the backs of animals: The valorization of reason in contemporary animal ethics. In J. Donovan & C. J. Adams (Eds.), *The feminist care tradition in animal ethics* (pp. 344–359). New York: Columbia University Press.

Botes, A. (2000). A comparison between the ethics of justice and the ethics of care. *Journal of Advanced Nursing, 32*, 1071–1075.

Compa, L., & Fellner, J. (2005). *Meat packing's human toll*. Human Rights Watch. Retrieved from http://www.hrw.org/en/news/2005/08/02/meatpackings-human-toll

Donovan, J. (1990). Animal rights and feminist theory. *Journal of Women in Culture and Society, 15*, 350–375.

Eisnitz, G. A. (1997). *Slaughterhouse*. New York: Prometheus Books.

Eisnitz, G. A. (2003). *Slaughterhouse*. Amherst, NY: Prometheus Books.

Elster, J. (1999). *Alchemies of the mind: Rationality and the emotions*. Cambridge: Cambridge University Press.

Espiritu, Y. L. (2000). *Asian American women and men: Labor, laws and love*. New York: Alta Mira Press.

Espiritu, Y. L. (2001). "We don't sleep around like white girls do": Family, culture, and gender in Filipina American lives. *Signs, 26*, 415–440.

Gaard, G. C. (1993). Living interconnections with animals and nature. In G. C. Gaard (Ed.), *Ecofeminism: Women, animals, nature*. Philadelphia: Temple University Press.

Gilligan, C. (1982). *In a different voice: Psychological theory and women's development*. Cambridge, MA: Harvard University Press.

Groves, J. M. (2001). Animal rights and the politics of emotion: Folk constructs of emotions in the animal rights movement. In J. Goodwin, J. M. Jasper, & F. Polletta (Eds.), *Passionate politics: Emotions and social movements* (pp. 212–229). Chicago, IL: University of Chicago Press.

Hall, L. (2005). Civil rights groups to PETA: 'You have used us enough', in Dissidentvoice on www.dissidentvoice.org. Retrieved on 1/15/08.

Herzog, H. A. (1993). "The movement is my life": The psychology of animal rights activism. *Journal of Social Issues, 49,* 103–119.

Herzog, H. A. (2007). Gender differences in human–animal interactions: A review. *Anthrozoos, 20,* 7–21.

Herzog, H. A., & Golden, L. L. (2009). Moral emotions and social activism: The case of animal rights. *New Perspectives on Human–Animal Interactions, 65,* 485–498.

Hondagneu-Sotelo, P., & Avila, E. (2007). 'I'm here but I'm there:' The meanings of Latina transnational motherhood. In D. A. Segura & E. P. Zavella (Eds.), *Migration in the U.S.-Mexico borderlands: A reader.* Durham: Duke University Press.

Human Rights Watch (HRW). (2004). *Blood, sweat and fear: Workers' rights in U.S. meat and poultry plants.* Washington, DC: Human Rights Watch.

Jamison, W. V., & Lunch, W. M. (1992). Rights of animals, perceptions of science, and political activism: Profile of American animal rights activists. *Science, Technology & Human Values, 17,* 438–458.

Jasper, J. M., & Nelkin, D. (1992). *The animal rights crusade: The growth of a moral protest.* New York: The Free Press.

Jerolmack, C. (2003). Tracing the profile of animal rights supporters: A preliminary investigation. *Society and Animals, 11,* 245–263.

Kelch, T. G. (2007 [1999]). The role of the emotional and the emotive in a theory of animal rights. In J. Donovan & C. J. Adams (Eds.), *The feminist care tradition in animal ethics* (pp. 259–300). New York: Columbia University Press.

Lowe, B. M., & Ginsberg., C. F. (2002). Animal rights as a post-citizenship movement. *Society & Animals, 10,* 203–215.

Luke, B. (2007 [1992]). Justice, caring, and animal liberation. In J. Donovan & C. J. Adams (Eds.), *The feminist care tradition in animal ethics* (pp. 125–152). New York: Columbia University Press.

Marcus, E. (2005). *Meat market.* Boston, MA: Brio Press.

Nibert, D. (2002). *Animal rights/human rights: Entanglements of oppression and liberation.* Boulder, CO: Rowman & Littlefield Publishers, Inc.

Plous, S. (1991). An attitude survey of animal rights activists. *Psychological Science, 2,* 194–196.

Plumwood, V. (1991). Nature, self, and gender: Feminism, environmental philosophy, and the critique of rationalism. *Hypatia, 6,* 3–27.

Prokhovnik, R. (2002). *Rational woman: A feminist critique of dichotomy.* New York: Manchester University Press.

Regan, T. (2004 [1983]). *The case for animal rights.* Los Angeles: University of California Press.

Schlosser, E. (2001). *Fast food nation: The dark side of the all-American meal.* Boston: Houghton Mifflin.

Serrato, C. (2010). *Race, class and veganism: A panel discussion.* Long Beach, CA: Animal Liberation Forum, 4/15–4/18/2010.

Shapiro, K. (2007 [1994]). The Caring Sleuth. In J. Donovan & C. J. Adams (Eds.), *The feminist care tradition in animal ethics* (pp. 153–173). New York: Columbia University Press.

Singer, P. (2009 [1975]). *Animal liberation.* New York: Harper Perennial.

Tong, R., & Williams, N. (2009). Feminist ethics. In E. Zalata (Ed.) *The stanford encyclopedia of ethics.* Retrieved from http://plato.stanford.edu/archives/fall2009/entries/feminism-ethics.

Torres, B. (2007). *Making a killing: The political economy of animal rights.* Oakland, CA: AK Press.

Chapter 19
Abusing the Human–Animal Bond: On the Making of Fighting Dogs

Linda Kalof and Maria Andromachi Iliopoulou

> *You became responsible, forever, for what you have tamed.*
> *(Little Prince by A. de Saint-Exupery)*

Introduction

Among the countless animals throughout history who have been tamed to serve humans, there is only one who serves by choice – the dog (Wilcox & Walkowicz, 1995). Dogs display "an inexhaustible willingness to form and sustain partnerships with humans" (Hart, 1995, p. 167), and they are the only species that assist humans in various social needs as police, therapy, and search and rescue animals (Udell & Wynne, 2008), sometimes to the endangerment of their own survival (Shewmake, 2002). It is well known that dogs have been selectively bred for socio-cognitive abilities and attachment to humans; they are thus strongly bonded to humans in relationships that consist of attachment behaviors similar to those found in child–parent and chimpanzee–human relations (Topál, Miklósi, Csányi, & Dóka, 1998). Humans have taken advantage of this bond of attachment to create ferocious, fighting dogs – animals who are intensely loyal and willing to fight to the death to protect humans and their property. Taking a creature with toddler psychology and behavior and making him an aggressive fighting dog creates an animal dominated by fear (Meisterfeld & Pecci, 2000) and one who participates in dogfighting out of intense loyalty to the bond he has with humans.

This chapter traces the history of the creation of fighting dogs and the contemporary terrain of dogfighting as an abuse of the human–animal bond. We begin with background on the domestication of the dog as companions and the breeding of dogs for specific characteristics useful to humans, particularly submissiveness. We then discuss the practice of using dogs to fight for sport and entertainment in the sixth century BC, proceed to a description of the use of dogs for bear- and bullbaiting

L. Kalof (✉)
Animal Studies Program, Department of Sociology, Michigan State University,
East Lansing, MI, USA
e-mail: lkalof@msu.edu

C. Blazina et al. (eds.), *The Psychology of the Human–Animal Bond*,
DOI 10.1007/978-1-4419-9761-6_19, © Springer Science+Business Media, LLC 2011

in the Middle Ages and Renaissance, and end with a discussion of the exploitation of canines in contemporary dogfighting contests. We next describe the process of creating a fighting dog and the essential characteristics of a good fighting dog: he must be reliably human friendly with a desire to please humans. Next, we discuss the use of animal blood sports as a means of validating masculinity, competitive sports as a source of manhood, and the practice of dogfighting as a sport uniquely centered on masculine values and sexuality. We conclude with a discussion of the misconceptions about dog aggression with an emphasis on the role of the media in creating a blaming-the-victim psychology that perpetuates the stereotype of fighting dogs as naturally vicious rather than abused animals enslaved by human males who need to prove their masculinity.

Background

Our first domesticated companion was probably the wolf, a wild animal brought into the human group as a hunting aid, a recipient of affection, and a useful forager of human debris (Kalof, 2007b). By the late Paleolithic, wolf descendants had evolved into fully domesticated companion species – 15,000-year-old burial sites have been uncovered with canidae carefully arranged in human graves (Clutton-Brock, 2011).[1] As the only "pre-agricultural domesticate," the dog's value was not based on his being a food source for humans, but rather dogs "paid dividends to their human companions who benefited from channeling the native predatory abilities and territorial proclivities of dogs to increase hunting success and be useful as sentries" (Driscoll & Macdonald, 2010, p. 4).

Over time humans learned how to breed animals to display specific desired physical traits and destroy those animals with undesirable characteristics, a process that resulted in the complete domination of humans over the domesticated dog. Selecting for specific behavioral traits played a major role in canine domestication. The favorable attributes of a domesticated animal included small size and morphologic and behavioral neotenic characteristics. Thus an adult dog was bred to resemble a wolf pup with a short muzzle (compared to his wild ancestors), hanging ears (for a submissive look), and short hair (Tuan, 1984). Desired behavioral traits included docility and active submission so that tameness could develop into domestication (Clutton-Brock, 1987). Undesired traits included behavioral and physical "misfits" (Coppinger & Coppinger, 2002, p. 247), particularly independence and dominance. Contemporary dogs are so behaviorally altered from their wild ancestors and so well integrated into human society that our relationship with them is considered to be "the closest we humans can ever get to establish a dialogue with another sentient life-form" (Serpell, 1995, p. 2).

One manifestation of the power and control humans had over dogs was the human penchant for deploying them in fighting and baiting spectacles. Using dogs to fight

---

[1] The archeological evidence is unclear as to whether the species was a wolf, dog or jackal (see Juliet Clutton-Brock, 1987, p. 58).

and bait other animals has a long cultural history closely linked to sport and entertainment. As early as 510 BC, Etruscan wall paintings from Tarquinia depict a masked Phersu,[2] the "beast-master," inciting a vicious dog to attack a human handicapped with a sack over his head and entangled in a rope. While usually considered a staged game of baiting as part of a funeral event (Kalof, 2007a), some scholars argue that the Phersu figure was an executioner responsible for exposing a doomed victim to a ferocious beast (Kyle, 1998). A sculpture from the wall of Themistocles shows that watching dogs fight small animals in baiting contests was also a popular pastime for young Athenian men in the sixth century BC, and Spartan youths also staged animal combats for entertainment (Kyle, 1998).

In the middle ages, training dogs to fight was useful in defending humans and their property. Mastiff-type dogs were set upon tethered bears who were ideal human substitutes because of their size and upright fighting stance (Kalof, 2007b). The training exercise was an elite pastime of the gentry – aristocrats would bet on their own dogs in fights with bears and chimpanzees riding horses (chimps were too small to fight a dog so, as surrogates for humans, they tested the dog's ability to attack a man on horseback) (Brownstein, 1969).

Mastiff dogs were an excellent canine choice to defend medieval humans. The Mastiff had long been known for his legendary devotion and as a superior guardian of human property and a war dog, not only because of his loyalty to humans but because of his acromegalic traits. Acromegalic traits in dogs are distinct due to the effect of growth hormones; increased bone growth (thus these dogs are massive), huge paws, bulky skull, heavy jaw and brows, wrinkled expression, large drop ears, abundant skin on the body, strong muzzle, and smooth coat (Wilcox & Walkowicz, 1995). The fiercest Mastiff dogs were the Molossus dogs, and, as a result, they were heavily exploited as war and combat dogs. They often wore "broad collars," fitted with huge curved blades, fiery torches and "spikes," and in medieval battles they wore a kind of protective armor made out of metal and light chain so that "they were armored as completely as the knights and their charging horses" (Davis, 1970, p. 175).

The medieval Mastiff was a descendant of the "bandogge," a dog who was collared or banded and tied up during the day and allowed to run loose at night (but only if his feet were maimed so he could not run fast enough to prey on deer). Roaming only his master's land, the intensely loyal mastiff was more useful as a protector of humans and their property than a village constable (Thomas, 1983). Since then, as now, the status of specific dog breeds was determined by the status of their owners (Thomas, 1983). The English Mastiff's strength and courage were symbolic displays of English masculine valor, both to the English themselves and their foreign visitors (MacInnes, 2003).

Animals were often used as entertainment during the medieval period. Bears and apes were trained to imitate humans (doing headstands, dancing, drinking ale, and smoking tobacco), horses were trained to dance on ropes and beat drums, and dogs

---

[2]The word "persona" comes from the Etruscan "phersu" or mask.

continued to be used in animal-baiting events (Strutt, 1903). Regular animal baitings were common amusement in late medieval London, and the most popular of all were bullbaitings. Medieval animal baiting was in fact associated primarily with festivals and the preparation for feasts because it was believed that the flesh of a baited animal (a bull, boar, or bear) who was exhausted from the frenzied exercise involved in fighting off a ferocious dog resulted in tender and digestible meat (Kalof, 2007b).

The medieval practice of baiting other animals with dogs (to protect people or produce tender meat) evolved into a full-scale blood sport during the Renaissance (Kalof & Taylor, 2007). Bearbaiting became a very popular event in the English countryside, enjoyed by all social classes and a moneymaker for local churches (bearbaitings at parish fund-raisers encouraged drinkers to spend their money on ale brewed by the church) (Stokes, 1996). Bearbaitings were also popular entertainment spectacles in London, where the baiting events occupied the same physical space as the London theaters and were attended by common Londoners, nobles, and monarchs (Dickey, 1991).

Just as the English Mastiff dog's strength and courage were symbolic of English masculinity, so also did the English identify with the baiting dog's courage and valor in the baiting ring, and the blood sport events became spectacular displays of masculine bravado (MacInnes, 2003). Indeed, the concept of baiting itself was deployed in a patriarchal symbolic system as a metaphor for the abuse of women, as in the recorded event from Somerset, England, of a man who threatened to tie his disobedient wife to a stake and set dogs on her (Stokes, 1996).

Creating a Fighting Dog

Dogs are not by their nature willing participants in violence; they must be carefully trained and conditioned to fight. Conditioning begins at an early age to make the animals develop the desirable level of "gameness" using a standard set of training techniques (Gibson, 2005, pp. 2–3):

Treadmill:	Dogs are run on the treadmills to increase cardiovascular fitness and endurance.
Catmill/Jenny:	Apparatus that looks like a carnival horse walker with several beams jetting out from a central rotating pole. The dogs are chained to one beam, and another small animal like a cat, small dog, or rabbit is harnessed to or hung from another beam. The dogs run in circles, chasing the bait. Once the exercise sessions are over, the dogs are usually rewarded with the bait they had been pursuing.
Springpole/Jumppole:	A large pole with a spring hanging down to which a rope, tire, or animal hide is affixed that the dogs jump to and dangle from for extended periods of time. This strengthens the jaw muscles and back

	legs. A variation of the springpole is a hanging cage, into which bait animals are placed. The dogs repeatedly lunge up toward the cage.
Flirtpole:	A handheld pole with a lure attached. The dogs chase the lure along the ground.
Chains:	Dogs have very heavy chains wrapped around their necks, generally in lieu of collars; they build neck and upper-body strength by constantly bearing the immense weight of the chains.
Weights:	Weights are often affixed to chains and dangled from the dogs' necks. This builds neck and upper-body strength. Generally, dogs are permanently chained this way. However, sometimes the trainers run them with their weights attached.
Bait:	Animals are tied up while the dogs tear them apart or sometimes they are confined in an area to be chased and mauled by the dogs.
Drugs/Vitamins/Supplements:	Dogs are given vitamins, supplements, and drugs (including cocaine) to condition them or to incite them to fight.

In spite of the rigorous, abusive training techniques humans use to create a fighting dog, there are losers in every dog fight. Some dogs refuse to fight, and they are immediately killed, thus allowing the owner to resurrect the status he lost because of the dog's poor performance in the ring (Evans et al., 1998). The losing dogs who survive the pit are also quickly dispatched or even tortured and mutilated if the owner is particularly embarrassed by the dog's lack of courage. Requiring young gang members to kill their own losing dog serves not only as a means of regaining lost respect but also as a mechanism to initiate young gang members into a culture of violence (Gibson, 2005).

The ideal breeding characteristic for a contemporary fighting dog is a quick, fearless animal who will attack other animals, but will be docile toward humans (Coile, 2005). During the late 1800s, the bull and terrier dogs were selectively bred for some new qualities, including a high pain threshold, resilience, a willingness to fight to the end, and, importantly, an increased affection for humans (Coile, 2005). Dogs who were not reliably human friendly could not be handled during fights and were euthanized. Thus, because aggressiveness toward humans was not part of the foundation of these new breeds, human aggressiveness is not a common behavioral trait of fighting dogs (Gallagher & Hunthhausen, 2006). Indeed, the common behavioral trait in fighting dogs is an intense desire to please humans.

Dogs have evolved mental processes over the course of their domestication that enable them to survive among humans, such as the ability to read and respond to human communication cues, including pointing, eye contact, and facial gestures (Morell, 2009). Dogs are not only willing and cooperative canine companions, but being around people and following their commands is enjoyable for them – so much so that scientists agree that domestication turned the dog into an animal who "yearns to be with a species other than its own" (Morell, 2009, p. 1065) The dog's ability for socialization and attachment to humans is so strong that experiments in a Budapest laboratory documented that four-month-old "puppies in a choice test always pre-ferred a human companion to a dog" (Morell, 2009, p. 1065). The coevolutionary process among humans and dogs has resulted in animals who tend to form stronger bonds with humans than their conspecifics; in other words, dogs have an innate ability for cooperation with humans that was enhanced by selective breeding during domestication (Naderi, Miklósi, Dóka, & Csányi, 2002). One aspect of this strong human–canine attachment is that both species have the capacity for a theory of mind, or the ability to understand the perspective of another.

The dog is unique in his ability to understand and respond to human social cues (Hare, Brown, Williamson, & Tomasello, 2002; Hare & Tomasello, 2005; Udell & Wynne, 2008). However, this ability is dependent on a successful period of social-ization during the dog's "critical period of social development" that occurs between two and sixteen weeks of age (compared to wolf pups who need to be socialized within the first two weeks of life) (Coppinger & Coppinger, 2002). However, wild dogs and feral dogs do not show the same affinity for humans; they survive without depending on humans, do not develop any social bonds with them, and avoid direct human contact, preferring to interact with canine members of their pack (Boitani, Francisci, Ciucci, & Andreoli, 1995).

While most domestic dogs have strong attachments to humans, there is wide variation in human attitudes toward dogs. For some humans, particularly those in Western culture, animals are personified or humanized in ways that allow us to understand and empathize with them – a reflexive consciousness of introspection and consideration of motives and reasons for action (Serpell, 1996). However, we tend to feel compassion only for those animals who share physical similarities with humans (such as mammals with upright stance and large size). Feelings of dis-tance and detachment from most animals might arise in the case of urban dwellers who may not be familiar with "pets" at all and whose experiences of other ani-mals are limited to negative interactions with pests such as flies, roaches, rats mice, and pigeons (Serpell, 1996). Thus, when animals do not play an important role in human lives, humans are often detached from or indifferent to animals, a detach-ment that often serves to justify abuse – "just as we have to depersonalize human opponents in wartime in order to kill them with indifference, so we have to create a void between ourselves and the animals on which we inflict pain and misery..." (Mirriam Rothschild cited in Serpell, 1996, p. 188).

It is reasonable to assume that part of the problem of contemporary dogfighting is the lack of empathy that comes from detachment from animals, which is common in urban areas. While some dogfighting takes place in rural areas of the US (Evans et al., 1998), the vast majority of these blood sport events occur in urban centers (Gibson, 2005). Indeed, most residents of high-crime areas have had some exposure to dog fighting, which are usually organized events that take place in abandoned buildings where street gang members gamble and traffic drugs (Kalof & Taylor, 2007). Further, it has been documented that the majority of dogfighters are men who use the sport and the dogs as a way to develop, express, and validate their masculinity (Evans et al., 2007; Kalof & Taylor, 2007).

Using Animal Blood Sports to Validate Masculinity

A similar connection between masculinity and the display of animal aggression has been documented in other combative blood sport rituals. For example, both bullfighting and cockfighting are male-focused activities in which masculine values including sexual potency and aggressiveness are played out in combative sport rituals. In bullfighting, the matador proves his superiority over the bull in a highly gendered performance that eventually emasculates the bull as the animal is worn to exhaustion and no longer able to exercise his wild and "willful maleness" (Marvin, 1988).

Substantial research has documented cockfighting as a ritualistic form of aggression used by men to recognize sexual potency among each other and in the larger community (Cook, 1994). Cockfighting is also used by men to express masculine identity and aggression in a "thinly disguised symbolic homoerotic masturbatory phallic duel, with the winner emasculating the loser through castration or feminization" (Dundes, 1994, p. 251). In another connection to masculinity, animal fighting has been compared to the recent surge of interest in paramilitary culture and games such as paintball, which allow males to prove their identities as men and build solidarity while not actually participating in violence (Evans et al., 1998).

Dogfighting is a blood sport similarly centered on sexuality, masculine values, and the deployment of animals as symbols of a culture infused with macho aggression and menacing violence. Both cockfighting and dogfighting are sport activities staged by humans in which animals are incited to fight, maim, and kill each other. Both are focused on *competition* without a survival-of-the-fittest component; *winning* as a singular goal with little interest in the process of fighting, only the outcome; *spectators* who watch the fights and validate the superiority of the winning animal's human handler; and *gambling* on one of the animals to win (Cashmore, 2005). Further, in both sports there is a clear juxtaposition between owning fighting animals and aggressive masculinity.

Traditional attributes of masculinity in US culture include assertiveness, aggressiveness, strength, and competitiveness (Evans et al., 1998). Competitive sports have long been a source of manhood, particularly as training in the virtues of fighting and the making of men (Evans et al., 1998); in antiquity competitive sports were used as a rite of passage and preparation for warfare for male youth (Kalof, 2007b). Since men from lower classes and the working class often lack opportunities to validate masculinity through occupational success, they tend to rely on a much more accessible route to the achievement of status – competitive dogfighting (Evans et al., 1998; Kalof & Taylor, 2007). In dogfighting, the dogs are the means through which their owners gain status; since the dog who fights in the pit is representing his owner and he is a reflection of his owner's masculine values; "cowards," "losers," and "curs" have to be executed by their macho owners in order to regain masculinity and status within their community (Evans et al., 2007; Kalof & Taylor, 2007). In the words of a clinical psychologist, for young unemployed men simply owning a pit bull is a way of gaining status (Kalof & Taylor, 2007, pp. 16–17):

> Remember it goes back to the time of (the) Roman Empire, the great warriors, soldiers, generals had wild animals as mascots, pets... animals so dangerous that mere mortals would cringe at the sight of some warrior-king walking with his lion, jaguar, or wild beast. Young boys see drug dealers with these killer dogs, expensive to purchase, expensive to maintain, train, and to bet on... These boys are imitating those macho kings, the dogs replace the lion. If you are poor, no job, many are impressed by the deadliness, the danger of being a thug, a gang represents work, money, and status. The dog is simply part of the image that distorted young boys applaud.

Thus blood sports are sustained by the "masculine neediness for blood, bond and brotherhood" (Kalof & Taylor, 2007, p. 22). In a patriarchal culture that perpetuates and exacerbates the domination, intimidation, and control over less powerful others (Kalof, Fitzgerald, & Baralt, 2004), the need to prove masculinity is not only linked to horrific animal abuse (Kalof & Taylor, 2007) but also to a vicious cycle of domestic violence, desensitization to violence, and animal cruelty (Siebert, 2010). For example, in cases of domestic violence, threats to torture or kill a pet are very commonly used as a means of intimidation in crimes of power and control over women and children (Siebert, 2010).

Conclusion: Blaming the Victim (the Dog)

The most unique and extraordinary interspecies relationship is the human–canine bond, and dogs are the only species who voluntarily ally themselves with humans (Serpell, 1995). Dogs relate to humans as members of the pack and as litter mates; they are easily trained and have a manageable physical size (Irvine, 2004). These precious attributes – trainability, size, and willingness to serve – have been taken advantage of for centuries by humans who have forced dogs into slavery by employing abusive training methods, using them as weapons to protect property, and pitting them against each other in combative blood sports (Kalof & Taylor, 2007).

The mass media rarely consider the fighting dog a victim of the human abuse of the human–animal bond. Instead news reports emphasize certain "fighting" breeds (primarily the American pit bull terrier or the pit bull) as evil predators who are unpredictable and kill and maim without discretion (Cohen & Richardson, 2002). In a review of 72 articles on pit bulls published in the *New York Times* between 1987 and 2000, Cohen and Richardson report that over one-third covered pit bull attacks on people, thus keeping the negative reputation of pit bull dogs "fresh in the minds of readers by simply assuming they are vicious" (2002, p. 287). Similar negative news reports on the aggressive "nature" of pit bulls have been documented outside the US (Kaspersson, 2008). Further, a "Pit Bull placebo" is perpetuated by media suggestions that the eradication of pit bull dogs is a cure for serious dog attacks

(Delise, 2002). This unfortunate argument is nothing more than an attempt to treat the symptoms of the aggressive dog problem (the pit bull and other "dangerous" breeds) rather than the causes (dog owners) – in other words, "the Pit Bull is made the scapegoat for the sins of (his) owners" (Kaspersson, 2008, p. 216). The reality is that pit bull dogs are extremely people oriented and loyal (Cohen & Richardson, 2002; Gibson, 2005), even after having suffered untold abuse.[3] Indeed, it is their fierce loyalty and gentleness toward humans that make pit bulls desirable for dog-fighting – he is a dog who is well known for his willingness to take substantial abuse and neglect but remain faithful and non-aggressive toward his owner (Gibson, 2005).

The media, however, attribute fighting dog behavior to genetics, lumping into one stereotyped category all breeds (and breed mixes) that resemble the pit bull dog. The false perception of a genetically based canine aggression is a problem of blaming the victim (the dog) rather than the perpetrator (the human). This misperception is a factor in the rise of a generalized antidog campaign in Western cultures (Serpell, 1995, p. 2) and associated legislative efforts to ban "aggressive" dog breeds (Delise, 2002). The argument that dogs regardless of breed are a menace to society is supported by public fears of health risks associated with dogs (such as the spread of disease, pollution, and dog bites), which contribute to a widespread and constantly growing hostility toward dogs (Serpell, 1995). Even though breed bans were initially directed toward a few specific breeds, the list of controlled breeds is constantly expanding, with Germany maintaining the broadest list. In some parts of Germany more than three dozen specific canine breeds are controlled by outright bans or muzzle/tether requirements, and in one German locality any dog who weighs more than 44 pounds and stands taller than 15.75 inches must be leashed (National Animal Interest Alliance, n.d.).

Unfortunately, the identification of an aggressive dog breed is not reliably assessed because the physical and behavioral characteristics are based on media reports. The news media increasingly report attacks by breeds falsely identified as pit bulls, and they show decreased interest in dog attacks by other breeds; thus attacks by almost any type of dog are falsely attributed to pit bulls (Delise, 2007). While this publicity negatively stereotypes pit bulls for the public, it has made the pit bull very desirable for criminals.

According to several scholars (AVMA, 2001; Delise, 2007; Serpell, 1995; Udell & Wynne, 2008), dog attacks occur as a result of irresponsible, abusive, and negligent dog ownership, and the majority of dog bites occur because the dogs are

---

[3]One of us (Iliopoulou) is a DVM who assesses animal cruelty cases for a local Animal Control organization. Of the 14 dogs she examined over a two-month period in 2010, 13 were pit bulls and 1 was a Rottweiler mix, all were starved, 7 had wounds suggestive of dogfighting, 3 had their ears cropped with scissors, 2 had been beaten by their owners, and 5 were tethered with heavy chains (one of whom had no teeth because of her efforts to chew through her tether). Eleven of the 14 dogs were submissive and exceptionally human friendly (one so scared that she urinated involuntarily every time she was touched) and wagged their tails frantically every time they were praised as good, sweet dogs.

starved, chained, and neglected and abused by their owners. However, the majority of aggressive dogs are portrayed by the media as naturally vicious, not the victims of abuse (Delise, 2007). It is a very common misconception to use "viciousness" as the reason for canine aggression (Overall, 1997, p. 90). Canine aggression is a highly misunderstood concept – dogs use growling, bared teeth, and biting as defensive behaviors when they feel scared, uncomfortable, or threatened, and certainly such behaviors do not manifest the state of mind that the term *vicious* suggests; it is impossible to evaluate and detect an emotional state such as viciousness in dogs (Overall, 1997). The prevention of dog attacks would be greatly enhanced with more stringent laws that prohibit animal cruelty and media coverage that educates the public about the problems of dog aggression rather than spreading panic with misconceptions.

Dogfighting is a male-focused activity in which masculine values such as sexual potency and aggressiveness are played out in combative sport rituals. The fascination with animal fighting has also been taken up by the media, which now provides frequent opportunities to observe brutal animal fights that emphasize violent natures, bloodbaths, and displays of animals depicted as vicious and threatening to human safety (Chris, 2006). Thus, in a culture where bloodshed and violence are considered fascinating, contemporary fighting dogs are victimized not only by a cultural history that prepared them for aggression but also by their stereotyping in the media as "naturally" vicious and aggressive toward humans. Fighting dogs are not portrayed in the media as the faithful, willing cooperative companions that they are. The steadfast loyalty of the fighting dog remains intact even after horrific mistreatment, torture, and torment – the most appalling of which is the abuse of the human–animal bond.

References

AVMA (American Veterinary Medical Association) Task Force on Canine Aggression and Human-Canine Interaction. (2001). A community approach to dog bite prevention. Retrieved from http://www.avma.org/public_health/dogbite/dogbite.pdf

Boitani, L., Francisci, F., Ciucci, P., & Andreoli, G. (1995). Population biology and ecology of feral dogs in central Italy. In J. Serpell (Ed.), *The domestic dog: Its evolution, behavior, and interaction with people* (pp. 217–244). New York: Cambridge University Press.

Brownstein, O. (1969). The popularity of baiting in England before 1600: A study in social and theatrical history. *Educational Theatre Journal, 21,* 237–250.

Cashmore, E. (2005). *Making sense of sports.* New York: Routledge.

Chris, C. (2006). *Watching wildlife.* Minneapolis, MN: University of Minnesota Press.

Clutton-Brock, J. (1987). *Animals as domesticates: A worldview through history.* East Lansing: Michigan State University Press.

Clutton-Brock, J. (2011). *Animals as domesticates: A worldview through history.* East Lansing: Michigan State University Press.

Cohen, J., & Richardson, J. (2002). Pit bull panic. *Journal of Popular Culture, 36,* 285–317.

Coile, D. C. (2005). *Encyclopedia of dog breeds.* Hauppauge, NY: Barron's Educational Series.

Cook, H. G. K. (1994). Cockfighting on the Venezuelan island of Margarita: A ritualized form of male aggression. In A. Dundes (Ed.), *The cockfight: A casebook* (pp. 232–240). Madison, WI: University of Wisconsin Press.

Coppinger, R., & Coppinger, L. (2002). *Dogs: A new understanding of canine origin, behavior, and evolution.* Chicago: University of Chicago Press.

Davis, H. P. (1970). *The new dog encyclopedia.* Harrisburg, PA: Stackpole Books.

Delise, K. (2002). *Fatal dog attacks: The stories behind the statistics.* Manorville, NY: Anubis Publishing.

Delise, K. (2007). *The pit bull placebo: The media, myths and politics of canine aggression.* Manorville, NY: Anubis Publishing.

Dickey, S. (1991). Shakespeare's mastiff comedy. *Shakespeare Quarterly, 42,* 255–275.

Driscoll, C. A., & Macdonald, D. W. (2010). Top dogs: Wolf domestication and wealth. *Journal of Biology, 9,* 10.

Dundes, A. (1994). Gallus as phallus: A psychoanalytic cross-cultural consideration of the cockfight as fowl play. In A. Dundes (Ed.), *The cockfight: A casebook* (pp. 241–282). Madison, WI: University of Wisconsin Press.

Evans, R., Kalich, D., & Forsyth, C. J. (1998). Dogfighting: Symbolic expression and validation of masculinity. *Sex Roles, 39,* 825–832.

Gallagher, C. P., & Hunthhausen, W. (2006). *The American pit bull terrier.* Neptune City, NJ: T.F.H. Publications.

Gibson, H. (2005). Dog fighting detailed discussion. Animal Legal and Historical Center, Michigan State University College of Law. Retrieved from www.animallaw.info/articles/ddusdogfighting.htm

Hare, B., Brown, M., Williamson, C., & Tomasello, M. (2002). The domestication of social cognition in dogs. *Science, 298,* 1634–1636.

Hare, B., & Tomasello, M. (2005). Human-like social skills in dogs? *Trends in Cognitive Sciences, 9,* 439–444.

Hart, L. A. (1995). Dogs as human companions: Review of the relationship. In J. Serpell (Ed.), *The domestic dog: Its evolution, behavior, and interaction with people* (pp. 161–177). New York: Cambridge University Press.

Irvine, L. (2004). *If you tame me: Understanding our connection with animals.* Philadelphia: Temple University Press.

Kalof, L. (Ed.). (2007a). *A cultural history of animals in antiquity.* Oxford: Berg.

Kalof, L. (2007b). *Looking at animals in human history.* London: Reaktion Books.

Kalof, L., Fitzgerald, A., & Baralt, L. (2004). Animals, women, and weapons: Blurred sexual boundaries in the discourse of sport hunting. *Society & Animals, 12,* 237–251.

Kalof, L., & Taylor, C. (2007). The discourse of dog fighting. *Humanity & Society, 31,* 319–333.

Kaspersson, M. (2008). On treating the symptoms and not the cause: Reflections on the dangerous dogs act. Papers from the British Criminology Conference. Retrieved from http://www.britsoccrim.org/volume8/13Kaspersson08.pdf

Kyle, D. G. (1998). *Spectacles of death in ancient Rome.* New York: Routledge.

MacInnes, I. (2003). Mastiffs and spaniels: Gender and nation in the English dog. *Textual Practice, 17,* 21–40.

Marvin, G. (1988). *Bullfight.* Urbana, IL: University of Illinois Press.

Meisterfeld, C. W., & Pecci, E. F. (2000). *Dog & human behavior: Amazing parallels, similarities.* Petaluma, CA: MRK Publishing.

Morell, V. (2009, August 28). Going to the dogs. *Science Magazine, 325,* 1062–1065.

Naderi, S. Z., Miklósi, A., Dóka, A., & Csányi, V. (2002). Does dog-human attachment affect their inter-specific cooperation? *Acta Biologica Hungarica, 53,* 537–550.

National Animal Interest Alliance. (n.d.). Germany bans breeds, reactions evoke holocaust memories. Retrieved from http://www.naiaonline.org/articles/archives/germany.htm.

Overall, K. L. (1997). *Clinical behavioral medicine for small animals.* St. Louis, MO: Mosby-Year Book, Inc.

Serpell, J. (Ed.). (1995). *The domestic dog: Its evolution, behavior, and interaction with people.* New York: Cambridge University Press.

Serpell, J. (1996). *In the company of animals.* New York: Cambridge University Press.

Shewmake, T. (2002). *Canine courage*. Portage, MI: PageFree Publishing, Inc.

Siebert, C. (2010, June 7). The animal-cruelty syndrome. *The New York Times*. Retrieved from http://www.nytimes.com/2010/06/13/magazine/13dogfighting-t.html?pagewanted=1&hp.

Stokes, J. (1996). Bull and bear baiting in Somerset: The gentles' sport. In A. F. Johnston & W. Husken (Eds.), *English parish drama* (pp. 65–80). Amsterdam: Rodopi.

Strutt, J. (1903). In J. C. Cox (Ed.), *The sports and pastimes of the people of England*. London; New York: Augustus M. Kelley.

Thomas, K. (1983). *Man and the natural world: A history of the modern sensibility*. New York: Pantheon.

Topál, J., Miklósi, A., Csányi, V., & Dóka, A. (1998). Attachment behavior in dogs (*Canis familiaris*): A new application of Ainsworth's (1969) strange situation test. *Journal of Comparative Psychology, 112*(3), 219–229.

Tuan, Y. F. (1984). *Dominance and affection: The making of pets*. New Haven, CT; London: Yale University Press.

Udell, M. A. R., & Wynne, C. D. L. (2008). A review of domestic dogs' (*Canis familiaris*) human-like behaviors: Or why behavior analysts should stop worrying and love their dogs. *Journal of the Experimental Analysis of Behavior, 89*, 247–261.

Wilcox, B., & Walkowicz, C. (1995). *The atlas of dog breeds of the world*. Neptune City, NJ: TFH Publishing.

Part V
Tests, Measurements, and Current Research Issues

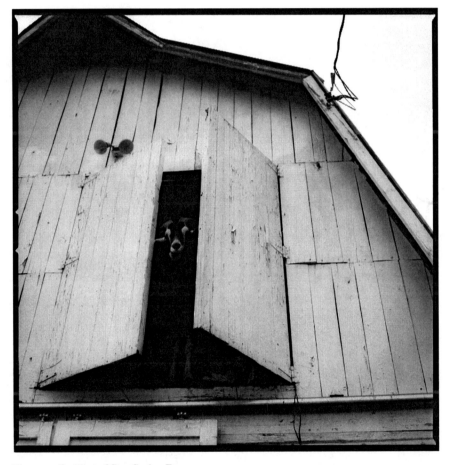

Newman, Resident of Star Gazing Farm
Newman, named after a character on the TV show *Seinfeld*, has been known to open car doors.

Chapter 20
The Pet Attitude Scale

Donald I. Templer and Hiroko Arikawa

The Pet Attitude Scale

It was the intention of the authors that this chapter be a resource of test and measures for the reader. The name of the Pet Attitude Scale (PAS) (Templer, Salter, Dickey, Baldwin, & Veleber, 1981), apparently the first published scale that measures human–animal bonding, reflects the fact that it was developed three decades ago. If it were constructed today, it would be more appropriately called the Companion Animal Attitude Scale. The word "pet" often implies subordinate status. The literature cited by Templer et al. (1981) also reflects the era in which it was written. For one thing, the quantity of literature cited was rather sparse. Since that time the literature on human–animal relationships has increased greatly. Second, the literature cited pertains to the benefits to the psychological and physical health of humans. Thirty years ago there was much less emphasis on animal welfare.

The intended purpose of the Pet Attitude Scale was to develop a psychometric instrument to measure this construct. The first part of this chapter pertains to the construction and validation of the instrument. The second part pertains to what has been learned about companion animal attitude on the basis of subsequent research with this instrument. There are numerous correlations and group differences that provide meaningful and coherent inferences. The third part of the chapter pertains to other animal attitude instruments. The fourth is the summary.

Construction and Validation

The first step in the construction of the Pet Attitude Scale was to devise 43 seven-point Likert Scale items that appeared to assess attitude toward pets. These items were intended to reflect both positive and negative cognition and emotion in a variety of contexts. These items were administered to 92 psychology class undergraduates

D.I. Templer (✉) (Retired)
Alliant International University, Fresno, CA, USA
e-mail: donaldtempler@sbcglobal.net

C. Blazina et al. (eds.), *The Psychology of the Human–Animal Bond*,
DOI 10.1007/978-1-4419-9761-6_20, © Springer Science+Business Media, LLC 2011

Table 20.1 The Pet Attitude Scale items

Key		
+	1.	I really like seeing pets enjoy their food
+	2.	My pet means more to me than any of my friends
+	3.	I would like a pet in my home
−	4.	Having pets is a waste of money
+	5.	House pets add happiness to my life (or would if I had one)
−	6.	I feel that pets should always be kept outside
+	7.	I spend time every day playing with my pets (or I would if I had one)
+	8.	I have occasionally communicated with a pet and understood what it was trying to express
−	9.	The world would be a better place if people would stop spending so much time caring for their pets and started caring more for other human beings instead
+	10.	I like to feed animals out of my hand
+	11.	I love pets
−	12.	Animals belong in the wild or in zoos, but not in the home
−	13.	If you keep pets in the house you can expect a lot of damage to furniture
+	14.	I like house pets
−	15.	Pets are fun, but it's not worth the trouble of owning one
+	16.	I frequently talk to my pet
+	17.	I hate animals
+	18.	You should treat your house pets with as much respect as you would a human member of your family

at a small liberal arts college in Mobile, Alabama. The seven items that correlated less than .35 with that score were deleted. Eighteen other items were deleted because they correlated excessively with a measure of social desirability. The 18 remaining items constitute the Pet Attitude Scale and are contained in Table 20.1. A Cronbach's alpha of .93 was found.

Criterion-oriented validity was carried out by contrasting two groups of participants, one working with animals and the other preparing for a people-helping career. The kennel workers scored significantly higher than the social work students on the Pet Attitude Scale, 112.88 and 97.72, respectively, $t = 3.53, p < .01$.

A principal component factor analysis with varimax rotation yielded three factors that had eigenvalues greater than 1.0. The first factor accounted for 84.6% of the variance and was labeled "love and interaction." The items with the highest loadings on this factor are item 16, "I frequently talk with my pet," item 8, "I have occasionally communicated with a pet and understood what it was trying to express," item 11, "I love pets," and item 7, "I spend time every day playing with my pet (or I would if I had one)." Factor 1 appears to assess degree of bonding. The second factor accounted for 8.6% of the variance and was labeled "pets in the home." The items with the highest loadings are item 6, "I feel that pets should always be kept outside," item 14, "I like housepets," item 12, "Animals belong in the wild or in zoos, but not in the home," and item 2, "I would like a pet in my home." Factor 2 appears to concern viewing the animal as a family member. The third factor accounted for 6.9% of the variance and was called "joy of pet ownership." The items with the highest loadings are 1, "I really like seeing pets enjoy their food," item 5, "Housepets add happiness to my life (or would if I had one)," and item 17, "I hate animals." Factor 3 seems to reflect mutual happiness.

It was decided to expand the construct validity of the PAS by correlating it with personality and psychopathology variables using college undergraduates. Table 20.2 contains the instruments that were employed and their scales. The Mini-Mult is an

Table 20.2 Correlations with Pet Attitude Scale score

Variable	Correlation
Mini-Mult ($N = 56$)	
L	.02
F	.08
K	−.21
Hypochondriasis	.23
Depression	.05
Hysteria	−.02
Psychopathic deviate	.09
Paranoia	.01
Psychasthemia	.05
Schizophrenia	.23
Hypomania	.20
Study of values ($N = 56$)	
Theoretical	.06
Economic	.15
Aesthetic	.03
Social	−.12
Political	.21
Religious	−.28*
Eysenck Personality Inventory ($N = 71$)	
Extraversion	.16
Neuroticism	.11
Lie	−.08
Personality Research Form ($N = 71$)	
Achievement	.08
Affiliation	.26*
Aggression	−.18
Autonomy	−.11
Dominance	−.20
Endurance	.26*
Exhibitionism	−.07
Harm avoidance	−.09
Impulsivity	.13
Nurturance	.21
Order	.07
Play	.20
Social recognition	−.03
Understanding	.03
Infrequency	−.10
Age ($N = 71$)	−.06
Sex ($N = 127$, 1 = male, 2 = female)	.03

*$p < .05$.

abbreviated version of the MMPI. Table 20.2 contains the product–moment correlation coefficients between those scales and the PAS. The PAS correlations with the Mini-Mult and the Neuroticism Scale of the Eysenck Personality Inventory are low and nonsignificant so as to infer very little relationship between pet attitude and psychopathology at least in the present college student participants. The PAS correlations with the Study of Values and Personality Research Form are also low. The three "significant" items out of a total of the combined 21 items of these two personality inventories should be interpreted with caution. The highest correlation suggests there may be a slight tendency for less religious people to have more favorable attitudes toward pets. (It is unlikely that this religious correlation is a chance occurrence. Subsequent research of Tangen (2008) found that frequency of religious attendance correlated negatively with Pet Attitude Scale total score, negatively with Factor 3, "pet-feeding enjoyment," and positively with Factor 5, "Pets cause damage.")

The appendix of this chapter contains the original format and the modified format items of the Pet Attitude Scale that are ready to administer to participants. The reader may feel free to copy these and use them for research purposes. The appendix also contains directions for scoring the PAS and the Animal–Human Continuity Scale that is described later in this chapter.

Subsequent Research

The Development of Pet Attitude in the Context of the Family

The impetus for the research on the family resemblance in pet attitude was the research of Templer, Ruff, and Franks (1971) that found family resemblance on the Death Anxiety Scale (DAS) (Templer, 1970). Templer et al. found the Death Anxiety Scale score of high school students correlated with scores of their parents, with the correlations being higher for the parent–adolescent dyad of the same sex. The highest correlation was between husband and wife. The authors inferred that level of death anxiety is determined in part by interpersonal relationships, perhaps especially in the family. The comparable study for pet attitude family resemblance was carried out by Schenk, Templer, Peters, and Schmidt (1994) with 118 high school students and 142 of their parents. Table 20.3 shows that all of the correlations are positive. It is apparent that the adolescent–mother correlations were higher than

Table 20.3 Correlations of parent's pet attitude with American adolescent's pet attitude

Parent Pet Attitude Scale score	Sons	Daughters	Combined
Father pet attitude	.08	.53***	.37***
Mother pet attitude	.33*	.61***	.51***

*$p < .05$.
***$p < .001$.

Table 20.4 Correlation coefficients between Kuwaiti family members

Family members	Kuwaitis (N)	r	Americans (r)
Father–daughter	102	.31**	.53**
Mother–daughter	124	.17*	.61**
Father–son	22	.25	.08
Mother–son	20	.30	.33*
Father–adolescent	124	.30**	.37**
Mother–adolescent	144	.18*	.51**
Father–mother	111	.35**	–

$*\, p < .05.$
$**\, p < .001.$

the adolescent–father correlations. The differences may be a function of children, especially when they are young, spending more time with their mothers while at home. It should be borne in mind that keeping pets in the home is essentially a domestic matter.

Al-Fayez, Awadalla, Templer, and Arikawa (2003) conducted a similar study with Kuwaiti high school students and their parents. Table 20.4 shows the correlations for the adolescent–parent dyads. It is apparent that in contrast to the pattern of correlations for American adolescents and their parents the father–adolescent correlations are higher than the mother–adolescent correlations. This difference was explained in terms of the more dominant role that Muslim fathers have in the family. The composite of the Kuwait and American findings suggest that attitudes toward pets are formed by interpersonal and, perhaps especially, family influences.

An incidental finding is that the adolescents, fathers, and mothers had lower Pet Attitude scores than are typically obtained with American participants. This may be at least in part a function of dogs being viewed as dirty in the Muslim religion. Many people from Muslim countries are greatly surprised that Americans tend to view dogs and other pets as family members and not infrequently sleep in the same bed.

Animal Fighting

Cock (male chicken) fighting is one of the more popular "sports" in the world, especially in Asia and Latin America. Cockfighting is such an integral part of the culture in the Philippines that politicians must be seen at the local cockfights in order to obtain votes. Cockfighting is now illegal in all the United States. It was legal in Oklahoma, Louisiana, and New Mexico until 2002. Cockfighting is especially popular among Latinos in the United States. It is most popular in Florida, Oklahoma, Texas, Kansas, Arizona, New Mexico, and Louisiana (Forsyth, 1996). The conviction and incarceration of professional football player Michael Vick for dogfighting and leading a national dogfighting ring brought this sort of animal abuse to the attention of the general public. Dogfighting appears to be more common in working-class males (Evans, Gauthier, & Forsyth, 1998).

Table 20.5 Questionnaire employed by Molina (2008)

		Animal research questionnaire			
		Please give your opinion about dogfighting and cockfighting			
		Please circle +3, +2, +1, –1, –2, or –3			
		Dogfighting is a good sport			
Strongly disagree	Disagree	Slightly disagree	Slightly agree	Agree	Strongly agree
–3	–2	–1	+1	+2	+3
		Cock- (male chicken) fighting is a good sport			
Strongly disagree	Disagree	Slightly disagree	Slightly agree	Agree	Strongly agree
–3	–2	–1	+1	+2	+3

Molina (2008) administered the Pet Attitude Scale, the Animal–Human Continuity Scale (AHCS), and the questionnaire contained in Table 20.5 to 209 community college students in the San Joaquin Valley (the rural agricultural region of California). The Animal–Human Continuity Scale will be described later in this chapter and assesses the degree that the respondent views humans and other animals on a continuum versus in a dichotomous fashion. A higher score indicates a greater dichotomous conceptualization.

Table 20.6 indicates the correlation between approval of dogfighting and cock-fighting scores on the Pet Attitude Scale and the Animal–Human Continuity Scale. It is apparent that disapproval of dogfighting was associated with more favorable pet attitude and with viewing humans and other animals in a less dichotomous fashion. It is acknowledged that the correlations are low. This is probably a function of the limited variability in the approval/disapproval questionnaire. The statement "Dogfights is a good sport" resulted in 81.1% strongly disagree, 13.6% disagree, 2.4% slightly disagree, 0.0% agree, and 1.9% strongly agree. The respective percentages for cockfighting are 71.4, 17.0, 5.3, 2.4, 1.9, and 1.9. It is recommended that the Pet Attitude Scale be used in other research and clinical situations in which approval/disapproval of other sorts of animal cruelty, and animal cruelty itself, are assessed.

Table 20.6 Correlations of PAS and AHCS with dogfighting approval and cockfighting approval

Independent variable	Dogfighting approval	Cockfighting approval
Pet Attitude Scale (PAS)	–.21**	–.09
Animal–Human Continuity Scale (AHCS)	–.14*	–.11
Sex (male = 1, female = 2)	–.04	–.21**

$^*p < .05$ (two-tailed test).
$^{**}p < .01$.

Japanese and United Kingdom Differences

Miura, Bradshaw, and Tanida (2002) determined similarities and differences between college students in Japan and the United Kingdom. British students had significantly higher scores on the Pet Attitude Scale. In both countries, females scored higher than males. Both Japanese and UK students who had more pets in their childhood home had higher scores on the Pet Attitude Scale. In both countries, participants who had considered childhood pets as friends had higher scores. It should be noted that in another study carried out in the United Kingdom, children who felt they had a pet of their own scored higher on the Pet Attitude Scale (Williams, Muldoon, & Lawrence, 2009).

Comrey Personality Scales

Morovati, Steinberg, Taylor, and Lee (2008) correlated the Pet Attitude Scale with the Comrey Personality Scales (Comrey, 2008) using college students. The highest correlations were not large but suggest that persons with a more positive attitude toward pets tend to be orderly, extraverted, emotionally stable, and rebellious.

Vegetarians

Dixon-Preylo and Arikawa (2008) found that male vegetarians had higher empathy toward humans and a higher Pet Attitude Scale mean score than did male nonvegetarians. The differences, however, were not significant with female vegetarians and nonvegetarians. There were positive correlations between Pet Attitude Scale score and empathy toward humans with both vegetarians and nonvegetarians.

Grief Following Loss of Companion Animal

Planchon and Templer (1996) determined the correlates of grief after the loss of a companion dog and that of a companion cat. Greater dog grief and cat grief were both associated with female gender, higher score on the Pet Attitude Scale, and higher score on the Templer, Lavoie, Chalguyian, and Thomas-Dobson (1990) Death Depression Scale. In a related study, Planchon, Templer, Stokes, and Keller (2002) found that general depression, death depression, the Pet Attitude Scale, and the Pet Attachment Survey correlated positively with dog grief and cat grief in both veterinary clients who recently lost a companion animal and college students with a history of such loss. The correlations tended to be higher with the veterinary clients.

Attitudes Toward People

Tangen (2008) determined the relationship between attitudes toward people and attitudes toward pets by the employment of the Pet Attitude Scale and the Trust and Cynicism Scale of the Revised Philosophy of Human Nature Scale (Wrightsman,

1974). The correlations were low, but the significant correlations tend to support the inference that more favorable attitudes toward companion animals are associated with more favorable attitudes toward people. Trust correlated with .18 with PAS score, .16, with PAS Factor 1, "General Pet Attitude," and PAS Factor 3, "Pet Feeding Enjoyment." The Cynicism Scale correlated .13 with PAS "Pet Feeding Enjoyment" and .16 with PAS Factor 5, "Pets Cause Damage." It should be noted that in the above-cited Prelo and Arikawa (2008) article, empathy toward humans correlated positively with the Pet Attitude Scale. Daly and Morton (2006) reported a correlation of .71 between a measure of empathy and the Pet Attitude Scale in Canadian children.

Use in Psychophysiological Research

Charnetski, Riggers, and Brennan (2004) reviewed the positive physiological effects of tactile contact with companion and other animals. Such contact can influence heart rate (e.g., Lynch, Thomas, Pastwitty, Katcher, & Weir, 1977), blood pressure (e.g., Vormbrock & Grossberg, 1988), cholesterol and triglycerides (Anderson, Reid, & Jennings, 1992), and skin conductance (Allen, Blascovich, Tomaka, & Kelsey, 1991). Charnetski et al. determined increase in immunoglobulin A from before to after petting a dog in one group, before and after petting a stuffed dog in another group, and before and after no relevant activity in the control group. There were no significant correlations between Pet Attitude Scale score and increase in immunoglobulin A in the petting live dog and control groups. There was a surprisingly high correlation of .62 ($p < .001$) in the petting stuffed dog group. The authors of this book chapter view this correlation as credible. Children are comforted by taking stuffed animals to bed with them.

Grossberg and Alf (1985) found that college students had lower blood pressure while petting a dog than during reading or conversation. There were significant negative correlations of Pet Attitude Scale score with mean arterial pressure and systolic pressure. The correlations of the Pet Attitude Scale with diastolic pressure and heart rate were negative but not significant.

Vormbrock and Grossberg (1988) reported that college undergraduates had blood pressure that was lowest while petting a dog, higher while talking with a dog, and highest when talking with an experimenter. The petting-of-dog effect was greatest in participants who scored higher on a modification of the Pet Attitude Scale. Implications for the treatment of hypertension were discussed.

In the research of Schuelke et al. (1991–1992), participants were selected on the basis of having high blood pressure and high scores on the Pet Attitude Scale. Systolic and diastolic blood pressures were lowered by participants petting their own dogs but not by petting a dog that was not their companion animal. Schuelke recommended companion animal petting as a treatment of hypertension.

Nursing Home Residents

Ruckdeschel and Van Haitsma (2001) studied the impact of introducing dogs, cats, birds, and plants in a program referred to as "Living Habitat" in a nursing home. After six weeks the residents more positively engaged in their environment. This improvement was greatest with residents with higher scores on the Pet Attitude Scale.

Family Functioning

Cox (1993) conducted a six-Southeastern-state survey with families in therapy. She found that Pet Attitude Scale correlated positively with both family cohesion and family adaptability. Cox suggested that therapists used the human–animal bond to help families adapt and improve health status.

Loneliness

Moroi (1984) administered the Pet Attitude Scale and the UCLA Loneliness Scale to Japanese undergraduates. The Pet Attitude Scale yielded three factors. Loneliness was negatively correlated with the pets-in-the-home factor and the affection factor. Loneliness was positively correlated with the interaction factor.

Reactions to Missing Dog

Crowley-Robinson (1998) reported on the reactions of staff to Heidi, a therapy dog in an Australian nursing home, being missing. The staff had previously filled out the Pet Attitude Scale. Those employees with high Pet Attitude Scale scores were more upset by the disappearance of Heidi and were more pleased when she returned. Those in the staff with higher Pet Attitude Scale scores were more likely to believe that having an animal-assisted therapy dog does not increase their workload.

Other Animal Attitude Scales

Animal–Human Continuity Scale

The Animal–Human Continuity Scale of Templer, Connelly, Bassman, and Hart (2006) is a distinct animal attitude scale in that it is related to philosophi-cal/religious/worldview assumptions about whether there is a qualitative difference between humans and other animals. The traditional Christian thought is that only humans have an immortal soul, a free will, and ability to think and reason. Experimental psychologists, however, have demonstrated that animals are capable of concept formation. Furthermore, some contemporary Catholic, Protestant, and Jewish theologians and clergy are questioning the traditional absolute dichotomy position. It was in this context and the context of animal and human emotional response similarity that the Animal–Human Continuity Scale was developed.

In the first step in the construction of the AHCS, 28 items that appeared to tap the dimension under consideration were devised. The next step was the rating of the adequacy of these items, which resulted in the deletion of nine items. The 19 remaining items were subjected to item–total score correlations, and 7 items were dropped because the correlations were too low. The surviving items constituting the AHCS are contained in Table 20.7. Items 1, 2, 3, 7, 9, 10, 11, and 12 are worded in the dichotomous direction. Items 4, 5, 6, and 8 are worded in the continuous direction. For the last four mentioned items, scoring is reversed. For the other eight items, the score circled by the participants is given. Total score is the sum of the 12 items. More detailed scoring directions are in the appendix. A higher score indicates greater dichotomous direction. The AHCS was subjected to an orthogonal factor analysis with varimax rotation. The three factors were labeled "rational capacity," "superiority vs. equality," and "evolutionary continuum." In the determination of external criterion validity, members of a conservative mountain community Methodist church scored more in the dichotomous direction than Unitarians.

Table 20.7 Format for Animal–Human Continuity Scale

Animal–Human Continuity Scale

Directions: Please answer each of the following questions as honestly as you can. Use the scale provided below. Choose only one answer and put the number on the line next to the question.

1	2	3	4	5	6	7
Strongly Disagree	Moderately Disagree	Slightly Disagree	Unsure	Slightly Agree	Moderately Agree	Strongly Agree

_____ 1. Humans have a soul but animals do not.

_____ 2. Humans can think but animals cannot.

_____ 3. People have a life after death but animals do not.

_____ 4. People are animals.

_____ 5. Animals are afraid of death.

_____ 6. People evolved from lower animals.

_____ 7. People are superior to animals.

_____ 8. Animals can fall in love.

_____ 9. People have a spiritual nature but animals do not.

_____ 10. The needs of people should always come before the needs of animals.

_____ 11. It's okay to use animals to carry out tasks for humans.

_____ 12. It's crazy to think of an animal as a member of your family.

Censhare Pet Attitude Survey

The Censhare Pet Attachment Survey (Holcomb, Williams, & Richards, 1988) is a 27-item, four-option Likert format, self-report instrument that is geared to respondents who already had a pet and assesses degree of bonding. It has relationship and intimacy subscales. Items pertaining to time spent with pet and being in close physical proximity to the pet or both are prominent in the instrument. Cronbach's alpha coefficients for the relationship maintenance and intimacy subscales are .83 and .74, respectively. It has correlated in a meaningful fashion with a number of psychometric instruments, including the Pet Attitude Scale.

Companion Animal Bonding Scale

The Poresky, Hendrix, Mosier, and Samuelson (1987) Companion Animal Bonding Scale consists of eight items with five options ranging from always to never and pertaining to one's childhood. These eight items pertain to (1) responsibility for care, (2) clean up, (3) hold, stroke, or pet, (4) sleep in your room, (5) animal was responsive, (6) close relationship, (7) travel, and (8) sleep near. Cronbach's alphas of .77 and .82 were obtained. The first factor appears to be one of bonding, the second related to animal size (inferred from sleeping arrangements), and the third related to the animal's responsiveness and autonomy. The Companion Animal Bonding Scale correlated .42 and .38 with the Pet Attitude Scale and is positively associated with the Companion Animal Semantic Differential. This scale has two forms: One is worded in the present tense and the other in the past tense. It is intended for older children and adults.

Lexington Attachments to Pets Scale

The Lexington Attachment to Pets Scale (LAPS) of Johnson, Garrity, and Stallones (1995) used items from other instruments, including the Pet Attitude Scale, the Companion Animal Bonding Scale, and the Pet Attitude Inventory (PAI). It is a 23-item instrument with good internal consistency, meaningful factor structure, and good construct validity with it having been used in a variety of settings. Persons with higher scores display behavior more beneficial toward companion animals.

Pet Attitude Inventory

The Pet Attitude Inventory of Wilson, Netting, and New (1987) consists of 36 questions. Six questions pertain to demographics. Eight questions pertain to childhood pet ownership. Fourteen questions pertain to present pets—their number, species, name, age, duration of ownership, and from where they were acquired. Five questions pertain to time and activities spent with the pet. Six questions pertain to talking to one's pet. There are a variety of other items, such as whether the pet is kept inside or outside, who would take care of the animal if owner is out of town or hospitalized, the burden of pet ownership, the reasons for having a pet, and degree of attachment to the pet.

Some persons may say that the PAI is not a psychometric instrument but more of an information sheet. Nevertheless, it is herein included because of its high quality and because it could very well complement what are clearly psychometric instruments. It is a well-designed and useful information sheet. There are aspects of the PAI that can be quantified and used in research. In fact, it was found that persons who owned pets in childhood and women had higher pet attachment. The PAI is good for obtaining information to be used with more quantifiable instruments. It can also be used in applied situations such as family counseling, religious exploration, and animal cruelty.

Pet Relationship Scale

The Pet Relationship Scale of Lago, Kafer, Delaney, and Connell (1988) appears to be a measure of love or companionship or bonding that the person has with the companion animal. The authors started out with 74 items: 12 Pet Attitude Scale items and 62 items culled from the human–animal literature or generated on from theory in the literature. The 22 items that had sufficient item–total score correlations constitute the Pet Relationship Scale. Very good internal consistency was found. There were three subscales—Affectionate Companionship, Equal Family Member Status, and Mutual Physical Activity. The subscales of the Pet Relationship Scale had meaningful correlation with owner characteristics. Women scored higher on all three subscales. The Pet Relationship Scale correlated positively with the Pet Attitude Scale.

The Companion Animal Semantic Differential

The Companion Animal Semantic Differential of Poresky, Hendrix, Mosier, and Samuelson (1988) has 18 bipolar items: (1) bad versus was good, (2) important versus unimportant, (3) not loving versus loving, (4) beautiful versus ugly, (5) hard versus soft, (6) friendly versus not friendly, (7) cuddly versus not cuddly, (8) cold versus warm, (9) pleasant versus unpleasant, (10) tense versus relaxed, (11) valuable versus worthless, (12) kind versus cruel, (13) bitter versus sweet, (14) happy versus sad, (15) sharp versus dull, (16) clean versus dirty, (17) distant versus close, and (18) trusting versus fearful. The participant is instructed to "check the mark along the scale that describes how you felt about the pet."

The Cronbach's alpha was .90. The median intercorrelation of items was .35. There were four factors: (1) perception of pet as loving animal, (2) monetary value of pet, (3) affective value, and (4) relating to the size of the animal. To obtain a one-dimensional instrument, only the items with loadings greater than .60 were retained. The factor analysis of this 9-item scale shows only one evaluative factor that accounted for 53% of the variance. The correlation between the 18-item and 9-item subset was .96. The Pet Attitude Scale correlated .31 with the 18-item scale and .23 with the 9-item scale.

The Miller-Rada Commitment to Pets Scale

This 10-item Likert-type format instrument (Staats, Miller, Carnot, Rada, & Turnes, 1996) is relatively unique in that it assesses the trouble or burden of companion animal ownership that one is willing to endure. When people get married, their vows include "for better or for worse." Just as adversity tolerance may be regarded as a strength of a marriage bond, it may also be regarded as the strength of the human–animal bond. Items pertain to getting rid of or not getting rid of an animal with circumstances such as destroying furniture, requiring extensive veterinary care, and housebreaking difficulty. Five of the ten items pertain to destructiveness. The instrument has a Cronbach's alpha of .89. Its validity was demonstrated by correlations with other companion animal attachment instruments.

Which Scale Is the Best?

None of them are better than the others. They are all good. The choice of instruments depends on the nature of the study or application. Each scale has strengths and limitations. We should use the scale that has the best fit for the situation. Using more than one of them adds depth to the findings. Please see the table in the appendix for the comparative advantages of the various scales.

Summary and Recommendations

The Pet Attitude Scale has been demonstrated to have good psychometric properties. Pet attitude apparently develops in the context of the family, with the Pet Attitude Scale scores of adolescents correlating with those of their family members. In the United States, the correlations are higher with the scores of the mother than scores of the father. In Kuwait the correlations are higher with scores of the father. Also pertaining to the importance of the family are research findings showing that persons who had companion animals in childhood have higher scores on the Pet Attitude Scale. There are definitely cross-cultural differences. Pet Attitude Scale score means are higher in the United States than in Kuwait. They are higher in the United Kingdom than in Japan. Pet attitude is related to religion. It certainly appears that pet attitude is related to interpersonal and social and cultural factors. Group-oriented intervention may be warranted for persons found guilty of cruelty to animals.

Pet attitude seems to be related to attitude toward other humans. Persons with higher scores on the Pet Attitude Scale tend to have greater empathy toward other people. This finding is consistent with the long-recognized fact that children who are cruel toward animals tend to be cruel toward other children. Persons with higher scores also tend to have more trust in other people. Although the research so far has not shown appreciable relationship between psychopathology and pet attitude, there may be certain individuals whose very negative attitudes toward people and pets are a function of chronic depression or inability to experience pleasure or pervasive anxiety.

Pet Attitude Scale score appears to be related to the treatment of animals and attitudes toward treatment of animals. Vegetarians have higher scores. It is possible that very low scores can be a sign of a person at risk for animal cruelty and indifference to the suffering of animals. A high score would appear to be a favorable indication for work in a veterinary clinic.

If two spouses or significant others or partners have very different pet attitudes, this could entail a compatibility problem. In couples counseling money, sex, rearing of children, and religion are matters that frequently have to be dealt with. Pet attitude may also be an important matter. If one spouse or partner can't stand animals and the other has a plethora of animals that share the bed and kitchen table, this is obviously a problematic matter.

Animal-assisted therapy did not begin with the construction of the Pet Attitude Scale. Nevertheless, research suggested that score on this instrument predicts potential to profit from such endeavors. It also appears to have value in predicting the potential to lower blood pressure and change other physiological measures. Companion animal attitude pertains to more than attitude. It pertains to behavior and health.

More research is needed not only on human–companion animal relationships but on the difference between human–companion animal and human–noncompanion animal relationships. The essence of the differences has more to do with human attitudes than with the physical characteristics or species of the animals. Raccoons are ordinarily regarded as "wild animals," but occasionally are found as pets in people's homes. There are a number of instances in which the status of an animal is not clear. Are the feral cats that come to one's house for food but do not allow people to pet them companion animals? Is the guard dog that is kept in the backyard but is ignored except for food and water a companion animal? The distinction between companion animals and noncompanion animals has more than academic interest implications. It pertains to the humane treatment of animals. Some people are kind to companion animals but cruel to noncompanion animals. The same person who poisons or traps or shoots a wolf or coyote would never cause his similar-looking German shepherd to suffer. There is often a distinction made between good animals and bad animals. The German shepherd is said to be good and the wolf is said to be bad. The same sort of distinction between categories of people is made during war. One can kill "gooks" because they are bad and demonized and dehumanized. Defense mechanisms should be viewed as pertaining to not only human–human relationships but to animal–human relationships as well. Defense mechanisms are involved not only in the harming of "bad" animals but in the eating of animals. People don't eat pigs. They eat pork. They don't eat birds. They eat poultry. They don't eat cattle. They eat beef. We are dealing with issues that are broader than attitudes toward companion animals.

Graduate students and young professionals are often looking for research ideas. We are here offering some suggestions. One of them is to compare persons with monotheistic religions to persons with Eastern religions such as Buddhism and Hinduism or Native American religions on the Animal–Human Continuity Scale. We predict that persons with monotheistic religions will score more in the dichotomous direction in contrast to adherents of the Eastern religions and Native American religion who would endorse more of a continuum point of view.

It was described earlier in this chapter how American and Kuwaiti families have different patterns of family resemblance on the Pet Attitude Scale. It is recommended that a study of family resemblance in a variety of cultures and religions on the various animal attitude scales be carried out.

It is recommended that the animal attitude scales be administered to farmers, ranchers, and various people who raise animals for food or actually do the butchering. We now know that the animals are too often treated in a cruel fashion for months or years prior to the actual killing. What are these people like? What do they feel or not feel? What do they think? Are they as evil and cruel as Adolf Hitler and Saddam Hussein? Are they farm laborers who send their wages back to Mexico to keep their families from starving? Are they people who were raised on farms and do what their parents taught them to do? Are they overwhelmed by guilt? Do they think animals have no feelings? Are they nice people whose good work feeds the nation? Do they view animals and humans in a completely dichotomous fashion?

There is a dearth of research on attitudes toward animals in gay men, lesbians, and transgendered persons. The animal attitude scales can help fill this vacuum. Are gay men and lesbians more likely to be against animal cruelty because they know what it is like to be on the receiving end of cruelty? Would they score more on the continuity direction on the Animal–Human Continuity Scale? Would gays and lesbians without children score higher on measures of bonding with animals? What is the animal attitude family resemblance pattern in two gay men with children and in two lesbians with children?

An Alternate Pet Attitude Scale Form

A perusal of Table 20.1 shows that all of the items are not ideally worded. Items 2, 8, and 9 could be viewed as implying that the respondent has a pet. Item 3 could be viewed as implying that the respondent does not have a pet. In order to address this issue, changes were made in four of the items by Munsell, Canfield, Templer, Tangen, and Arikawa (2004) as indicated in Table 20.8. Questionnaires were handed out to 203 undergraduate participants with half receiving the original format and half receiving a format with four of the items revised as contained in Table 20.8. The revised items did not improve the internal consistency with the PAS. Cronbach's

Table 20.8 Item–total score correlations for original and modified 4 items

Item	Original	Correlation	Modified	Correlation	Z-score
2	My pet means more to me than any of my friends	.555**	My pet means more to me than any of my friends (or would if I had one)	.692**	1.58
3	I would like to have a pet in my home	.634**	I would like a pet, or to continue to have a pet, in my home	.390**	2.97*
8	I have occasionally communicated with my pet and understood what it was trying to express	.682**	I have occasionally communicated with my pet and understood what it was trying to express (or would if I had one)	.681**	.01
16	I frequently talk to my pet	.666**	I frequently talk to my pet (or would if I had one)	.652**	.173

*$p < .05$ (two-tailed test).
**$p < .01$ (two-tailed test).

alpha is a very favorable .92 with both formats. As indicated in Table 20.8, the correlation with total score did not differ significantly for three of the items. For item 3, the correlation was significantly higher with the original wording.

Munsell et al. inferred that the findings of their study provide reassurance about the original wording of the original format. Even though the original wording is not scientifically precise, the participants apparently intuited the intended meaning of the item. Although the basic integrity of the previous research may be assumed, the modified format would appear to provide greater credibility to at least some participants, patients, researchers, and clinicians. Munsell et al. recommended that if one wishes to use the modified wording, it should be for items 2, 8, and 16. It is here recommended that the reader decide whether to use the original or revised format. There are no overwhelming arguments for choosing one over the other.

Appendix

Age_____
Sex_____

The Pet Attitude Scale (Original Format)

Please answer each of the following questions as honestly as you can, in terms of how you feel right now. This questionnaire is anonymous and no one will ever know which were your answers. So, don't worry about how you think others might answer these questions. There aren't any right or wrong answers. All that matters is that you express your true thoughts on the subject.

Please answer by circling one of the following seven numbers for each question:

1	2	3	4	5	6	7
strongly disagree	moderately disagree	slightly disagree	unsure	slightly agree	moderately agree	strongly agree

For example, if you slightly disagree with the first item, you would circle 3.

Thank you for your assistance.

---

1. I really like seeing pets enjoy their food.

1	2	3	4	5	6	7
strongly disagree	moderately disagree	slightly disagree	unsure	slightly agree	moderately agree	strongly agree

2. My pet means more to me than any of my friends.

1	2	3	4	5	6	7
strongly disagree	moderately disagree	slightly disagree	unsure	slightly agree	moderately agree	strongly agree

3. I would like a pet in my home.

1	2	3	4	5	6	7
strongly disagree	moderately disagree	slightly disagree	unsure	slightly agree	moderately agree	strongly agree

4. Having pets is a waste of money.

1	2	3	4	5	6	7
strongly disagree	moderately disagree	slightly disagree	unsure	slightly agree	moderately agree	strongly agree

5. Housepets add happiness to my life (or would if I had one).

1	2	3	4	5	6	7
strongly disagree	moderately disagree	slightly disagree	unsure	slightly agree	moderately agree	strongly agree

6. I feel that pets should always be kept outside.

1	2	3	4	5	6	7
strongly disagree	moderately disagree	slightly disagree	unsure	slightly agree	moderately agree	strongly agree

---

7. I spent time every day playing with my pet (or I would if I had one).

1	2	3	4	5	6	7
strongly disagree	moderately disagree	slightly disagree	unsure	slightly agree	moderately agree	strongly agree

8. I have occasionally communicated with my pet and understood what it was trying to express.

1	2	3	4	5	6	7
strongly disagree	moderately disagree	slightly disagree	unsure	slightly agree	moderately agree	strongly agree

9. The world would be a better place if people would stop spending so much time caring for their pets and started caring more for other human beings instead.

1	2	3	4	5	6	7
strongly disagree	moderately disagree	slightly disagree	unsure	slightly agree	moderately agree	strongly agree

10. I like to feed animals out of my hand.

1	2	3	4	5	6	7
strongly disagree	moderately disagree	slightly disagree	unsure	slightly agree	moderately agree	strongly agree

11. I love pets.

1	2	3	4	5	6	7
strongly disagree	moderately disagree	slightly disagree	unsure	slightly agree	moderately agree	strongly agree

12. Animals belong in the wild or in zoos, but not in the home.

1	2	3	4	5	6	7
strongly disagree	moderately disagree	slightly disagree	unsure	slightly agree	moderately agree	strongly agree

13. If you keep pets in the house you can expect a lot of damage to the furniture.

1	2	3	4	5	6	7
strongly disagree	moderately disagree	slightly disagree	unsure	slightly agree	moderately agree	strongly agree

14. I like housepets.

1	2	3	4	5	6	7
strongly disagree	moderately disagree	slightly disagree	unsure	slightly agree	moderately agree	strongly agree

15. Pets are fun but it's not worth the trouble of owning one.

1	2	3	4	5	6	7
strongly disagree	moderately disagree	slightly disagree	unsure	slightly agree	moderately agree	strongly agree

16. I frequently talk to my pet.

1	2	3	4	5	6	7
strongly disagree	moderately disagree	slightly disagree	unsure	slightly agree	moderately agree	strongly agree

17. I hate animals.

1	2	3	4	5	6	7
strongly disagree	moderately disagree	slightly disagree	unsure	slightly agree	moderately agree	strongly agree

18. You should treat your housepets with as much respect as you would a human member of your family.

1	2	3	4	5	6	7
strongly disagree	moderately disagree	slightly disagree	unsure	slightly agree	moderately agree	strongly agree

Pet Attitude Scale

Page 1

Age_____

Sex_____

The Pet Attitude Scale (Modified)

Please answer each of the following questions as honestly as you can, in terms of how you feel right now. This questionnaire is anonymous and no one will ever know which were your answers. So, don't worry about how you think others might answer these questions. There aren't any right or wrong answers. All that matters is that you express your true thoughts on the subject.

Please answer by circling one of the following seven numbers for each question:

1	2	3	4	5	6	7
strongly disagree	moderately disagree	slightly disagree	unsure	slightly agree	moderately agree	strongly agree

For example, if you slightly disagree with the first item, you would circle 3.

Thank you for your assistance.

---

1. I really like seeing pets enjoy their food.

1	2	3	4	5	6	7
strongly disagree	moderately disagree	slightly disagree	unsure	slightly agree	moderately agree	strongly agree

2. My pet means more to me than any of my friends (or would if I had one).

1	2	3	4	5	6	7
strongly disagree	moderately disagree	slightly disagree	unsure	slightly agree	moderately agree	strongly agree

3. I would like a pet or continue to have a pet in my home.

1	2	3	4	5	6	7
strongly disagree	moderately disagree	slightly disagree	unsure	slightly agree	moderately agree	strongly agree

4. Having pets is a waste of money.

1	2	3	4	5	6	7
strongly disagree	moderately disagree	slightly disagree	unsure	slightly agree	moderately agree	strongly agree

5. Housepets add happiness to my life (or would if I had one).

1	2	3	4	5	6	7
strongly disagree	moderately disagree	slightly disagree	unsure	slightly agree	moderately agree	strongly agree

6. I feel that pets should always be kept outside.

1	2	3	4	5	6	7
strongly disagree	moderately disagree	slightly disagree	unsure	slightly agree	moderately agree	strongly agree

7. I spent time every day playing with my pet (or I would if I had one).

1	2	3	4	5	6	7
strongly disagree	moderately disagree	slightly disagree	unsure	slightly agree	moderately agree	strongly agree

8. I have occasionally communicated with my pet and understood what it was trying to express (or would if I had one).

1	2	3	4	5	6	7
strongly disagree	moderately disagree	slightly disagree	unsure	slightly agree	moderately agree	strongly agree

9. The world would be a better place if people would stop spending so much time caring for their pets and started caring more for other human beings instead.

1	2	3	4	5	6	7
strongly disagree	moderately disagree	slightly disagree	unsure	slightly agree	moderately agree	strongly agree

10. I like to feed animals out of my hand.

1	2	3	4	5	6	7
strongly disagree	moderately disagree	slightly disagree	unsure	slightly agree	moderately agree	strongly agree

11. I love pets.

1	2	3	4	5	6	7
strongly disagree	moderately disagree	slightly disagree	unsure	slightly agree	moderately agree	strongly agree

12. Animals belong in the wild or in zoos, but not in the home.

1	2	3	4	5	6	7
strongly disagree	moderately disagree	slightly disagree	unsure	slightly agree	moderately agree	strongly agree

13. If you keep pets in the house you can expect a lot of damage to the furniture.

1	2	3	4	5	6	7
strongly disagree	moderately disagree	slightly disagree	unsure	slightly agree	moderately agree	strongly agree

14. I like housepets.

1	2	3	4	5	6	7
strongly disagree	moderately disagree	slightly disagree	unsure	slightly agree	moderately agree	strongly agree

15. Pets are fun but it's not worth the trouble of owning one.

1	2	3	4	5	6	7
strongly disagree	moderately disagree	slightly disagree	unsure	slightly agree	moderately agree	strongly agree

16. I frequently talk to my pet (or would if I had one).

1	2	3	4	5	6	7
strongly disagree	moderately disagree	slightly disagree	unsure	slightly agree	moderately agree	strongly agree

17. I hate animals.

1	2	3	4	5	6	7
strongly disagree	moderately disagree	slightly disagree	unsure	slightly agree	moderately agree	strongly agree

18. You should treat your housepets with as much respect as you would a human member of your family.

1	2	3	4	5	6	7
strongly disagree	moderately disagree	slightly disagree	unsure	slightly agree	moderately agree	strongly agree

PET ATTITUDE SCALE AND ANIMAL–HUMAN CONTINUITY SCALE
SCORING INSTRUCTIONS

To Whom It May Concern:

You have my permission to use my Pet Attitude Scale and my Animal–Human Continuity Scale. No payment is needed. Enclosed find the scales and relevant articles.

For the Animal–Human Continuity Scale, score the number the participant indicates for items 4, 5, 6, and 8. For example, if the participant indicates 6 on item 5, score 6. For items 1, 2, 3, 7, 9, 10, 11, and 12, reverse the scoring. For example, if a participant indicates 6 on item 3, score 2. Add the scores for each of the 12 items. The higher the score, the higher the participant is in the dichotomous direction.

For the Pet Attitude Scale, score the number circled for items 1, 2, 3, 4, 7, 8, 10, 11, 14, 16, and 18. For example, if a participant circles 7 on item 1, score 7. For items 4, 6, 9, 12, 13, 15, and 17, reverse the scoring. For example, if a participant circles 5, score 3. Total score is the sum of all 18 items.

It is probably not important whether one uses the original format of the Pet Attitude Scale or the revised format with the wording of three items changed. The latter has the advantage of more precise wording but without demonstrated psychometric superiority.

Sincerely,

Donald I. Templer
donaldtempler@sbcglobal.net
(559)431-1886

Comparative Properties of Animal Attitude Studies

	No. of items	Bonding	General pet attitude	Human qualities	Burden/ expenses	Family members	History	Face validity	Times cited
Animal–Human Continuity Scale	12	Low	Low	Very high	Low	Low	Low	High	Medium
Censhare Pet Attitude Survey	27	Very high	High	High	Medium	High	Low	High	High
Companion Animal Bonding Scale	8	Very high	High	Medium	Medium	Medium	High[a] Low[b]	High	High
Companion Animal Semantic Differential	18	High	High	Low	Low	Low	High	Low	Medium
Lexington Attachment to Pets Scale	23	Very high	High	High	Low	High	Low	High	Medium
The Miller-Rada Commitment to Pets Scale	10	Medium	Medium	Low	Very high	Low	Low	High	Medium
Pet Attitude Inventory	36	High	High	Medium	Low	Low	High	High	High
Pet Attitude Scale	18	High	Very high	Medium	High	Medium	Low	High	High
Pet Relationship Scale	14	Very high	High	High	Low	Very high	Low	High	High

[a]High (past form)
[b]Low (present form)

References

Al-Fayez, G., Awadalla, A., Templer, D. I., & Arikawa, H. (2003). Companion animal attitude and its family pattern in Kuwait. *Society & Animals, 11*, 17–28.

Allen, K. M., Blascovich, J., Tomaka, J., & Kelsey, R. M. (1991). Presence of human friends and pet dogs as moderators of autonomic responses to stress in women. *Journal of Personality and Social Psychology, 61*, 582–589.

Anderson, W. P., Reid, C. M., & Jennings, G. L. (1992). Pet ownership and risk factors for cardiovascular disease. *Medical Journal of Australia, 157*, 298–301.

Charnetski, C. J., Riggers, S., & Brennan, F. X. (2004). Effect of petting a dog on immune system function. *Psychological Reports, 95*, 1087–1091.

Comrey, A.L. (2008). The Comrey Personality Scales. In G. J. Boyle, G. Matthews, & D. H. Saklofske (Eds.), *The SAGE Handbook of Personality Theory and Assessment: Personality Measurement and Testing* (Vol. 2, pp. 113–134). Thousand Oaks, CA, USA: Sage Publications, Inc.

Cox, R. P. (1993). The human/animal bond as a correlate of family functioning. *Clinical Nursing Research, 2(2)*, 224–231.

Crowley-Robinson, P. (1998). Nursing home staffs' empathy for a missing therapy dog, their attitudes to animal-assisted therapy programs and suitability of dog breeds. *Anthrozoos, 11*, 101–104.

Daly, B., & Morton, L. L. (2006). An investigation of human–animal interactions and empathy as related to pet preference, ownership, attachment, and attitudes in children. *Anthrozoos, 19(2)*, 113–127.

Dixon-Preylo, B., & Arikawa, H. (2008). Comparison of vegetarians and non-vegetarians on pet attitude and empathy. *Anthrozoos, 21*, 387–395.

Evans, R., Gauthier, D., & Forsyth, C. (1998). Dogfighting: Symbolic expression and validation of masculinity. *Sex Roles, 39*, 835–838.

Forsyth, C. (1996). A pecking disorder: Cockfighting in Louisiana. *International Review of Modern Sociology, 26*, 15–25.

Grossberg, J. M., & Alf, E. F., Jr. (1985). Interaction with pet dogs: Effects on human cardiovascular response. *Journal of the Delta Society, 2*, 20–22.

Holcomb, R., Williams, R. C., & Richards, P. S. (1988). The elements of attachment: Relationship to maintenance and intimacy. *Journal of the Delta Society, 2*, 28–34.

Johnson, T. P., Garrity, T. F., & Stallones, L. (1995). Psychometric evaluation of the Lexington Attachment to Pets Scale (LAPS). *Anthrozoos, 5*, 160–175.

Lago, D., Kafer, R., Delaney, M., & Connell, C. (1988). Assessment of favorable attitudes towards pets: Development and preliminary validation of self-report pet relationship scales. *Anthrozoos, 1*, 240–284.

Lynch, J. J., Thomas, S. A., Pastwitty, D. A., Katcher, A. H., & Weir, L. O. (1977). Human contact and cardiac arrhythmia in a coronary care unit. *Psychosomatic Medicine, 39*, 188–192.

Miura, A., Bradshaw, J. W. S., & Tanida, H. (2002). Childhood experiences and attitudes towards animal issues: A comparison of young adults in Japan and the UK. *Animal Welfare, 11*, 437–448.

Molina, M. (2008). *Psychological correlates for the approval of animal fighting*. Doctoral dissertation, Alliant International University, Fresno, CA.

Moroi, K. (1984). Loneliness and attitudes toward pets. *Japanese Journal of Experimental Social Psychology, 24*, 93–103.

Morovati, D. R., Steinberg, A. L., Taylor, L. C., & Lee, H. B. (2008). Further validation evidence for the Pet Attitude Scale. *North American Journal of Psychology, 10*, 543–552.

Munsell, K. L., Canfield, M., Templer, D. I., Tangen, K., & Arikawa, H. (2004). Modification of the pet attitude scale. *Society and Animals: Journal of Human–Animal Studies, 12*, 137–142.

Planchon, L. A., & Templer, D. I. (1996). The correlates of grief after death of pet. *Anthrozoos, 9,* 107–113.

Planchon, L. A., Templer, D. I., Stokes, S., & Keller, J. (2002). Bereavement experience following the death of a companion cat or dog. *Society & Animals, 10,* 94–105.

Poresky, R. H., Hendrix, C., Mosier, J. E., & Samuelson, M. L. (1987). The companion animal bonding scale: Internal reliability and construct validity. *Psychological Reports, 60,* 743–746.

Poresky, R. H., Hendrix, C., Mosier, J. E., & Samuelson, M. L. (1988). The companion animal semantic differential: Long and short form reliability and validity. *Educational and Psychological Measurement, 48,* 255–260.

Ruckdeschel, K., & Van Haitsma, K. (2001). The impact of live-in animals and plants on nursing home residents: A pilot longitudinal investigation. *Alzheimer's Care Quarterly, 2*(4), 17–27.

Schenk, S., Templer, D. I., Peters, N. B., & Schmidt, M. (1994). The genesis and correlates of attitudes toward pets. *Anthrozoos, 7,* 60–68.

Schuelke, S. T., Trask, B., Wallace, C., Baun, M. M., Bergstrom, N., & McCabe, B. (1991–1992). Physiological effects of the use of a companion animal dog as a cue to relaxation in diagnosed hypertensives. *The Latham Letter, 13,* 14–17.

Staats, S., Miller, D., Carnot, M. J., Rada, K., & Turnes, J. (1996). The Miller-Rada commitment to Pets Scale. *Anthrozoos, 9(2/3),* 88–93.

Tangen, K. A. (2008). *The relationship between attitudes toward animals and attitudes toward people.* Doctoral dissertation, Alliant International University, Fresno, CA.

Templer, D. I. (1970). The construction and validation of a Death Anxiety Scale. *Journal of General Psychology, 82,* 165–177.

Templer, D. I., Connelly, H., Bassman, L., & Hart, J. (2006). Construction and validation of an animal-human continuity scale. *Social Behavior and Personality, 34,* 769–776.

Templer, D. I., Lavoie, M., Chalgujian, H., & Thomas-Dobson, S. (1990). The measurement of death depression. *Journal of Clinical Psychology, 46*(6), 824–839.

Templer, D. I., Ruff, C. F., & Fanks, C. M. (1971). Death anxiety: Age, sex, and parental resemblance in diverse populations. *Developmental Psychology, 4*(1), 108.

Templer, D. I., Salter, C. A., Dickey, S., Baldwin, R., & Veleber, D. (1981). The construction of a pet attitude scale. *Psychological Record, 31,* 343–348.

Vormbrock, J. K., & Grossberg, J. M. (1988). Cardiovascular effects of human–pet dog interactions. *Journal of Behavioral Medicine, 11,* 509–517.

Williams, J. M., Muldoon, J., & Lawrence, A. (2009). Children and their pets: Exploring the relationships between pet ownership, pet attitudes, attachments to pets and empathy. *Education and Health, 28,* 12–15.

Wilson, C. C., Netting, F. E., & New, J. C. (1987). The Pet Attitude Inventory. *Anthrozoos, 1,* 76–84.

Wrightsman, L. S. (1974). *Assumptions about human nature: A social-psychological analysis.* Monterey, CA: Brooks/Cole.

Chapter 21
Qualitative Directions in Human–Animal Companion Research

David Shen-Miller

> *Tschuang-Tse and Hui-Tse were standing on the bridge across the Hoa river. Tschuang-Tse said: "Look how the minnows are shooting to and fro! That is the joy of fishes."*
> *"You are not a fish," said Hui-Tse, "how can you know in what the joy of the fishes consists?"*
> *"You are not I," answered Tschuang-Tse, "how can you know I do not know in what the joy of the fishes consists?"*
> *"I am not you," Hui-Tse conceded, "and I do not know you. All I know is that you are not a fish; therefore you cannot know the fishes."*
> *Tschuang-Tse answered: "Let us return to your question. You ask me: 'How can you know in what the joy of the fishes consists?' Essentially you knew that I know, and yet you asked me. No matter: I know it from my own joy of the water"*
> *(Burghardt, 1985, p. 908).*[1]

Qualitative Directions in Human–Animal Companion Research

Researcher inquiries into topics such as animal welfare, animal affect, and human experiences of the human–animal bond have historically been rooted in positivist epistemologies and reliant on quantitative measures and experiments, rather than naturalistic observations and individual experiences (Fraser, 2009). In this chapter, I target several topic areas within human–animal and animal research to explore the existence and benefits of qualitative research approaches. I begin with an overview of qualitative research with humans, including the benefits of using qualitative

---

[1]From "The Old Chinese Tschuang-Tse," in Bierens de Haan, 1947, p. 7, as cited in Burghardt, (1985, p. 908). Burghardt noted, "Bierens de Haan (1947) translated this story from Hempelmann (1926, p. 1), who in turn cited Martin Buber as the source" (p. 908).

D. Shen-Miller (✉)
Tennessee State University, Nashville, TN, USA
e-mail: dmiller20@tnstate.edu

C. Blazina et al. (eds.), *The Psychology of the Human–Animal Bond*,
DOI 10.1007/978-1-4419-9761-6_21, © Springer Science+Business Media, LLC 2011

research to explore topics such as understanding perspectives on animal abuse and neglect, human–animal companionship, grief and loss issues, and the benefits of animal-assisted therapy. Following this, I explore qualitative research endeavors into the subjective experiences of animals (e.g., Minero, Tosi, Canali, & Wemelsfelder, 2009), as well as methodological relations between quantitative behavioral observations and qualitative categories of animal affect, welfare, and experience (e.g., Wemelsfelder, Hunter, Mendl, & Lawrence, 2001). I conclude with an overview of the challenges to using qualitative methods, evaluative criteria specific to qualitative research on human–animal connections, and ethical considerations for both animal and human–animal qualitative inquiry.

Qualitative Research Methods with Humans

The Role of Qualitative Research

When considering a qualitative approach to scientific inquiry, a number of questions arise, including the topics one wishes to explore, the goals of the research, and the researcher's beliefs about the nature of science and knowledge. Researchers who use qualitative methods typically do so when wanting to explore topics that are new, not well understood, and need more in-depth examination. In addition, some choose qualitative methods to study topics or answer questions that are difficult or impossible to explore using traditional methods. Researchers also choose qualitative methods to explore discrepancies, contradictions, and nuances that exist in the empirical literature (Creswell, 2007; Morrow, 2007; Morrow, Rakhsha, & Castaneda, 2001).

In other instances, qualitative research is used to extend existing research and add to existing knowledge. For example, in their review of epidemiological studies on relations between owning a pet and human health, Friedmann, Thomas, and Eddy (2000) raised questions for future research, including attention to links between individuals' "meaning of specific types and even breeds of animals... (and) differences in their responses to animals" (p. 138). Although the authors did not mention qualitative research in this discussion, their emphasis on the *meaning* that individuals attribute to different animals and on the perceptions of danger and beliefs about innate characteristics of animals that differ by culture could be explored through qualitative investigation.

Below, I discuss the characteristics and defining features of qualitative research, including the differences between qualitative and quantitative approaches. I also provide an overview of the major methods common to qualitative approaches before shifting into discussion of qualitative research on the human–animal bond and with animals.

Characteristics and Defining Features

Qualitative research with humans consists of a set of empirical procedures designed to describe and interpret the experiences of research participants in a context-specific setting (Creswell, 2007; Ponterotto, 2005). Typically, qualitative researchers hold relatively similar beliefs about the process of scientific inquiry, including beliefs about (a) the nature of being, or *ontology* (i.e., reality can best be understood through exploring different views and perspectives), (b) the nature of knowing, or *epistemology* (i.e., proximity to the individuals and/or phenomenon under study is an invaluable part of inquiry), and (c) the role of language, or *rhetoric* (i.e., research results should include participants' terms and language; Creswell, 2007; Morrow, 2007). Additionally, qualitative researchers often make clear their *axiology* (values that inform the study) and use *methods* that are shaped by the data collection and analysis that emerge during the inquiry, rather than by theory or predetermined design (Creswell, 2007; Morrow, 2007).

A number of characteristics are typical of qualitative research, such as (a) focus on studying individuals (or groups) in their natural, context-laden world (vs. a lab or otherwise "controlled" environment), (b) attending to the meaning people make of their lived experiences, and (c) maintaining people's stories as a whole and centralizing the contexts of participants' lives in understanding the data. In addition, qualitative researchers (d) locate investigations in social interactions and contexts, (e) use language as both a tool for understanding and a focus of inquiry, (f) begin with questions rather than hypotheses, and (g) work inductively using an emergent research design (Morrow, 2007; Morrow et al., 2001). Haverkamp and Young (2007) added that creating a research question is not a one-time act, but rather a circular process that evolves with the researcher's understanding.

Further, data collection, analysis, and presenting results are considered inseparable parts of the inquiry process, as researchers cycle between inductive and deductive reasoning as they develop, test, and refine theories throughout the research project (Morrow, 2005). Finally, subjectivity is thought to play an important role in qualitative research designs. Because the researcher frequently serves as the primary instrument for data collection and analysis, researchers tend to acknowledge that some level of bias or personal influence (i.e., subjectivity) affects the kinds of questions being asked, interactions with participants, and data analysis (Morrow, 2005; Morrow et al., 2001; Peshkin, 1988). As a result, researchers typically include processes of self-awareness and self-reflection in their work (e.g., Beckstead & Morrow, 2004).

Differences Between Qualitative and Quantitative Approaches

Based on the above discussion, major differences between traditional qualitative and quantitative approaches are apparent. Differences begin with the approaches to research and in the relationship between the researcher and participants. Because data collection in qualitative research often involves interviews and/or joining activities with the community or person under study, researchers and participants often form bonds that are tighter than those formed during quantitative studies. Moreover, the distance from participants that quantitative researchers might require (to maintain objectivity) is typically not considered essential in qualitative research. In some cases, maintaining this distance is actually seen as detrimental to the process. In fact, getting close to participants enables qualitative researchers to uncover and understand participants' experiences and the meanings they make of them from participants' points of view, rather than exclusively from the researchers' point of view. As part of this focus, qualitative data tend to be verbal, visual, and language based, rather than the number based.

A final set of differences involves the research design. Qualitative researchers typically design their inquiries with the idea that the research methods should be flexible enough to make changes if needed based on findings that emerge during the study. Often, findings emerge during a project that require the researcher to ask additional questions, gather additional information, or head in a new direction entirely to follow leads and/or add context for better understanding. For example, researchers may need to conduct follow-up interviews with participants, seek participants with specific types of experiences, and/or use new methods of data collection (e.g., reading journal entries, looking at participants' artwork). Because qualitative researchers typically use a blend of inductive (data driven) and deductive (hypothesis driven) approaches to understanding the data, designs that allow for such flexibility enable moving back and forth among these methods of analysis.

To engage in the back-and-forth process between inductive and deductive data analysis, qualitative researchers frequently write, reflect, and analyze data during data collection, rather than waiting until all data have been gathered. Qualitative studies typically include relatively small numbers of individuals, groups, or institutions, rather than the large population samples often sought in quantitative studies. Qualitative researchers typically seek participants with particular types of experiences to meet the specific goals of an inquiry. This focus reflects a difference in terms of research questions and goals; qualitative researchers typically focus on understanding results in the context of participants' lives, rather than seeking explanations or developing theories that will apply broadly beyond their sample of participants. Finally, qualitative studies are often evaluated on the basis of the sufficiency and redundancy of the data, with the goal of reaching *saturation* (finding no new additive information or categories), rather than reaching a predetermined number of participants, level of significance, or power (Morse, 1995; Sandelowski, 1995).

Overview of Qualitative Methods

These differences are actualized in the genres or traditions of qualitative research. Each tradition enables a different approach to inquiry, truth seeking, data analysis, presentation of results, and evaluation (Creswell, 2007). Studies may rely on one method (e.g., interviews) of data collection, although researchers often combine multiple methods and seek different forms of data in their work. For example, in their study of the effects of integrating service dogs into families with an autistic child, Burrows, Adams, and Spiers (2008) combined participant observation, video recordings of family and dog interactions, and semi-structured interviews with parents.

A full account of qualitative research traditions and methods is beyond the scope of this chapter. However, in this section I cover several topics that are relevant to most of the methods used across different traditions. Specifically, I will discuss *researcher subjectivity, insider/outsider status, sampling, data collection and analysis,* and *evaluative criteria* (i.e., *rigor and trustworthiness*). Readers interested in gaining an in-depth overview of qualitative methods and traditions should refer to John Creswell's excellent *Qualitative Inquiry and Research Design* (2007), and those interested in the specifics of a particular genre or tradition are encouraged to seek primary sources (e.g., Glaser & Strauss, 1967; Moustakas, 1994). Further, there exists excellent information on specific methods that are used across genres, such as Kvale and Brinkmann's (2009) highly insightful and widely used text on crafting quality interviews.

Researcher Subjectivity. Because the researcher typically plays a central role in data collection and analysis, qualitative studies are particularly vulnerable to the potential for researchers to influence data collection, analysis, or presentation, that is, *researcher subjectivity* (Charmaz, 2006; Morrow & Smith, 2000; Peshkin, 1988). This type of concern has often been a criticism of qualitative methods, and qualitative researchers frequently go to great lengths to minimize the potential for researcher subjectivity. Some methods used to manage subjectivity include spending lengthy amounts of time in the field gathering data, communicating regularly with participants, maintaining a record of methodological, analytical, and conceptual decisions made during the study, and writing and presenting results. In general, maintaining a record of all of these decisions and procedures is described as a researcher journal or an *audit trail*. Peshkin (1988) also urged researchers to monitor subjectivity throughout the process of inquiry by attending to the feelings aroused during fieldwork (e.g., excitement, distress, disgust, amazement) and their responses to being in different settings and situations.

One reason that attention to subjectivity is so important is that unexamined biases that influence the process present significant challenges to the quality of the work—which is particularly troubling in studies with the potential for significant social and/or individual impact. Several researchers (e.g., Sandøe, Christiansen, & Forkman, 2006; Würbel, 2009b) have noted that science plays a strong role in discussions of animal welfare, answering questions about animal suffering and treatment, and helping set standards of care regarding conditions in zoos, farms, research environments, circuses, homes, and many other settings. For example, questions about sentience that inevitably arise during discussions of animal welfare and animal rights (Singer, 1975). In his discussion of Romanes' (1883) analogy postulate, Bermond (1997) reviewed neuroanatomical literature and concluded that researchers' inability to ask questions of their subjects posed significant limitations to studies of the emotional and mental states of animals. Bermond identified researcher assumptions of animal emotionality and consciousness that should be considered as additional threats to such studies, including beliefs that (a) if an animal experiences physiological responses in an emotion-inducing situation, emotional responses will co-occur, (b) emotion plays a role in behavioral reinforcement among animals, and (c) advanced cognitive processes imply the presence of consciousness.

Similarly, Würbel (2009b) discussed Levine, Mills, and Houpt's (2005) finding that despite an absence of pain differences between the groups of animals, more than half of a sample of veterinary students considered using a rubber ring for castration acceptable for cattle and sheep but not dogs or cats, and commented that "the different ratings merely reflect the students' prejudice about the different animals' abilities to experience pain and the animals' relative moral status" (Würbel, 2009b, p. 122).

Insider/Outsider Status. Some researchers have also written about the importance of considering one's own status with regard to a given community being studied and whether one is an *insider* (i.e., having the same or similar experiences with participants, such as a dog owner studying other dog owners) or an *outsider* in relation to the population of interest. Researchers from a wide variety of fields including psychology (e.g., Morrow, 2007), cross-cultural research (e.g., Banks, 1998), feminist research (e.g., Fine, 1994; Traustadottir, 2001), and anthropology (e.g., Geertz, 1977) have pointed out that being an insider or outsider affects one's level of understanding throughout the duration of the study—and beyond. Whether one is an insider or outsider can lead to differences in understanding and can affect the focus of the researcher's attention (i.e., what one does and does not notice when conducting field observations) and the design of the study (e.g., what kinds of questions one thinks to ask and the kinds of data one seeks to collect). Such differences can also affect the quality of the data made available from participants (i.e., the level of trust established between researchers and participants), the kinds of assumptions one makes about the data, and overall awareness and insight into the contexts of participants' lives. From an ethical vantage point, differences in terms of one's status as an insider/outsider can raise concerns such as loyalty (e.g., whether to "protect" participants or other motivations related to presenting results) and other issues (e.g., confidentiality) in terms of the overall study and presentation of results. When one is an insider, this status can also create dilemmas about where to stand on the continuum of being an observer or whether to participate in group activities and shift to being a *participant observer.*

Sampling. As mentioned above, qualitative researchers typically work with small numbers of participants, and often gather participants using what is described as *purposive* sampling. In purposive or theoretical sampling, researchers seek participants to meet the specific goals of a study, or to gather more information about a theory that may be forming during the course of the study (Creswell, 2007; Miles & Huberman, 1994). Purposive sampling might include seeking participants who (a) have intense experiences of a particular phenomenon, (b) exemplify a person from a particular type of background, and/or (c) have had extreme variations of an experience. For example, researchers exploring pet loss might seek participants who have had first-hand experience witnessing violent deaths of their pet companions (i.e., intense experiences), participants who are from low and high social class backgrounds (i.e., specific types of background), or participants who have lost pets as a result of domestic violence *and* those who have lost pets but are unsure whether their pets are still living (i.e., extreme variations of an experience). In another example, researchers interested in how emotions change over time in response to pet loss might seek to work with retrospective and in vivo accounts of individuals dealing with pet loss to identify a process of change. In such an inquiry, purposive sampling could include seeking participants with recent and long-time losses, as well as participants from specific cultural, gender, and socioeconomic backgrounds to explore the effects of those types of contexts on pet loss.

There are numerous other kinds of purposive sampling, all with a specific purpose. Some examples include *snowball* (i.e., finding participants through recommendations or contacts of existing participants), *typical* (seeking participants based on their normal or average experience of a phenomenon), and *confirming/disconfirming* case sampling (seeking participants whose experiences confirm, disconfirm, or nuance a theory in development). Qualitative researchers may use these and other types of sampling based on the study goals as well as what emerges during data analysis.

Data Collection. Data in qualitative research are collected through a variety of methods including in-person, phone, or Web-based interviews, observations (including *field observations* and/or *participant observation*), analysis of electronic data (e.g., Website information, discussion groups, forums), or physical data (e.g., documents, artifacts). In observation-based data, researchers work to capture as much contextual information about the participants as possible, including verbal and nonverbal behavior and notes about the setting (e.g., noise, lighting, temperature, movement, positions of people). Although interviews can range from open (i.e., unstructured discussion in which the participant sets the topics to be explored) to fully structured formats, many researchers use semi-structured formats, in which they have a few predetermined questions as well as freedom to follow up topics of interest that emerge during the interview. This format allows some uniformity across participants while creating the flexibility necessary to follow a participant's unique experience. Many researchers also include as data any thoughts, feelings, insights, hunches, and reactions that they experience during the research process (Morrow & Smith, 2000).

Data Analysis. Data analysis is typically considered inseparable from data collection and results writing. In their analyses, typically qualitative researchers work with large amounts of data from a wide variety of sources. Although the types of methods vary by genre, data are typically compared to each other and organized through grouping small bits of data into categories. This "constant comparison" method was developed and presented by Glaser and Strauss (1967) in their foundational text on grounded theory. In some genres (e.g., grounded theory), these categories are then analyzed and organized in successively abstract ways to establish relations among them and develop a theory. In other approaches, data may be grouped into a contextually laden, coherent story about a participant and her or his actions (e.g., narrative analysis), reduced to the universal essence of a phenomenon (e.g., phenomenology), or compiled into detailed descriptions of a case or several cases that focus on a few key themes or contexts (e.g., case study).

Miles and Huberman (1994) presented one of the most detailed accounts of methods of data analysis. Their three-part analysis begins with a conceptual framework that includes tentative categories (created prior to data collection). Both categories and the framework are analyzed and reformatted throughout the inquiry as needed. The initial categories are used as "bins" in which data are organized; these bins are updated (or split into more bins) as data do or do not fit. Later in the analysis, as they continue to refine their results, the researchers continue to refine their results by using a wide variety of techniques and models. In this stage, researchers test ways in which the categories that have developed relate to one another and develop visual displays of these potential relations.

Although their model may seem to rely on predetermined hypotheses (rather than working solely with ideas as they emerge from the data), Miles and Huberman's approach provides an excellent example of working with an inductive and deductive approach to data analysis. Also, as they and other authors (e.g., Glaser & Strauss, 1967) have pointed out, rare is the case in which a researcher does not have any preconceived ideas about what they will find in their inquiry. Rather, most researchers have experience in their line of study and find it difficult to impossible to avoid hunches about what concepts might be involved. Some approaches (e.g., phenomenology) advocate for setting all such preexisting notions aside (through the technique of *bracketing assumptions*), whereas others acknowledge that establishing preconceived categories provides a means to organize data in a preliminary way. In either way, researchers often check later in the study to ensure that through their methods they did not "force" the data in directions that were not authentic (Glaser, 1992).

Evaluation. Evaluative criteria for qualitative studies are both similar and different from criteria for quantitative studies. Several authors (e.g., Guba & Lincoln, 2004; Haverkamp & Young, 2007; Whittemore, Chase, & Mandle, 2001) have pointed out that differences in the philosophical assumptions that underlie specific qualitative traditions have consequences for the ways in which researchers conduct inquiry, interpret results, and disseminate findings. As a result, they have suggested that evaluation of qualitative research should be based on both the specific criteria of the method and paradigmatic assumptions underlying the study. For example, Haverkamp and Young (2007) pointed out that counting the number of times that participants used a particular response as a way to establish important themes would be justified in a positivist approach to research, but perhaps less justified in a constructivist approach.

Erickson (1986) pointed out that one must consider whether there are sufficient amounts, types and interpretation of evidence, whereas Denzin (2004) suggested that research studies be evaluated on the basis of representation—that is, how participants' lived experiences are represented in the text—including how the researcher's perspective is included and/or discussed. Morrow et al. (2001) added that readers should consider the social impact of a study in their evaluation, considering the contribution of a study to participants' lives (e.g., education, consciousness raising, creating social change) an important aspect of qualitative research.

In conjunction with this discussion, the term *trustworthiness* is typically used in qualitative research. Trustworthiness is the extent to which the findings of a study are worth attending to and considering as true (Lincoln & Guba, 1985; Morrow, 2005). The degree to which a study is considered "trustworthy" is based on the researchers' adherence to standards of (a) truth value, (b) applicability, (c) consistency, and (d) neutrality (Lincoln & Guba, 1985; Morrow, 2005). Lincoln and Guba (1985) developed one of the most widely used discussions of evaluative criteria associated with trustworthiness, suggesting criteria that parallel those used to evaluate quantitative studies and that fit with the four standards noted above. These include *credibility* (internal validity, or truth value), *transferability* (external validity, or applicability), *dependability* (reliability, or consistency), and *confirmability* (objectivity, or neutrality). Credibility refers to the degree to which the results accurately represent participant perspectives, and transferability refers to the degree to which findings may be externalized or generalized beyond the context of the original participants. Dependability refers to the degree to which findings would be replicated if the study were to be done again using similar elements (e.g., participants, contexts), and confirmability refers to the degree to which findings are rooted in the data and not driven by researcher biases.

Although these criteria tend to serve as the "gold standard" for qualitative researchers, Whittemore and colleagues suggested that "explicitness, vividness, creativity, thoroughness, congruence, and sensitivity" should be considered secondary criteria that provide additional means to increase the quality of a study (Whittemore et al., 2001, pp. 527–529). Those authors pointed out that while credibility, transferability, confirmability, and dependability are criteria that are required of all studies, secondary criteria such as those noted above will be differently important based on the focus, nature, and philosophical approach of individual studies.

Rigor and Trustworthiness. Specific methods are often used to establish trustworthiness and address concerns about credibility, transferability, dependability, and confirmability. These methods increase the methodological rigor of qualitative studies and include (a) using multiple data sources, (b) maintaining a researcher journal that tracks methodological and conceptual processes and changes—and the rationale for doing so (also known as an *audit trail*). Additional methods include (c) checking data and analyses with participants for accuracy, (d) immersing oneself (i.e., collecting data and/or reading the data) in the field and in the data long enough to establish depth of understanding, (e) exploring cases for any information that might disconfirm or nuance the results, (f) providing contextually rich information about the events under study (i.e., "thick description"; Geertz, 1977), and (g) providing information about the social, historical, and cultural contexts of the participants, the researchers, and the project (Erickson, 1986; Lincoln & Guba, 1985; Morrow et al., 2001). Seeking *saturation* of data (i.e., continuing to gather data until one is unable to find new information or insights), *triangulating* among multiple sources of data regarding a phenomenon (i.e., seeing if participants' experiences converge—or how they are different), managing researcher subjectivity, and using audit trails are all marks of sound qualitative research methods (Erickson, 1986; Lincoln & Guba, 1985; Morrow, 2005).

Qualitative Topics and Traditions in Human–Animal Research

Topics. Researchers have often employed these methods to explore a wide range of topics related to the human–animal bond. Different inquiries have focused on the experiences of having companion animals (with particular attention to the social significance of pets and the processes by which they are anthropomorphized; e.g., Anderson, 2003; Ellson, 2008; Fidler, 2003; Greenebaum, 2004; Morrow, 1998; Wiggett-Barnard & Steel, 2008); the benefits of animal-assisted therapy (AAT) and/or the impact of pet ownership on human health and well-being (e.g., Burgon, 2003; Burrows et al., 2008; Castel et al., 2008; Conniff, Scarlett, Goodman, & Appel, 2005; Kato, Atsumi, & Yamori, 2004; Turner, 1997); the role of pets in humans' mental health and gender identity (e.g., Mueller, 2003; Ramirez, 2006); the role of pets in recovery from natural disasters (Orr, 2006); the role of pets in community and social/mental health (e.g., Wood, Giles-Corti, Bulsara, & Bosch, 2007); the impact of moral issues and animal welfare on decision making about treatment of animals (e.g., Atwood-Harvey, 2005); and the importance of internal psychic relations between humans and animals (e.g., Brown, 2007).

Researchers have also used qualitative methods to explore grief and loss issues (e.g., Connell, Janevic, Solway, & McLaughlin, 2007; Gilbert, 2008; Kellehear & Fook, 1997) and links between domestic violence and animal abuse (e.g., Allen, Gallagher, & Jones, 2006; Pagani, Robustelli, & Ascione, 2007). Others have used qualitative methods to evaluate or refine existing measures (e.g., Castel et al., 2008), to evaluate mental or physical health programs that involve animals (e.g., Darrah, 1996), or in consumer research (e.g., Ellson, 2008).

In these investigations researchers used qualitative inquiry to uncover depth and contexts in participants' lived experiences as they explored processes that affect the human–animal bond. For example, Atwood-Harvey (2005) examined how veterinarians and their staff coped with feelings of discomfort and moral ambiguity when participating in animal declawing procedures. In her study, Atwood-Harvey found a complex set of interactions among personal beliefs and self- and occupational identity that involved coping mechanisms in which participants relied on organizational structures and the language of veterinary medicine to resolve feelings of discomfort and ambiguity. Atwood-Harvey found that participants used both the depersonalized, dispassionate language used in veterinary texts and existing organizational structures to "protect their own self-identity as people who work toward the best interest of animals, and paradoxically support action toward felines that they find morally objectionable" (p. 315).

In a similar exploration with a different focus, Greenebaum (2004) documented anthropomorphizing practices among pet owners through the dynamics of a local dog bakery. In her study, Greenebaum explored how the interpersonal processes involved in regular visits to the bakery reinforced pet owners' relationships with their dogs and created community, friendships, and self-identity among human participants. In both instances, the qualitative approaches allowed the researchers to examine in depth the processes by which such shifts occurred.

Traditions. A wide range of qualitative traditions or genres have been used in studies of the human–animal bond including phenomenology (e.g., Wiggett-Barnard & Steel, 2008), case studies (e.g., Burgon, 2003), ethnography (e.g., Atwood-Harvey, 2005), grounded theory (e.g., Adams, 1997), naturalistic inquiry (e.g., Gilbert, 2008), and content analysis (e.g., Anderson, 2003; Connell et al., 2007; Kellehear & Fook, 1997; Tannen, 2004). Many researchers have also combined quantitative and qualitative research in their investigations. For example, researchers have used both types of analysis on survey questions (e.g., Conniff et al., 2005), combined quantitative data with participant observation (e.g., Kato et al., 2004), and used focus groups to assess the validity of quantitative outcome measures (Castel et al., 2008; Wood et al., 2007). Yang and Chen (2002) employed a multi-method qualitative study in which they asked children to draw impressions of the word "death" of significant individuals in their lives, including pets, and to provide a brief written commentary explaining their pictures. The researchers used a phenomenographic method combined with chi-square and descriptive statistical analyses to analyze participants' drawings and explanations and a hierarchical category system to develop both categories around metaphysical, psychological, and biological concepts of death.

Qualitative Topics and Traditions in Animal Research

Inquiry into the Mental Lives of Animals

Turning to research on animals' experiences, qualitative methods look somewhat different. Modern inquiries into the mental lives of nonhuman animals (henceforth "animals") were initially driven by beliefs that the study of instinct was both psychological and subjective in nature (Burkhardt, 1997). In the late nineteenth and early twentieth centuries, some researchers (e.g., Darwin, Romanes, Yerkes) used qualitative methods such as observer accounts to understand animals' mental power (Fraser, 2009). At the time, researcher methods for understanding the minds of animals were based on the observation of animals coupled with *introspection* and *projection* (i.e., searching inwardly to understand one's own internal experiences, and extending those same experiences and processes to animals). For example, Morgan (1894) stated that investigations of *any* mind other than one's own (whether human or nonhuman) utilized a "doubly inductive method" (p. 49) in which an individual first analyzed his or her own conscious experience and then used it to understand another organism's behavior and reasoning.

Over the course of time, however, researchers of animals have wrestled with internal and external critiques that their methods were compromised experimenter subjectivity and *anthropomorphism* (i.e., assigning human traits or forms to nonhuman animals). These struggles have included internal debates over the necessity of understanding the subjective experiences of animals to the science of animal behavior, sparked by a shift in the early to middle twentieth century toward positivist approaches (Burghardt, 1985; Burkhardt, 1997). Both internal and external concerns were rooted in beliefs that processes such as animals' consciousness, souls, or affective states were unable to be measured or observed and thus were unsuitable for scientific inquiry. Consequently, inquiries into topics such as animal welfare and affect moved away from introspection toward more empirically measurable approaches. Inquiries began to be measured using positivist approaches such as physiological and quantitative measures and controlled experiments rather than naturalistic observations and individual experiences (Fraser, 2009).

Current Methodological Conventions in Animal Research

Currently, most investigations into animals' experiences continue to rely on quantitative approaches that include controlled experimental conditions that rely on numerical evaluations of behavior and can be easily observed and replicated (Fraser, 2009). Most researchers view individual differences as "noise" and focus their attention on findings that can be generalized across animals and species. Affective responses in animals are considered to be epiphenomena (i.e., not real phenomena in themselves) of underlying observable processes, rather than explanatory or causative phenomena—and as such are often excluded from analysis (Fraser, 2009). Even animal welfare researchers, whose methods specifically target animals' affective states, continue to use mainly quantitative approaches of behavioral and physiological measures (Fraser, 1999). Würbel (2009b) suggested that such approaches may be necessary to avoid diminishing the impact of their findings in debates about the scientific credibility of their methods:

> Biologically meaningful behavioural and physiological measures of integrity of form and function may provide powerful indicators of animal welfare. . .importantly, this may relieve scientists from solving the 'hard problem' of consciousness and may thus provide an opportunity for applied ethology to strengthen its impact on ethical and legal decisions, thereby advancing animal welfare without compromising scientific credibility (p. 126).

Critiques of Quantitative Approaches

Methods. Fraser (2009) noted that these conventions reflect beliefs among researchers that animals' affective states are unimportant, as well as emphasis on the pursuit of *internal validity* (i.e., the belief that changes can be attributed to a particular intervention or experiment) at the expense of *external validity* (i.e. the belief that the results of a study can be generalized to populations beyond the laboratory and/or participants). Some researchers (e.g., Balcombe, 2009; Fraser, 2009; Würbel, 2009a) have suggested that the sole use of quantitative approaches to explore animal affect places significant constraints on studies (and conclusions) about animal suffering and animal behavior, missing the complexity of phenomena as they occur in natural environments.

Wemelsfelder and Farish (2004) pointed out that the use of behavioral or physiological (i.e., quantitative) measures to assess qualitative categories (e.g., well-being, suffering, distress, panic) of animals' experiences provides only indirect measurement. As a result, they suggested, researchers may provide single interpretations when multiple ones are needed, or miss causal connections entirely. For example, the same behavior (e.g., running) could indicate a wide range of different emotional states (e.g., fear, aggression, excitement), and a stressful event could result in multiple physiological changes in the same animal (Wemelsfelder & Farish). Similarly, combinations of quantitative measurements of behaviors (e.g., pacing, bleating, defecating, flattening ears) may not capture the full gestalt of behavior as experienced by an observer; in some cases a qualitative label (e.g., "fearful") may provide a more accurate and holistic integration of behaviors and physical symptoms. Wemelsfelder and Farish (2004) noted in fact that researchers using quantitative methods seem to rely on qualitative description when summarizing the behaviors that they observe: "it is striking how, with the evaluation and summing up of quantitative results, qualitative characterisations (sic) of an animal's state seem to just spontaneously emerge" (p. 261).

Alternate Research Paradigms for Understanding Animals' Experiences

As noted above, critiques of qualitative investigations are rooted in notions that any investigations into animals' affective and mental states include bias due to researcher subjectivity, the vagaries of anthropomorphism, and debates about whether animal affect and mental states exist. To address these and other concerns, animal researchers have designed methods such as Wemelsfelder, Hunter, Mendl, and Lawrence's (2000) Free Choice Profiling and Burghardt's (1991) critical anthropomorphism. Fraser (2009) also described a more general alternative paradigm used by Goodall, Smuts, and other researchers when capturing the complexity of animal behavior. According to Fraser, this type of approach to capturing the complexity of animals' lives is characterized by (a) combining qualitative and quantitative data, (b) focusing on individual differences, and (c) using naturalistic observation rather than controlled experimental conditions. Fraser (2009) stated that the use of these combined quantitative and qualitative data changes the landscape of our understanding of animals' behavior in compelling ways, as the "narrative detail, individual differences, and unique social relations that Goodall and others described almost force us to postulate insight, desire and emotion simply to make sense of the (animals') behavior" (p. 114).

Some researchers have explored qualitative topics such as the subjective experiences of animals (e.g., Minero et al., 2009) and animal welfare (e.g., Mazurek, Marie, & Desor, 2007). Typically qualitative assessment of animal behavior involves attention to the animal's dynamic interaction style with the environment and includes terms such as "calm," "friendly," "hostile," or "curious" (Wemelsfelder et al., 2000). Minero et al. (2009) pointed out that many of these studies integrate measurement with interpretation and can be highly context dependent or context sensitive along with the risks of engaging in anthropomorphism.

Critical Anthropomorphism. Along with a number of other authors, Balcombe (2009) argued that anthropomorphizing is inevitable because of our inability to ask animals what they are feeling. Several authors (e.g., Balcombe, 2009; Burghardt, 1991; Minero et al., 2009) have noted however that there is a difference between being unaware that one is anthropomorphizing and engaging in *critical* anthropomorphism. In fact, Burghardt (1985, 1991) developed *critical anthropomorphism,* in which researchers draw on existing scientific data and knowledge about animals when making assumptions about animals' affective and sentient experiences. He argued that drawing on available knowledge about animals (e.g., biology, social interactions, ecological needs, history) when engaging in anthropomorphism enables researchers to make educated guesses about animals' experiences:

> Anthropomorphism can be a pragmatic strategy... in describing animal behavior to other knowledgeable people, and even to ourselves, utilizing the rich, ordinary language with which we are familiar... what I am calling for is a critical anthropomorphism and predictive inference that encourages the use of data from many sources (prior experiments, anecdotes, publications, one's thoughts and feelings, neuroscience, imagining being the animal, naturalistic observations, insight from observing one's maiden aunt, etc.). But however eclectic in origin, the product must be an inference that can be tested or, failing that, can lead to predictions supportable by public data (Burghardt, 1985, pp. 916–917).

An important component of this method is to consider the animals being studied as active participants in the process (Rivas & Burghardt, 2002). Burghardt and colleagues (Burghardt, 2007; Rivas & Burghardt, 2002) cautioned researchers to be vigilant in terms of subjective biases, encouraging researchers to explore how our status as animals affects our thoughts and behaviors, including our understanding of other animals. These authors also warned against uncritically generalizing our perceptions of the world to animals (Rivas & Burghardt, 2002).

Free Choice Profiling. Wemelsfelder and her colleagues (e.g., Minero et al., 2009; Wemelsfelder et al., 2000) have proposed a different response to critiques of the subjectivity inherent in qualitative approaches to animals' experiences, arguing that the assessment of animal behavior should integrate many pieces of information (e.g., behavioral events, posture and movement subtleties, contexts, interaction styles). Wemelsfelder and colleagues noted that researchers use qualitative assessments of animal behavior and terms such as *confident, nervous, calm, and excitable* to summarize an animal's dynamic interaction style and describe changes in behavior and physiology. Doing so, they suggested, provides unique insight into understanding the "whole animal" across various contexts (Wemelsfelder et al., 2001). For example, Minero et al. (2009) noted that the use of qualitative methods in combination with quantitative methods uncovered significant differences in horses' demeanors (e.g., "calm" and "reactive") during handling that were not captured using quantitative measures alone.

Wemelsfelder and her colleagues have pursued these assessments using Free Choice Profiling, an approach that allows researchers to quantify qualitative descriptors used in their evaluations. This approach to observing animal behavior evaluates specific qualitative terms through a process of inter-rater reliability as part of analysis of animals' welfare, behavioral organization, and behavioral expression.

Across a number of studies, Wemelsfelder and her colleagues have worked with untrained observers who are given "complete freedom" (rather than using a pre-determined list of categories) to generate their own labels and categories for the behavioral expressions of animals in different environments (Wemelsfelder et al., 2000). Wemelsfelder and her colleagues argue that observers must be "free and unbiased" when choosing terms (e.g., "bold/shy," "sociable/solitary") to allow for true flexibility in perceiving the details of behavior and context and integrating these elements into summaries of expression.

After generating their labels, observers compile a list of those descriptors and quantify the animal behaviors using those descriptors on a numerically or categori-cally organized scale (often ranging from "minimum" to "maximum"). Generalized Procrustes Analysis (a multivariate statistical analysis) is used to transform all configurations of observation patterns into one multidimensional, cross-observer, *consensus profile,* using principal component analysis to determine the main axes of the profile and the extent to which animal behaviors vary on those axes. The seman-tic meaning for each of the axes is then developed by returning to individual profiles to assess which of the terms best fits with each axis. Typically the consensus profile includes two main factors or axes (e.g., "factor 1 was labeled as ranging from 'explo-rative/ social' to 'suspicious/nervous' and factor 2 as ranging from 'calm/apathetic' to 'impatient/ reactive'") (Minero et al., 2009, p. 79).

This process also evaluates the extent of inter-rater agreement among descrip-tors and meanings and provides an additional validity check (Minero et al., 2009). Each individual rater's profile is assessed in relation to its fit with the consensus profile in quantitative terms, with the most highly correlated labels or categories used as descriptors for the main factors in the consensus profile (Minero et al., 2009). Finally, experimenters can explore convergence across individual word charts on different labels (e.g., confidence) to interpret qualitative differences between individual animals.

Findings across studies using Free Choice Profiling show significant agreement across observers' assessments and descriptions of animals' expressions, despite their lack of training and their freedom of choice for descriptors. Wemelsfelder et al. (2000) suggested that such findings supported the existence of "com-monly perceived and systematically applied criteria" (p. 194) and noted that the process of determining the consensus profile transformed multiple series of observational terms into "meaningful and subtle transitions of expression (e.g., 'friendly-inquisitive-playful-bold-forceful-irritated-agitated-restless' or 'friendly-relaxed-gentle-calm-tense-careful-cautious-restless')," which ultimately provided coherent frameworks to use in capturing animals' behavioral expression (p. 207).

Ethical Considerations and Challenges

In this next section, I discuss ethical issues that pertain to qualitative research with both humans and animals. Several authors (e.g., Cieurzo & Keitel, 1999; Haverkamp, 2005) have pointed out that although the American Psychological

Association's ethical principles and code of conduct (e.g., American Psychological Association, 2000) provides significant direction for the conduct of research, the unique aspects of qualitative research (e.g., close relationships between researchers and participants, flexible design, and changes in data collection) sometimes translate into increased ambiguity in the application of those guidelines. In such cases, additional ethical consideration is needed. Considerations of qualitative research ethics in the human–animal bond and in animal research may draw on perspectives from general guidelines on animal research ethics and general qualitative research ethics. When reviewing differences between ethics for research with humans and research with animals, readers are encouraged to consider the extent to which guidelines for research with animals extend to research with humans, and vice versa.

General Ethical Guidelines on Animal Research. The Association for the Study of Animal Behaviour and the Animal Behavior Society produced guidelines for the treatment of animals in behavioral research and teaching (Anonymous, 2006). In these guidelines, the authors recommend that researchers be knowledgeable of and follow local laws related to care and well-being of animals, especially considering that some studies are invasive or involve manipulation of animals (e.g., confinement, disrupting natural ecology). These guidelines suggest that when possible, researchers follow principles of *replacement* (replacing animals with nonanimal subjects, more sentient with less sentient animals, animals on farms rather than animals caught in the wild), *reduction* (using the lowest number of animals possible for sufficient statistical power),[2] and *refinement* (maximizing the scientific rigor and benefits of the study while minimizing harm to animals) (Anonymous, 2006; Sherwin et al., 2003). Sherwin et al. (2003) also urged researchers to consider factors such as effects of handlers, duration of the study, capture and/or procurement and transport of animals, care and housing of animals during experiments, design and implementation of the study, and thinking not only about the effects of enduring what is painful but also the effects of being denied what is pleasurable. Experimental designs that require isolation and overcrowding or that involve social disruption or deprivation should be evaluated carefully, as should the inducement of disease or introduction of harmful chemicals. Animals in such studies should be monitored frequently, and all studies should include consultation with experts on early detection of disease and distress (Sherwin et al., 2003).

Sherwin et al. (2003) encouraged researchers to be as noninvasive as possible in natural ecosystems, to attend to the potential impact (e.g., drawing blood samples, marking, and recapturing) of interactions with animals in terms of their reproductive capacity and physical survival, and to consider whether "reward" strategies, aversive stimulation, and/or deprivation or restriction of resources cause unnecessary pain or distress to animal subjects. Morton and Griffiths (1985) similarly

---

[2]Sherwin et al. (2003) suggested that these numbers could be reduced by relying on previous work, heightened attention to research and statistical designs, inclusion of naturally occurring events (i.e., epidemiological approach).

encouraged researchers to be alert to pain, distress, and discomfort in experimental animals by looking for changes in their appearance, food and water intake, behavior, physiology (e.g., muscle tone, weight) throughout the research process. These authors emphasized the importance of assessing these criteria at the onset of experimentation.

Although focused on documentaries rather than qualitative research, Pollo, Graziano, and Giacoma's (2009) discussion of ethics is relevant in terms of depictions of animal life and conveyance of research with animals. Their discussion is particularly relevant in terms of the mediation of reality that is presented; the authors suggested that ethical decisions are involved in all aspects of presenting material through film to an audience, including shot selection, ordering events and images, presenting information, and using narrative comments and music.

General Qualitative Research Ethics. Qualitative research with humans is bound by the same research ethics as quantitative research, as well as potential additional requirements. For example, the evolving nature of research designs and potential for intense and unexpected affect during interviews make gaining truly informed consent difficult to establish at the beginning of qualitative studies (Cieurzo & Keitel, 1999; Haverkamp, 2005). As such, researchers may need to anticipate such shifts in process at the outset of the project and inform participants (and Institutional Review Boards) of this possibility. In addition, informed consent may need to be revisited multiple times during an inquiry. Considering how the closeness of the researcher–participant relationship may influence interpersonal dynamics during data collection and throughout the study, some authors (e.g., Haverkamp, 2005; Morrow, 2007) have raised questions about participants' freedom to withdraw from a study. Although this freedom certainly exists, frequent interactions between researchers and participants may cause participants to feel pressure to continue in a study despite significant need to withdraw. The closeness of the bond can also have ramifications when ending the research relationship, in terms of emotional difficulty for both researchers and participants (Haverkamp, 2005; Morrow, 2007). Haverkamp (2005) also commented on the unique types of ethical concerns raised when the qualitative researcher is a clinician, including needing to be clear about one's boundaries and responsibilities when participants become psychologically distressed during interviews or other aspects of the research process. Haverkamp (2005) continued that in addition to these concerns, researchers should attend to confidentiality issues in multiply layered ways. She suggested that researchers protect the confidentiality not only of participants but also of those people that participants mention during their interviews.

Morrow et al. (2001) listed additional ethical issues with which qualitative researchers need to be concerned. For example, when gathering data with minority populations, researchers need to be respectful of cultural norms, taking photos, handling artifacts, attending special (i.e., possibly sacred) events, confidentiality issues (including important cases that add a great deal of dimension to the study but might be easily identifiable), and the potential impact on the community of reporting results. Morrow et al. (2001) also recommended that researchers consider what participants will gain through their participation and the impact of the research on participants' lives. Such considerations have ramifications for research with animals as well, particularly in the context of animal welfare discussions as noted below.

Concluding Remarks

In this chapter I presented an overview of qualitative research and methods including attention to how researchers approach inquiry with humans and with animals. A number of similarities are apparent across inquiry with humans and animals. In both fields, qualitative research is driven by desire for a holistic approach to inquiry and desire to understand "the whole phenomenon" or "the whole animal" as each exists in their natural contexts. Authors of qualitative endeavors seek relevance and applicability of the findings to individual cases and local contexts (e.g., Fraser, 2009; Guba & Lincoln, 2004).

At the same time, researchers who are interested in undertaking qualitative inquiry on either topic face critiques and concerns about the influence of researcher subjectivity. Within animal research several have developed methods to address subjectivity, including the approaches of *critical anthropomorphism* and *free choice profiling*. Within research with humans, methodologists have developed genres and methods that include attention to researcher subjectivity such as maintaining researcher journals, using auditors to assess their work, and checking with participants for accuracy.

In addition, a number of overlaps exist with regard to ethical considerations between the two fields of study. For example, topics such as careful treatment of research subjects/participants, attention to the quality of the study design, and attention to impact on participants in the study and on their lives afterward are discussed in research in both areas of study.

Clinicians may consider how to apply these approaches to their own work in terms of conducting both research and clinical practice. Morrow and Smith (2000) suggested that there is significant overlap between being a clinician and being a researcher in terms of the reliance on reflexivity (self-examination around subjectivity), use of narrative and storytelling, centrality of client/participant constructions, communication of results (or feedback), and the use of interviews. Similarly, Hoshmond (1991) stated that inquiry around *how* one comes to clinical decisions and impressions is an essential component of clinical practice. In either instance, attention to the data one receives about a client, the way in which those data are managed and organized (e.g., through clinical judgment), and how those data are interpreted (i.e., the role of clinician subjectivity) are all of utmost importance in clinical work. On a final note, clinicians who are interested in conducting qualitative research either through single case studies or studies with greater numbers of participants can consider how to apply the above techniques to their practices and areas of interest.

Acknowledgment I would like to thank Deborah Olson, Ph.D., for thoughtful and very helpful comments on an earlier version of this chapter.

References

Adams, C. L. (1997). *Owner grieving following companion animal death.* Unpublished doctoral dissertation, University of Guelph, Canada.

Allen, M., Gallagher, B., & Jones, B. (2006). Domestic violence and the abuse of pets: Researching the link and its implications in Ireland. *Practice, 18,* 167–181.

American Psychological Association. (2000). *Ethical principles of psychologist and code of conduct.* Washington, DC: Author. Retrieved, from http://www.apa.org/ethics/code/index.aspx.

Anderson, P. K. (2003). A bird in the house: An anthropological perspective on companion parrots. *Journal of Human-Animal Studies, 11,* 393–418.

Anonymous (2006). Guidelines for the treatment of animals in behavioural research and teaching. *Animal Behaviour, 71,* 245–253.

Atwood-Harvey, D. (2005). Death or Declaw: Dealing with moral ambiguity in a veterinary hospital. *Journal of Human-Animal Studies, 13,* 315–342.

Balcombe, J. (2009). Animal pleasure and its moral significance. *Applied Animal Behaviour Science, 118,* 208–216.

Banks, J. A. (1998). The lives and values of researchers: Implications for educating citizens in a multicultural society. *Educational Researcher, 27,* 4–17.

Beckstead, A. L., & Morrow, S. L. (2004). Mormon clients' experiences of conversion therapy: The need for a new treatment approach. *The Counseling Psychologist, 32,* 651–690.

Bermond, B. (1997). The myth of animal suffering. In M. Dol, S. Kasanmoentalib, S. Lijmbach, E. Rivas, & R. van den Bos (Eds.), *Animal consciousness and animal ethics* (pp. 125–143). Assen: Van Gorcum.

Brown, S. (2007). Companion animals as selfobjects. *Anthrozoös, 20,* 329–343.

Burghardt, G. M. (1985). Animal awareness: Current perceptions and historical perspective. *American Psychologist, 40,* 905–919.

Burghardt, G. M. (1991). Cognitive ethology and critical anthropomorphism: A snake with two heads and hognose snakes that play dead. In C. A. Ristau (Ed.), *Cognitive ethology: The minds of other animals: Essays in honor of Donald R. Griffin* (pp. 53–90). Hillsdale, NJ: Lawrence Erlbaum Associates.

Burghardt, G. M. (2007). Critical anthropomorphism, uncritical anthropocentrism, and naïve nominalism. *Comparative Cognition and Behavior Reviews, 2,* 136–138.

Burgon, H. (2003). Case studies of adults receiving horse-riding therapy. *Anthrozoös, 16,* 263–276.

Burkhardt, R. W. (1997). The founders of ethology and the problem of animal subjective experience. In M. Dol, S. Kasanmoentalib, S. Lijmbach, E. Rivas, & R. van den Bos (Eds.), *Animal consciousness and animal ethics* (pp. 1–13). Assen: Van Gorcum.

Burrows, K. E., Adams, C. L., & Spiers, J. (2008). Sentinels of safety: Service dogs ensure safety and enhance freedom and well-being for families with autistic children. *Qualitative Health Research, 18,* 1642–1649.

Castel, L. D., Williams, K. A., Bosworth, H. B., Eisen, S. V., Hahn, E. A., Irwin, D. E., et al. (2008). Content validity in the PROMIS social-health domain: A qualitative analysis of focus-group data. *Quality of Life Research, 17,* 737–749.

Charmaz, K. (2006). *Constructing grounded theory: A practical guide through qualitative analysis.* London: Sage.

Cieurzo, C., & Keitel, M. A. (1999). Ethics in qualitative research. In M. Kopala & L. A. Suzuki (Eds.), *Using qualitative methods in psychology* (pp. 63–76). Thousand Oaks, CA: Sage.

Connell, C. M., Janevic, M. R., Solway, E., & McLaughlin, S. J. (2007). Are pets a source of support or added burden for married couples facing dementia? *Journal of Applied Gerontology, 26,* 472–485.

Conniff, K. M., Scarlett, J. M., Goodman, S., & Appel, L. D. (2005). Effects of a pet visitation program on the behavior and emotional state of adjudicated female adolescents. *Anthrozoös, 18,* 379–395.

Creswell, J. W. (2007). *Qualitative inquiry and research design: Choosing among five approaches* (2nd ed.). Thousand Oaks, CA: Sage.

Darrah, J. P. (1996). A pilot survey of animal-facilitated therapy in Southern California and South Dakota nursing homes. *Occupational Therapy International, 3,* 105–121.

Denzin, N. K. (2004). The art and politics of interpretation. In S. H. Hesse-Biber & P. Leavy (Eds.), *Approaches to qualitative research* (pp. 447–472). New York: Oxford Press.

Ellson, T. (2008). Can we live without a dog? Consumption life cycles in dog-owner relationships. *Journal of Business Research, 61,* 565–573.

Erickson, F. (1986). Qualitative methods in research on teaching. In M. Wittrock (Ed.), *Handbook of research on teaching* (3rd ed., pp. 119–161). New York: Macmillan.

Fidler, M. (2003). Animal status as a response to pet owner experience. *Anthrozoös, 16,* 75–82.

Fine, M. (1994). Working the hyphens: Reinventing self and other in qualitative research. In N. K. Denzin & Y. S. Lincoln (Eds.), *The Sage handbook of qualitative research* (pp. 70–82). Thousand Oaks, CA: Sage.

Fraser, D. (1999). Animal ethics and animal welfare science: Bridging the two cultures. *Applied Animal Behaviour Science, 65,* 171–189.

Fraser, D. (2009). Animal behaviour, animal welfare and the scientific study of affect. *Applied Animal Behaviour Science, 118,* 108–117.

Friedmann, E., Thomas, S. A., & Eddy, T. J. (2000). Companion animals and human health: Physical and cardiovascular influences. In A. L. Podberscek, E. S. Paul, & J. A. Serpell (Eds.), *Companion animals and us: Exploring the relationships between people and pets* (pp. 125–142). New York: Cambridge University Press.

Geertz, C. (1977). *The interpretation of cultures.* New York: Basic Books.

Gilbert, K. R. (2008). Loss and grief between and among cultures: The experience of third culture kids. *Illness, Crisis, & Loss, 16,* 93–109.

Glaser, B. G. (1992). *Emergence vs forcing: Basics of grounded theory analysis.* Mill Valley, CA: Sociology Press.

Glaser, B. G., & Strauss, A. L. (1967). *The discovery of grounded theory: Strategies for qualitative research.* New York: Aldine.

Greenebaum, J. (2004). It's a dog's life: Elevating status from pet to 'Fur Baby' at Yappy hour. *Journal of Human-Animal Studies, 12,* 117–135.

Guba, E. G., & Lincoln, Y. S. (2004). Competing paradigms in qualitative research: Theories and issues. In S. H. Hesse-Biber & P. Leavy (Eds.), *Approaches to qualitative research* (pp. 17–38). New York: Oxford Press.

Haverkamp, B. E. (2005). Ethical perspectives on qualitative research in applied psychology. *Journal of Counseling Psychology, 52,* 146–155.

Haverkamp, B. E., & Young, R. A. (2007). Paradigms, purpose, and the role of the literature: Formulating a rationale for qualitative investigation. *The Counseling Psychologist, 35,* 265–294.

Hoshmand, L. L. T. (1991). Clinical inquiry as scientific training. *The Counseling Psychologist, 19,* 431–453.

Kato, K., Atsumi, T., & Yamori, K. (2004). Generating process of stories in robot assisted activity: A case study of Robot Assisted Activity with pet-type robot at a for-profit nursing home. *Japanese Journal of Experimental Social Psychology, 43,* 155–173.

Kellehear, A., & Fook, J. (1997). Lassie come home: A study of 'lost pet' notices. *Journal of Death and Dying, 34,* 191–202.

Kvale, S., & Brinkmann, S. (2009). *InterViews: Learning the craft of qualitative research interviewing* (2nd ed.). Thousand Oaks, CA: Sage.

Levine, E. D., Mills, D. S., & Houpt, K. A. (2005). Attitudes of veterinary students at one US college toward factors relating to farm animal welfare. *Journal of Veterinary Medical Education, 32,* 481–490.

Lincoln, Y. S., & Guba, E. G. (1985). *Naturalistic inquiry.* Beverly Hills, CA: Sage.

Mazurek, M., Marie, M., & Desor, D. (2007). Potential animal-centred indicators of dairy goat welfare. *Animal Welfare, 16*, 161–164.

Miles, M. B., & Huberman, M. (1994). *Qualitative data analysis: An expanded sourcebook.* Thousand Oaks, CA: Sage.

Minero, M., Tosi, M. V., Canali, E., & Wemelsfelder, F. (2009). Quantitative and qualitative assessment of the response of foals to the presence of an unfamiliar human. *Applied Animal Behaviour Science, 116*, 74–81.

Morgan, C. L. (1894). *An introduction to comparative psychology.* London: Walter Scott.

Morrow, S. (2005). Quality and trustworthiness in counseling psychology. *Journal of Counseling Psychology, 52*, 250–260.

Morrow, S. L. (2007). Qualitative research in counseling psychology: Conceptual foundations. *The Counseling Psychologist, 35*, 209–235.

Morrow, S. L., Rakhsha, G., & Castaneda, C. L. (2001). Qualitative research methods for multicultural counseling. In J. G. Ponterotto, J. M. Casas, L. A. Suzuki, & C. M. Alexander (Eds.), *Handbook of multicultural counseling* (2nd ed., pp. 575–603). Thousand Oaks, CA: Sage.

Morrow, S. L., & Smith, M. L. (2000). Qualitative research for counseling psychology. In S. D. Brown & R. W. Lent (Eds.), *Handbook of counseling psychology* (3rd ed., pp. 199–230). New York: Wiley & Sons.

Morrow, V. (1998). My animals and other family: Children's perspectives on their relationships with companion animals. *Anthrozoös, 11*, 218–226.

Morse, J. (1995). The significance of saturation. *Qualitative Health Research, 5*, 147–149.

Morton, D. B., & Griffiths, P. H. M. (1985). Guidelines on the recognition of pain, distress, and discomfort in experimental animals and an hypothesis for assessment. *Veterinary Record, 116*, 431–436.

Moustakas, C. (1994). *Phenomenological research methods.* Thousand Oaks, CA: Sage.

Mueller, S. A. (2003). *Boys of divorce and their dogs: The role of the pet dog in helping to manage some gender role conflict issues.* Unpublished doctoral dissertation, University of Hartford, West Hartford, CT.

Orr, A. E. (2006). *The role of pets in the experience of Hurricane Charley victims: A phenomenological study (Florida),* Unpublished doctoral dissertation, Capella University.

Pagani, C., Robustelli, F., & Ascione, F. R. (2007). Italian youths' attitudes toward, and concern for, animals. *Anthrozoös, 20*, 275–293.

Peshkin, A. (1988). In search of subjectivity—one's own. *Educational Researcher, 17*, 16–21.

Pollo, S., Graziano, M., & Giacoma, C. (2009). The ethics of natural history documentaries. *Animal Behaviour, 77*, 1357–1360.

Ponterotto, J. G. (2005). Qualitative research in counseling psychology: A primer on research paradigms. *Journal of Counseling Psychology, 52*, 126–136.

Ramirez, R. (2006). 'My dog's just like me': Dog ownership as a gender display. *Symbolic Interaction, 29*, 373–391.

Rivas, J., & Burghardt, G. M. (2002). Crotalomorphism: A metaphor for understanding anthropomorphism by omission. In M. Bekoff, C. Allen, & G. M. Burghardt (Eds.), *The cognitive animal: Experimental and theoretical perspectives on animal cognition* (pp. 9–17). Cambridge, MA: MIT Press.

Romanes, G. J. (1883). *Mental evolution in animals.* London: Kegan Paul, Trench & Co.

Sandelowski, M. (1995). Sample size in qualitative research. *Research in Nursing and Health, 18*, 179–183.

Sandøe, P., Christiansen, S. B., & Forkman, B. (2006). Animal welfare: What is the role of science? In J. Turner & J. D'Silva (Eds.), *Animals, ethics, and trade: The challenge of animal sentience.* London: Earthscan.

Sherwin, C. M., Christiansen, S. B., Duncan, I. J., Erhard, H. W., Lay, D. C., Mench, J. A., et al. (2003). Guidelines for the ethical use of animals in applied ethology studies. *Applied Animal Behaviour Science, 81*, 291–305.

Singer, P. (1975). *Animal liberation.* New York: Harper Perennial.

Tannen, D. (2004). Talking the dog: Framing pets as interactional resources in family discourse. *Research on Language and Social Interaction, 37*, 399–420.

Traustadottir. (2001). Research with others: Reflections on representation, difference, and othering. *Scandinavian Journal of Disability Research, 3*, 9–28.

Turner, W. G. (1997). Evaluation of a pet loss support hotline. *Anthrozoös, 10*, 225–230.

Wemelsfelder, F., & Farish, M. (2004). Qualitative categories for the interpretation of sheep welfare: A review. *Animal Welfare, 13*, 261–268.

Wemelsfelder, F., Hunter, E. A., Mendl, M. T., & Lawrence, A. B. (2000). The spontaneous qualitative assessment of behavioural expressions in pigs: First explorations of a novel methodology for integrative animal welfare measurement. *Applied Animal Behaviour Science, 67*, 193–215.

Wemelsfelder, F., Hunter, T. E. A., Mendl, M. T., & Lawrence, A. B. (2001). Assessing the "whole animal": A free choice profiling approach. *Animal Behavior, 62*, 209–220.

Whittemore, R., Chase, S. K., & Mandle, C. L. (2001). Validity in qualitative research. *Qualitative Health Research, 11*, 522–537.

Wiggett-Barnard, C., & Steel, H. (2008). The experience of owning a guide dog. *Disability and Rehabilitation: An International, Multidisciplinary Journal, 30*, 1014–1026.

Wood, L. J., Giles-Corti, B., Bulsara, M. K., & Bosch, D. A. (2007). More than a furry companion: The ripple effect of companion animals on neighborhood interactions and sense of community. *Journal of Human-Animal Studies, 15*, 43–56.

Würbel, H. (2009a). The state of ethological approaches to the assessment of animal suffering and welfare. *Applied Animal Behaviour Science, 118*, 105–107.

Würbel, H. (2009b). Ethology applied to animal ethics. *Applied Animal Behaviour Science, 118*, 118–127.

Yang, S. C., & Chen, S. (2002). A phenomenographic approach to the meaning of death: A Chinese perspective. *Death Studies, 26*, 143–175.

Chapter 22
Pet Loss and Grief: An Integrative Perspective

Güler Boyraz and Michael E. Bricker

> *Your grief for what you've lost holds a mirror*
> *up to where you're bravely working*
> *Expecting the worst, you look and instead,*
> *here's the joyful face you've been wanting to see...*
> Jalaluddin Rumi

As the role of pets in human life has increased substantially in the past 20 years, increasing attention has been given to human–animal bonds in the psychology literature (e.g., Brown, 2002, 2004, 2007; Gilbey, McNicholas, & Collis, 2007; Kurdek, 2008). Recent research suggests that people develop strong affectional bonds with their pets and experience a significant amount of distress when faced with their loss (e.g., Field, Orsini, Gavish, & Packman, 2009; Planchon & Templer, 1996; Wrobel & Dye, 2003). Despite the growing body of literature on the human–animal bond, research remains limited that examines both the nature of the relationship between human beings and animals and individuals' response to the loss of a pet. Further, while some studies suggest that the grief experienced following a pet's loss is comparable in intensity to that of losing a loved one (Field et al., 2009; Gerwolls & Labott, 1994), other findings (Wrobel & Dye, 2003) indicate that not all bereaved pet owners experience grief symptoms. Clearly, variations exist in the meaning that humans attribute to the pets in their lives, as well as the level of distress experienced following their loss. Therefore, it is important to understand the variables that account for the differences in individuals' response to pet loss.

In order to further an understanding of the components of bereavement among pet owners, one purpose of this chapter is to provide a theoretical discussion on pet loss by integrating different theoretical perspectives on bereavement and discussing the applicability of these theories in conceptualizing this phenomenon. Most of the previous research in this area used Bowlby's (1982) Attachment theory when conceptualizing grief following the loss of a pet. Although Cognitive Stress Theory (CST, Lazarus & Folkman, 1984) and others recent theories (e.g., constructivist and

G. Boyraz (✉)
Department of Psychology, Tennessee State University, Nashville, TN, USA
e-mail: gboyraz@gmail.com

C. Blazina et al. (eds.), *The Psychology of the Human–Animal Bond*,
DOI 10.1007/978-1-4419-9761-6_22, © Springer Science+Business Media, LLC 2011

trauma perspectives) are not cited in the previous pet loss literature, we suggest that these theories may provide a useful framework for understanding why people show differing reactions to the loss of a pet. Further, integrating different perspectives may help mental health practitioners to develop a broader understanding of the variables that may impact individuals' adjustment to the loss of a pet, allowing them to intervene more effectively. The second purpose of this chapter is to discuss the challenges in designing human–animal bond research (e.g., theoretical issues, study design, and sampling issues) and to provide a review of recent studies on pet loss.

Attachment Theory

Attachment theory emphasizes people's tendency to develop strong emotional bonds with others and provides a way to understand various forms of psychological distress (e.g., anxiety, anger, and depression), related to separation from attachment figures (Bowlby, 1980). Attachment behavior is defined as "any form of behavior that results in a person attaining or retaining proximity to some other differentiated and preferred individual" (Bowlby, 1980, p. 39). However, Bowlby (1982) also noted that "it is inaccurate to describe attachment behavior solely in terms of attaining and maintaining proximity to a particular individual" (p. 374). Thus, individuals may form various forms of bonds (e.g., caregiving bond, attachment bond) with others during their life, although not all of these bonds are considered attachment bonds. While individuals may seek proximity to a companion, or a child may seek proximity to a playmate, these behaviors are not considered attachment behaviors unless the goal of the behavior is to regain a sense of security or safety (Bowlby, 1982).

In distinguishing attachment bonds from other types of affectional bonds, it is important to clarify the theoretical constructs thought to comprise the formation of an attachment bond. An attachment bond is hypothesized to involve four behavioral features toward attachment figures: *proximity maintenance* (seeking closeness), *separation distress* (experiencing distress when the attachment figure is absent), *safe haven* (turning to attachment figure to alleviate distress), and *secure base* (using the attachment figure as a base of security when facing challenges; Ainsworth, 1991; also see Kobak, 2009). Proximity seeking and separation distress are not limited to attachment bonds; but rather, these types of behaviors are thought to be observed in other types of affectional bonds as well (see Kobak, 2009 for a discussion). Therefore, affectional bonds are not considered to be an attachment bond unless an individual relies on the other as a source of comfort (safe haven) or security (secure base). For example, a mother's bond with her baby is not considered an attachment bond because she does not rely on her child for security and comfort (see Collis & McNicholas, 1998). On the other hand, individuals in romantic relationships may turn to their partners for security and comfort in times of distress; thus, many romantic love relationships can be considered to involve a bond of attachment (Hazan & Shaver, 1987).

There has been an ongoing debate in the psychology literature regarding whether the bond between humans and pets meets the criteria for attachment bonds. Some researchers (e.g., Collis & McNicholas, 1998; Kobak, 2009) have suggested these bonds do not meet the criteria for attachment bonds. However, other researchers have asserted that individuals develop attachment bonds with their pets and turn to them for security and comfort (e.g., Kurdek, 2008, 2009). In two different studies, Kurdek (2008, 2009) noted that pet owners rated key attachment-related components of "proximity maintenance" and "secure base" as the most salient features of their human–animal relationship. For example, some of the participants in this study reported that they were more likely to turn to their pets than to relatives or friends in times of distress. While these findings seem to offer preliminary support for the idea that people may turn to animal companions for security and comfort in times of distress, existing literature does not offer enough empirical support regarding whether pets can serve as attachment figures. In addition, the methodological challenges, which will be discussed later in this chapter (e.g., difficulty measuring safe haven and secure base behaviors, see Kobak, 2009 for a discussion), help to clarify the complicated nature of determining the relationship between pets and their human owners.

Attachment and Loss

Bowlby's (1982) Attachment theory has largely been based on the observations of human and primate infants. Bowlby and other researchers' findings suggest that both human and primate infants show some universal, common reactions when they are separated from their mothers. For example, infants' initial response to separation tended to involve crying, active searching, and resisting others (*protest*), followed by intense sadness and realization that the attachment figure will not return (*despair*). When the attachment figure returned, infants typically demonstrated a defensive disregard for and avoidance of the mother (*detachment* – which has been discussed only in reference to human mother–infant separation; see Hazan & Shaver, 1987).

Bowlby and others have also extended Attachment theory to provide an understanding of attachment and loss in adults (see Mikulincer & Shaver, 2007, for a review). In furthering this framework, they proposed that striking similarities exist between the response of young children following the loss of a mother and the responses of bereaved adults following the loss of a loved one. For example, Bowlby (1982) suggested that grief following the loss of a loved one is characterized by protest responses and intense sadness and realization that the deceased person will not return (despair and disorganization). These responses are followed by a reorganization or redefinition phase during which bereaved individuals redefine the self and the situation (Bowlby, 1982). Bowlby (1982) noted that this redefinition phase involves bereaved individuals' cognitive efforts to reshape internal representational models by reorganizing the attachment configuration. During this redefinition phase, most bereaved individuals continue to feel a sense of connection with their deceased loved one (i.e., persistence of the relationship or continuous bonds), which has been found to foster adjustment in many bereaved persons (see Bowlby, 1982).

In the recent literature, several researchers further extended Attachment theory in an attempt to understand individuals' reactions to pet loss. These researchers suggested that patterns of grief reactions following the loss of a pet are similar to grief reactions following the loss of a loved one (Field et al., 2009). For example, Field and his colleagues (2009) explored the mediating role of the continuous bond with the deceased pet by examining its association with the relationship between the strength of the past attachment with the pet, attachment anxiety, and severity of grief. Their findings indicated that participants experienced distress in response to separation from their pets (as indicated by participants complicated grief scores). Participants also reported an attempt to maintain proximity with the deceased pet (as indicated by participants' mean scores on a continuous bonds scale). In addition, higher levels of pet attachment were associated with higher scores on the continuous bonds scale, which, in turn were associated with higher levels of grief. It has been suggested in the literature that the losses that activate the attachment system of the individuals typically trigger an effort to continue to have a connection with the deceased (Field, Gao, & Paderna, 2005; also see Neimeyer, 2005–2006). Therefore, based on their findings (e.g., participants' scores on continuous bonds scale), Field and his colleagues concluded that humans do develop attachment bonds with their animals. While Field and his colleagues' findings can offer a preliminary understanding of the applicability of Attachment theory to human–animal bond, as well as grief following the pet loss, it appears that this is the only study that has examined the role of attachment styles and continuous bonds in complicated bereavement. Thus, more research is needed to support and extend their findings.

Stress, Trauma, and Constructivist Theories

Cognitive Stress Theory

Although Cognitive Stress Theory (Lazarus & Folkman, 1984) has not been used in the previous literature to understand individuals' response to pet loss, it may provide a useful framework for further understanding this phenomenon and may also serve to clarify how bereaved individuals may be helped in coping with the loss of their pets. CST integrates principles of coping that may work well in explaining aspects of the grieving process. According to CST perspective, loss of a loved one is considered a stressor that may impose demands on the individual. Unlike traditional theories of grief that assume that all bereaved persons respond similarly to loss, CST instead focuses on the relationship between a person's subjective evaluations of the loss and his or her emotional response to it. Therefore, according to this perspective, a pet owner's subjective interpretation of the loss, rather than the loss itself, determines his/or her reaction to loss.

According to CST, the coping process starts with an individual's evaluation of (1) the personal meaning or significance of the event (primary appraisal) and (2) his or her assessment of their available resources for coping with the event (secondary appraisal). The degree to which an event is perceived as stressful depends on the level of personal significance of the event, as well as the extent to which the event is appraised as exceeding one's coping resources and, in conjunction with this, the threat that this poses to his or her well-being (Lazarus & Folkman, 1984). Primary and secondary appraisals are thought to affect the type and intensity of emotion that the individual will experience (Folkman, 2001). Therefore, in the context of a pet loss, the significance of distress appears dependent upon a pet owner's subjective appraisals of the personal significance of the loss and his or her coping resources.

Empirical research provides support for the role of cognitive appraisals of loss in adjustment to loss (see Bonanno & Kaltman, 1999, for a review). More importantly, it has been found that positive appraisals (e.g., perceiving loss as a catalyst for personal growth) are more common than negative appraisals of loss, suggesting that grieving is not an exclusively negative event (see Bonanno & Kaltman, 1999 and Gillies & Neimeyer, for a review). Further, those who appraise loss positively have been found to adjust better to loss (see Bonanno & Kaltman, for a review). However, it appears that there is no study in the literature examining the role of cognitive appraisals in pet bereavement, to date.

From a CST perspective, should a pet owner appraise the loss as stressful, he or she is then thought to engage in an evaluation of their coping resources and to use various coping mechanisms (e.g., problem-focused coping or emotion-focused coping) in an attempt to cope with the loss. Coping efforts of individuals are typically directed at either changing the environment or reframing the meaning of the event. Any subsequent change in the person–environment relationship is suggested to lead to reappraisal of the situation that, in turn, influences future coping efforts (Folkman, 2001). In addition, Folkman (2001) also proposed that bereavement is a combination of several stressors (rather than a single focal stressor) that may require use of several coping strategies over time.

Trauma Theories

Similar to Cognitive Stress Theory, the trauma perspective (e.g., Janoff-Bulman, 1992; Parkes, 1988) of bereavement focuses on the individual's subjective evaluations of loss and its relation to the person's adjustment. According to Parkes (1988), each individual has an "assumptive world" that includes his or her beliefs about the world. Janoff-Bulman (1992), who expanded on the assumptive world concept of Parkes (1988), argued that in the core of their assumptive world, most individuals believe that they are worthy and that the world is a benevolent and meaningful place. Individuals are thought to develop these personal and societal assumptions based on their past experiences and use them to interpret past events, as well as to plan for and predict the future. These beliefs give individuals a sense of invulnerability and reflect a general optimism that things will work out well. According to Janoff-Bulman (1992), although most individuals accept the fact that negative things happen to people; these same individuals tend to underestimate the likelihood of these events happening to them and often feel personally protected from misfortune. In other words, these beliefs make individuals feel safe, secure, and protected. Janoff-Bulman (1992) uses the following example (i.e., an internal dialogue) when explaining how these assumptions may serve to convey protection:

> My world is benevolent. Even in such a good world, negative events happen, even if relatively infrequently. Yet, when they occur, they are not random, but rather are meaningfully distributed. They happen to people who deserve them either because of who they are or what they did or failed to do. I am a good, competent, careful person. Bad things couldn't happen to me. (p. 19).

Parkes (1988) argued that the death of a loved one is an event that can invalidate these assumptions and create a discrepancy between one's internal representation of the world (i.e., assumptive world) and their perception of the "real", external world. For example, an individual who has experienced a trauma or loss may no longer perceive the world as a benevolent and meaningful place and may question their previous assumptions of a simple cause and effect nature to the experience of negative events (Janoff-Bulman, 1992). Therefore, according to trauma perspective, the amount of distress experienced as a result of the loss of a pet is directly influenced by the extent to which an individual's fundamental assumptions are invalidated. Indeed, empirical research suggests that bereaved individuals who are unable to make sense of loss are likely to experience higher levels of distress than those who explain loss with their existing meaning structures (Currier, Holland, Coleman, & Neimeyer, 2006).

Many pet owners may not experience the loss of a pet as traumatic; therefore, they may not experience a questioning of their assumptions. However, others, especially those who lose their pets as a result of an unexpected or traumatic loss, may find that the experience of a pet's death has served to call into question their core beliefs. For these individuals, Trauma Theory holds that successful adjustment to bereavement requires a readjustment of their assumptive world. Thus, individuals who have experienced loss may need to engage in a process of rebuilding assumptions in order to minimize the discrepancy between the previously held positive assumptions and the new reality that the loss brings. This rebuilding process may result in the development of more flexible assumptions that are more durable and resistant to being shattered in the future (Janoff-Bulman, 1992).

According to Janoff-Bulman and Yopyk (2004), the experience of trauma or loss may not only shatter the current assumptions of individuals but also increase awareness of potential tragedies and losses that may occur in the future. Therefore, when conceptualized from trauma perspective, losing a pet may not only create distress for some pet owners but also act as a catalyst for an increased awareness of the inevitability of loss and the fragility of life. Empirical literature (e.g., Yalom & Liberman, 1991) suggests that losing a loved one is associated with an increased existential awareness (i.e., an engagement in existential quests related to meaning of life and death) for some bereaved individuals, which, in turn, has been associated with personal growth. Therefore, it is possible that the death of a pet may also promote a process of reexamination of purpose and meaning in life by increasing some pet owners' awareness of the finiteness of life, which may result in personal benefits and a reprioritization of goals for some bereaved individuals.

According to trauma perspective, individuals who are engaged in a search for meaning following invalidation of their assumptions may attempt to use a variety of cognitive and affective tasks to make sense of the event and determine its value in his or her life (Janoff-Bulman & Frantz, 1997). An individual's immediate reaction to a traumatic event or loss usually involves searching for answers to questions related to the reasons for the event. The person often tries to attribute a cause to the event and make sense of what happened through engaging in such questioning (i.e., meaning as comprehensibility). As months pass, an individual's meaning-related search starts to center around the significance or value of the event in his or her life (i.e., meaning as significance). Engaging in such "existential quests" may lead to the acquisition of positive meaning by the individual related to the event (Janoff-Bulman & Yopyk, 2004). Empirical research (e.g., Davis, Nolen-Hoeksama, & Larson, 1998; Gamino & Sewell, 2004; Michael & Synder, 2005) suggests that most bereaved individuals are able to find positive meaning and personal benefits (e.g., increased personal strength, increased spirituality, deeper appreciation of life, and increased compassion, forgiveness, and tolerance for others) from their experience. What's more, those who find benefits from their experience also demonstrate better adjustment to loss (Davis et al., 1998).

Constructivist Perspective

The constructivist perspective offers a broad perspective of bereavement by integrating several theories (e.g., Personal Construct Theory, Attachment theory, Trauma Theories, CST). Similar to CST and trauma perspective, and unlike traditional theories of grief that presume that all bereaved persons respond similarly to loss at an emotional level, the constructivist perspective (Gillies & Neimeyer, 2006; Neimeyer & Raskin, 2000) emphasizes the uniqueness of an individual's response to loss. A constructivist view emphasizes the person's tendency to create and maintain a meaningful self-narrative (Neimeyer, Burke, Mackay, & van Dyke Stringer, 2010), which is defined by Neimeyer (2004) as "an overarching cognitive-affective-behavioral structure that organizes the 'micro-narratives' of everyday life into a 'macro-narrative' that consolidates our self-understanding, establishes our characteristic range of emotions and goals, and guides our performance on the stage of the social world" (pp. 53–54). Individuals are thought to establish their identities by constructing and sharing these narratives with others (Neimeyer et al., 2010). Drawing from Janoff-Bulman (1992), Neimeyer et al. (2010) suggested that, at the center of our self-narratives are our core beliefs and assumptions about the world and ourselves (e.g., the belief that self is worthy and deserves good things and that the world is a benevolent, just place).

According to the constructivist perspective, loss is an event that can profoundly challenge our ways of construing life and the coherence of our self-narratives (Neimeyer, 1999; Neimeyer et al., 2010). Accordingly, the process of grieving is suggested to involve a reconstruction of the meaning that has been challenged by the loss (Neimeyer, 2000). Similar to trauma perspective, the constructivist view argues that losses that are seen by the individual as consistent with their preloss meaning structures are often less disruptive than are losses that are more incongruous, since they do not challenge the bereaved person to reexamine or reconstruct their preloss meaning structures. Therefore, according to constructivist perspective, the loss of a pet can be seen as an event that can challenge an individual's way of understanding life and undermine his or her self-narrative. Therefore, the intensity of the grief following the loss of pet may be determined both by the significance and role of one's pet in his or her self-narrative and the degree to which the experience of loss is consistent with preloss meaning structures of the individual.

According to constructivist perspective, bereaved individuals whose loss experience is inconsistent with his or her preloss meaning structures appear to engage in a process of searching for meaning in attempt to reconstruct meaning structures that can incorporate the current loss (Gillies & Neimeyer, 2006). Individuals may do so by engaging in two general meaning-making processes: by attempting to assimilate the experience of loss into their preloss meaning structures and self-narratives – *assimilation* (e.g., an individual may develop familiar religious explanations of loss), or by adjusting, deepening, or expanding their self-narratives and beliefs to comprehend the reality of loss – *accommodation* (see Neimeyer et al., 2010, for a discussion). Neimeyer and his colleagues (2010) emphasized the relational aspect of the meaning making–making process and suggested that individuals often seek support and validation (e.g., validation for the changed narrative) from others during this process. According to constructivist perspective, bereaved individuals who successfully assimilate or accommodate the loss achieve a meaningful transition in their self-narrative; in contrast, a failure to achieve this is thought to result in complicated grief and fragmented self-narratives (Neimeyer et al., 2010).

Similar to trauma perspective, constructivist perspective suggests that (1) making sense of the death and (2) finding benefits or positive meaning from it are two important tasks that most bereaved individuals engage in following loss (Gillies & Neimeyer, 2006). Further, Gillies and Neimeyer (2006) suggested that the process of meaning reconstruction following loss usually leads to changes in the bereaved person's identity. In other words, the process of meaning reconstruction may also involve a reconstruction of identity, as well. In their article, Neimeyer, Prigerson, and Davies (2002) provided the following example when discussing the process of meaning following the loss of a loved one:

> One mother whose child died after years of intensive caregiving for his congenital heart problem exemplified this response, seeking answers to the urgent question of why this tragedy had befallen her family. Feeling as if the loss were a violation of the entire belief system that had given her life meaning, she reformulated a wiser, if darker, view of the universe, seeing the death as a spiritual wake-up call from a demanding god who forced her to reappraise the materialism and superficiality of her previous life. The result was a great deal of pain and soul searching but also growth. (p. 240)

As illustrated in this example, despite the grief and distress the experience of loss brings, the process of meaning making following the loss of a loved one can be a catalyst for personal growth and wisdom for some bereaved individuals. It is important to note that, although the experience of loss can create a crisis of meaning for some bereaved individuals, not all individuals who encounter loss experience an invalidation of their meaning structures. Therefore, some individuals may not engage in a search for meaning when faced with loss. Carnelley, Wortman, Bolger, and Burke's (2006) study with 768 widows indicated that more than half of the individuals (59%) accepted the death of their spouse and, in turn, did not engage in a search for meaning, while the remaining individuals (41%) did engage in a meaning search following their loss. Further, research has also seemed to indicate that bereaved individuals who never search for meaning following the loss of their loved one tend to show better adjust better to the loss (e.g., Davis, Wortman, Lehman, & Silver, 2000).

The literature on pet loss has mainly focused on the distress and grief that the loss of a pet may bring. However, as both theoretical and empirical literature suggests, individuals may construe the loss in a positive way and may find benefits from their experience. Therefore, it may be important for further research to explore the process of meaning making following the loss of a pet as a way to help further our understanding of individuals' differing adjustment to such an event.

Integration and Recommendations

Each of the theories reviewed above provide valuable insights into our understanding of pet loss. Attachment theory focuses on individuals' attachment histories, as well as the nature of the bond between the bereaved person and the deceased loved one, and how these factors affect individuals' response to loss. CST, Constructivist Theory, and Trauma Theories focus on the role of individuals' subjective interpretations of the loss, contextual factors, and coping responses and the influence these factors have on the grieving process. Further, it appears that these theories share some ideas by viewing grieving as a process of meaning making through which individuals develop an understanding of the loss and make meaningful sense of it. While the main emphasis in Bowlby's (1982) Attachment theory seems to be on attachment bonds, he also focused on the process of meaning making and suggested that during the redefinition phase of grief, bereaved individuals engage in cognitive efforts to reshape internal representational models and to reorganize the attachment configuration (i.e., internal working model).

Integrating the above-reviewed theories may help both clinicians and researchers develop a broader understanding of the variables that impact individuals' subjective response to pet loss. Existing empirical literature on bereavement (i.e., losing a loved one) suggests that several variables can complicate the process of bereavement and may even explain why some individuals present with symptoms that mirror post-traumatic stress disorder (PTSD). Some of these variables include the attachment history of the individual (e.g., Fraley & Bonanno, 2004), specific circumstances related to death (e.g., violent death vs. natural death), and an inability to make sense of death (Currier et al., 2006; Neimeyer, Prigerson, & Davies, 2002). Therefore, using a broader, more integrative approach to conceptualizing pet loss can assist researchers and mental health clinicians in achieving a broader understanding of the variations involved in individuals' response to loss.

It is also important to note that the theories reviewed above emphasize the role of context in understanding individuals' responses to the loss of a pet. These contextual factors may include personality, attachment history of the individual, previous history of losses, social support networks of the individual, family, and cultural history. All of these factors may have significant influence on the ways individuals respond to loss. For example, cultural meanings and attitudes toward death are likely to influence the ways an individual construes death, as well as how they respond to it. For example, as Aiken (2001) suggested, some cultures, such as Tlingit people of Alaska or Basques of Northern Spain, view death as a natural phenomenon and respond to death calmly and even joyfully. Similarly, cultural attitudes toward animals in a given society may have significant influences on the meaning that an individual attributes to his or her relationship with companion animals. In addition, constructivist theory emphasizes that the grieving and meaning-making process is not an exclusively private event; rather, social support and validation from others play an important part in the meaning-making process (Neimeyer et al., 2010).

Until now, existing empirical research has largely focused on the level of pet owners' attachment to their pets and the intensity of grief they experience following the pet's death. However, no studies have been conducted, to date, that examine the process of meaning making following a pet's loss. Empirical research on bereaved individuals who have experienced the loss of a loved one suggest that making sense of the death and finding positive meaning in the death are two important processes that impact the grieving process (e.g., Currier, Holland, & Neimeyer, 2006; Davis et al., 1998). No studies appear to exist that examine whether survivors of pet loss engage in these tasks and how these processes affect their adjustment. Therefore, researchers may focus on exploring these areas, as well.

One additional area that more recent research has focused on is clarifying a distinction between normal (uncomplicated) grief and complicated grief as a way to understand adjustment to a loss. For those individuals who may not have had their assumptions about the world questioned, it is still common for them to present with normal grief symptoms that mirror major depressive disorder for a period of time, such as feelings of sadness, loss of appetite, sleep difficulties, and weight loss (4th ed.; *DSM-IV-TR*; American Psychiatric Association; 2000). On the other hand, persons who experience the loss as traumatic may present with symptoms of complicated grief that mirror posttraumatic stress disorder. Some of these symptoms include intrusive thoughts about the deceased, disbelief, loss of a sense of security and meaning, isolation, separation distress, and nightmares; these symptoms typically last for longer periods of time than in the case of normal bereavement and usually impair the functioning of the individual (Horowitz et al., 1997; Prigerson et al., 1999).

Only a few studies (i.e., Field et al., 2009; Luiz Adrian, Deliramich, & Frueh, 2009) have examined complicated grief among bereaved pet owners. For example, Field and colleagues (2009) used the Inventory of Complicated Grief (Prigerson et al., 1995) to assess the complicated grief among bereaved pet owners and reported a mean complicated grief score of 2.15 ($SD = 0.82$) for their participants. They noted that this value is slightly lower than findings for human loss within the first year of bereavement using the same instrument (e.g., $M = 2.55$; $SD = 1.07$; Filanosky, 2004). Another recent study by Luiz Adrian et al. (2009) indicated that only about 20% of bereaved pet owners report significant grief reactions following the loss of a pet, and a smaller of percentage of them (<5–12%) report pathological grief reactions, suggesting that pathological grief occurs rarely among bereaved pet owners. While these findings are preliminary, they seem to suggest that although most pet owners may be resilient to loss of a pet, a small group of individuals may experience long-term adjustment difficulties following their pet's loss.

Empirical findings indicate that variables such as the cause of death (e.g., natural death vs. euthanasia), living conditions (living alone vs. living with others), availability of supportive others, and gender and age of the bereaved pet owner (Davis, Irwin, Richardson, & O'Brien-Malone, 2003; McCutcheon & Fleming, 2001) can influence the level of grief experienced following the loss of a pet. However, research regarding the variables that lead to pathological or complicated grief is limited. As previously discussed, Field et al. (2009) findings indicate that one of the variables that contributes to complicated grief is the attachment history of the individual. Also, other variables may provide insights into what complicates the grieving process, including: cause of death, prior losses that the individual has experienced, individuals' beliefs and assumptions about the world and themselves, personality factors, and the meaning that individuals ascribe to their relationships with pets. Existing empirical research on bereavement (i.e., human loss) as well as grief theories listed above and elsewhere can provide clinicians with valuable insights into the variables that may complicate the bereavement process and can also guide researchers who are conducting future research on pet loss. In addition, a review of these data can help to inform practitioners' conceptualizations of the bereavement experienced by pet owners and may also aid these clinicians in tailoring interventions that are more effective at fostering adjustment to the loss.

The following section of this chapter includes a review of the recent studies on pet loss and a discussion on the methodological issues and challenges in designing human–animal bond research.

Methodological Issues and Recommendations

Study Design

Table 22.1 presents a summary of the recent studies that have been conducted on pet loss. As can be seen from the table, most of the existing empirical studies have used cross-sectional research designs. While these studies do not permit causal inferences, they provided valuable information about the correlations among the variables of interest and add support for the assertion that a relationship exists between the loss of a pet and the experience of significant distress for some pet

Table 22.1 Recent studies on pet loss

Study	Sample	Subject recruitment method	Time since loss	Design
Archer and Winchester (1994)	$n = 88$ no demographic information is provided	Convenience sampling and adds (veterinary surgeries, a local hairdresser, and a social services department)	Within the year previous the study	Cross-sectional
Brown, Richards, and Wilson (1996): pet bereavement among adolescents	$n = 55$ 51% females 97% Caucasian	Convenience sampling (through high schools and referrals)	Within the year previous the study	Cross-sectional
Planchon, Templer, Stokes, and Keller (2002)	$n = 63$ veterinary clients (76% female and 94% Caucasian) and 391 undergraduate psychology students (55% female and 27% Caucasian)	Convenience sampling (veterinary clients and undergraduate psychology students)	Not reported	Cross-sectional
Davis et al. (2003)	$n = 68$ 71% female	Through advertisements and the personal contact	Time since loss ranged from 2 months to 15 years	Qualitative cross-sectional
Wrobel and Dye (2003): cat and dog loss	$n = 174$ 64% females 90.2% Caucasian	Participants were recruited from a college campus, from a local business setting, and by referrals from various veterinarians in the area	Lost a pet sometime in the past (time since loss is not reported)	Cross-sectional (retrospective reports)
Hunt, Al-Awadi, and Johnson (2008): pet loss following Hurricane Katrina	$n = 65$ 95% women 95% Caucasian	Internet recruitment through various Internet message boards	Not reported	Cross-sectional
Field et al. (2009): cat and dog loss	$n = 71$ 86% women 91% Caucasian	Death notices (a computer-generated file of pet loss survivors)	Within 12 months of loss	Cross-sectional

Table 22.1 (continued)

Study	Sample	Subject recruitment method	Time since loss	Design
Luiz Adrian et al. (2009): complicated grief and PTSD among bereaved pet owners	$n = 106$ (of 106 participants, 69 reported the loss of a pet) 76% female 44% Caucasian	Participants were recruited from a veterinary clinic	Not reported	Cross-sectional
Lowe, Rhodes, Zwiebach, and Chan (2009): the impact of pet loss on hurricane survivors	$n = 365$ (women) 81.9 African American 17.3% lost a pet	Participants were part of an educational intervention in New Orleans	Not reported	Longitudinal

owners. One of the areas that future research may focus on is developing a more comprehensive understanding of pet loss through longitudinal studies. As mentioned earlier in this chapter, individuals may engage in several different tasks at different stages of grief. Therefore, cross-sectional study designs alone are inadequate, as they do not allow researchers to understand the developmental trajectories that could be accounted for in longitudinal research.

Further, most of the researchers who have conducted studies in this area have collected retrospective data from participants, in their attempt to understand the intensity and type of grief symptoms that bereaved individuals experience at different stages of grief. For example, in their study, Wrobel and Dye (2003) developed and used a Pet Death Survey, which is based on questions developed by Fogle and Abrahamson (1990). Using this survey, they asked participants who had experienced the loss of a pet anytime in the past to recollect grief-related symptoms they experienced at the time of loss, 6 months after loss, and 12 months after loss. However, the use of the measure in this way seems problematic, as no information appears to exist in the literature regarding the validity of the Pet Death Survey when collecting retrospective data about grief symptoms. For example, it is possible that participants do not accurately recall the symptoms they experienced in the past. In addition, participants who experienced the loss more recently may be likely to recall their symptoms more accurately than those who experienced the loss further in the past. Therefore, collecting data from recently bereaved pet owners and following up with them at set time intervals may serve to increase the accuracy of the data being collected.

Finally, researchers have tended to exclusively use quantitative study designs when exploring grief among bereaved pet owners. It appears that, there is only one qualitative study (Davis et al., 2003) in the recent literature that focuses on grief following a pet's loss. As discussed earlier in the chapter, several theories suggest that the meaning an individual attributes to a loss plays a significant role in the grieving process. Therefore, future research may benefit from using qualitative methods when exploring the meaning that individuals ascribe to their pets, as well as to the pet's loss. Further, existing research on bereavement suggests that some bereaved individuals engage in a search for meaning process following the loss of a loved one and that many bereaved individuals are able to find positive meaning in their loss (e.g., Wheeler, 2001); however, no research has been conducted to examine this meaning-making process. Therefore, future qualitative research may focus on examining whether the loss of a pet leads to an engagement in search for meaning as well as how the process of meaning making occurs following the loss.

Measures

One of the significant challenges of conducting research on human–animal bond is the difficulty involved in measuring a number of the constructs. As discussed earlier, Kurdek (2008, 2009) examined whether the bonds between human beings and animals involve the features of attachment bonds. Kurdek (2009) adapted the Emotional Reliance Scale (Ryan, La Guardia, Solky-Butzel, Chirkov, & Kim,

2005) to measure safe haven and secure base behaviors. However, as Kobak (2009) suggested, measuring these constructs in adults requires multiple methods that examines the convergent and divergent validity of these constructs. Kobak (2009) noted that "one of the difficulties in measuring safe haven behavior in older children and adults is that they rarely experience the degree of fear that would result in seeking safety with a protective figure." (p. 448).

Similarly, it appears that there are no valid instruments in the literature to measure continuous bonds with the deceased pet. In their study, Field et al. (2009) used the following four items to assess the continuous bond (or persistence of the relationship with the deceased) with the deceased pet: (1) focused on fond memories of deceased, (2) shared fond memories with others of deceased, (3) positive influence of the deceased on who I am today, and (4) looking at photographs or pictures of the deceased. While these items emphasize the importance of pet in their owners' lives as well as the significance of the loss, they may fail to measure the construct of "continues bonds" with the deceased comprehensively. In his book, Bowlby used the following examples when describing participants' continuous bonds to their deceased loved one:

> ... half or more of the widows and widowers reach a state of mind in which they retain a strong sense of the continuing presence of their partner without the turmoils of hope and disappointment, search and frustration, anger and blame that are present earlier. (Bowlby, 1982, p. 96)
>
> Dreams of the spouse still being alive share many of the characteristic features of the sense of presence: they occur in about half of widows and widowers, they are extremely vivid and realistic, and in a majority of cases are experienced as comforting. (Bowlby, 1982, p. 97).

He used the following examples from previous empirical studies to describe widows and widowers' continuous bonds with their deceased spouse:

> Twelve months after their loss two out of three of the Boston widows continued to spend much time thinking of their husband and one in four of the 49 described how there were still occasions when they forgot he was dead. So comforting did widows find the sense of the dead husband's presence that some deliberately evoked it whenever they felt unsure of themselves or depressed. (Bowlby, 1982, p. 97).
>
> More than one in ten widows and widowers reported having held conversations with the dead spouse; ... Two-thirds of those who reported experiences of their dead spouse's presence, either with or without some form of sensory illusion or occasionally hallucination, described their experiences as being comforting and helpful. Most of the remainder were neutral about them and only eight of the total of 137 subjects who had such experiences disliked having them. (Bowlby, 1982, p. 97).

Therefore, continuing bond with the deceased attachment figure may involve not only focusing on the memories of the deceased, looking at his/her pictures, or thinking about positive aspects of the relationship with the deceased but also feeling the presence of the deceased loved one and, in some cases, having conversations with the deceased or forgetting that he/she is dead. Therefore, future research may build on the existing findings to develop valid and reliable scales and approaches (e.g., using multiple methods to measure a construct) for measuring these constructs.

Sampling Method

Another issue in bereavement research involves issues around sampling. Most of the participants in existing studies were recruited from undergraduate courses or from veterinary clinics through referrals. Participants who volunteer to participate in these studies are likely to be different than those who did not; thus, using a convenience sampling method introduces potential sampling bias.

Although random sampling may prove difficult when exploring pet loss and grief, researchers are encouraged to make strides in recruiting more representative samples as a way to increase the validity of their findings. As seen in Table 22.1, most of the participants in previous research studies were Caucasian and female, suggesting that the samples of the majority of these studies were not representative of the total population of survivors of pet loss. Therefore, it is important for future researchers to make attempts to gather more representative samples and to use less-biased sampling methods as a way to further contribute to the expanding literature in this area.

Conclusion

Empirical research on human loss suggests that variations exists in individuals' response to loss: some individuals adjust to loss in a very short period of time and return to their original level of functioning shortly after the death of a loved one; others move beyond their previous level of functioning and report personal growth and wisdom in addition to grief and distress; and some individuals experience long-term adjustment difficulties and impairment in their functioning. It is also important to note that the results of empirical research (Bonanno, Wortman, & Nesse, 2004) show that most individuals show resilience to loss; only between 10 and 20% of bereaved individuals report intense grieving that significantly impairs the quality of their lives.

In this chapter, our goal was to emphasize the subjective and contextual nature of the human–animal bond and, therefore, highlight the unique patterns of grieving. Thus, we challenge clinicians and researchers to pursue and develop a more comprehensive understanding of these patterns, which includes a variety of different individual and contextual variables (e.g., attachment history, previous losses, the meaning attributed to the relationship with companion animals, the personal significance of loss, cultural attitudes toward death). It is also important to note that grieving is an intrapersonal phenomenon. As constructivist theory emphasizes, the process of grieving and the meaning reconstruction is an interpersonal one, as well. We propose that our identities and meaning structures are social constructions, and that the process of meaning reconstruction following the loss of a loved one will be influenced from our social environments. More simply, as Gillies and Neimeyer (2006) suggested, "What we believe about what happens to our lost one after death, our new positions in the world in their absence, and even how to go about grieving, are informed by our social and cultural environments" (p. 58).

While it may seem daunting to draw from existing theory in defining new conceptualizations that more precisely explain the components involved in bereavement and adjustment to a pet's loss, we believe that researchers and clinicians alike are ideally equipped to take on this challenge. Future researchers can provide a unique contribution to our understanding of this phenomenon by shedding light on the aspects involved in the loss of pet, as well as helping to deepen our understanding of the unique and shared experiences that differentiate one's adjustment to, and sense making of the loss. Further, we believe that the development of a more comprehensive framework will allow practitioners to more effectively meet the needs of the bereaved, as it relates both generally and specifically to adjustment to their animal companion's loss.

References

Aiken, L. R. (2001). *Dying, death, and bereavement* (4th ed.). Mahwah, NJ: Lawrence Erlbaum Associates, Inc.

Ainsworth, M. D. S. (1991). Attachments and other affectional bonds across the life cycle. In: C. M. Parkes, J. Stevenson-Hinde, & P. Marris (Eds.), *Attachment across the life cycle* (pp. 33–51). New York: Routledge.

American Psychiatric Association. (2000). *Diagnostic and statistical manual of mental disorders: DSM-IV-TR* (4th ed., text revision). Arlington: Author.

Archer, J., & Winchester, G. (1994). Bereavement following the death of pet. *The British Journal of Psychology, 85,* 259–271.

Bonanno, G. A., & Kaltman, S. (1999). Toward an integrative perspective on bereavement. *Psychological Bulletin, 125,* 760–776.

Bonanno, G. A., Wortman, C. B., & Nesse, R. M. (2004). Prospective patterns of resilience and maladjustment during widowhood. *Psychology and Aging, 19,* 260–271.

Bowlby, J. (1980). *Loss: Sadness & depression. Vol. 3: Attachment and loss.* London: Hogarth Press (International psycho-analytical library no.109).

Bowlby, J. (1982). *Attachment and loss. Vol. 1: Attachment* (2nd ed.). New York: Basic Books (new printing, 1999, with a foreword by Allan N. Schore; originally published in 1969).

Brown, B. H., Richards, H. C., & Wilson, C. A. (1996). Pet bonding and pet bereavement among adolescents. *Journal of Counseling & Development, 74,* 505–509.

Brown, S. E. (2002). Ethnic variations in pet attachment among students at an American school of veterinary medicine. *Society & Animals, 10,* 455–456.

Brown, S. E. (2004). The human–animal bond and self psychology: Toward a new understanding. *Society & Animals, 12,* 67–86.

Brown, S. E. (2007). Companion animals as selfobjects. *Anthrozoös, 20,* 329–343.

Carnelley, K. B., Wortman, C. B., Bolger, N., & Burke, C. T. (2006). The time course of grief reactions to spousal loss: Evidence from a national probability sample. *Journal of Personality and Social Psychology, 91,* 476–492.

Collis, G. M., & McNicholas, J. (1998). A theoretical basis for health benefits of pet ownership: Attachment versus psychological support. In C. C. Wilson & D. C. Turner (Eds.), *Companion animals in human health* (pp. 105–122). Thousand Oaks, CA: Sage.

Currier, J., Holland, J., Coleman, R., & Neimeyer, R. A. (2006). Bereavement following violent death: An assault on life and meaning. In R. Stevenson & G. Cox (Eds.), *Violence.* Amityville, NY: Baywood.

Currier, J. M., Holland, J. M., & Neimeyer, R. A. (2006). Sense-making, grief, and the experience of violent loss: Toward a mediational model. *Death Studies, 30,* 403–428.

Davis, C., Nolen-Hoeksama, N., & Larson, J. (1998). Making sense of loss and benefiting from the experience: Two construals of meaning. *Journal of Personality and Social Psychology, 75,* 561–574.

Davis, C. G., Wortman, C. B., Lehman, D. R., & Silver, R. C. (2000). Searching for meaning in loss: Are clinical assumptions correct? *Death Studies, 24,* 497–540.

Davis, H., Irwin, P., Richardson, M., & O'Brien-Malone, A. (2003). When a pet dies: Religious issues, euthanasia and strategies for coping with bereavement. *Anthrozoös, 16,* 57–74.

Field, N. P., Gao, B., & Paderna, L. (2005). Continuing bonds in bereavement: An attachment theory based perspective. *Death Studies, 29,* 277–300.

Field, N. P., Orsini, L., Gavish, R., & Packman, W. (2009). Role of attachment in response to pet loss. *Death Studies, 33,* 334–355. doi: 10.1080/07481180802705783.

Filanosky, C. A. (2004). The nature of continuing bonds with the deceased and their effect on bereavement outcome. *Dissertation Abstracts International: Section B: The Sciences and Engineering, 65*(2-B), 1027.

Fogle, B., & Abrahamson, D. (1990). Pet loss: A survey of the attitudes and feelings of practicing veterinarians. *Anthrozoös, 3,* 143–150.

Folkman, S. (2001). Revised coping theory and the process of bereavement. In M. Stroebe, R. Hansson, W. Stroebe, & H. Schut (Eds.), *Handbook of bereavement research: Consequences, coping, and care* (pp. 563–584). Washington, DC: American Psychological Association.

Fraley, R. C., & Bonanno, G. A. (2004). Attachment and loss: A test of three competing models on the association between attachment-related avoidance and adaptation to bereavement. *Personality and Social Psychology Bulletin, 30,* 878–890.

Gamino, L. A., & Sewell, K. W. (2004). Meaning constructs as predictors of bereavement adjustment: A report from the Scott & White grief study. *Death Studies, 28,* 397–421.

Gerwolls, M. K., & Labott, S. M. (1994). Adjustments to the death of a companion animal. *Anthrozoös, 7,* 172–187.

Gilbey, A., McNicholas, J., & Collis, G. (2007). A longitudinal test of the belief that companion animal-ownership can help to reduce loneliness. *Anthrozoös, 20,* 345–353.

Gillies, J., & Neimeyer, R. A. (2006). Loss, grief, and the search for significance: Toward a model of meaning reconstruction in bereavement. *Journal of Constructivist Psychology, 19,* 31–65.

Hazan, C., & Shaver, P. R. (1987). Romantic love conceptualized as an attachment process. *Journal of Personality and Social Psychology, 52,* 511–524.

Horowitz, M. J., Siegel, B., Holen, A., Bonanno, G. A., Milbrath, C., & Stinson, C. H. (1997). Diagnostic criteria for complicated grief disorder. *American Journal of Psychiatry, 154,* 904–910.

Hunt, M., Al-Awadi, H., & Johnson, M. (2008). Psychological sequelae of pet loss following Hurricane Katrina. *Anthrozoös, 21,* 109–121.

Janoff-Bulman, R. (1992). *Shattered assumptions: Towards a new psychology of trauma.* New York: Free Press.

Janoff-Bulman, R., & Frantz, C. M. (1997). The impact of trauma on meaning: From meaningless world to meaningful life. In M. Power & C. Brewin (Eds.), *The transformation of meaning in psychological therapies: Integrating theory and practice.* Sussex: Wiley & Sons.

Janoff-Bulman, R., & Yopyk, D. (2004). Random outcomes and valued commitments: Existential dilemmas and the paradox of meaning. In J. Greenberg, S. L. Koole, & T. Pyszczynski (Eds.), *Handbook of experimental existential psychology.* New York: Guilford.

Kobak, R. (2009). Defining and measuring of attachment bonds; comment on Kurdek (2009). *Journal of Family Psychology, 23,* 447–449.

Kurdek, L. A. (2008). Pet dogs as attachment figures. *Journal of Social and Personal Relationships, 25,* 247–266.

Kurdek, L. A. (2009). Pet dogs as attachment figures for adult owners. *Journal of Family Psychology, 23,* 439–446.

Lazarus, R. S., & Folkman, S. (1984). *Stress, appraisal, and coping*. New York: Springer.

Lowe, S. R., Rhodes, J. E., Zwiebach, L., & Chan, C. S. (2009). The impact of pet loss on perceived social support and psychological distress among Hurricane Katrina survivors. *Journal of Traumatic Stress, 22*, 244–247.

Luiz Adrian, J. A., Deliramich, A. N., & Frueh, B. C. (2009). Complicated grief and posttraumatic stress disorder in humans' response to the death of pets/animals. *Bulletin of the Menninger Clinic, 73*(3), 176–187. doi: 10.1521/bumc.2009.73.3.176.

McCutcheon, K. A., & Fleming, S. J. (2001). Grief resulting from euthanasia and natural death of companion animals. *Journal of Death and Dying, 44*, 169–188.

Michael, S. T., & Synder, C. R. (2005). Getting unstuck: The roles of hope, finding meaning, and rumination in the adjustment to bereavement among college students. *Death Studies, 29*, 435–458.

Mikulincer, M., & Shaver, P. R. (2007). *Attachment in adulthood: Structure, dynamics, and change*. New York: Guilford Press.

Neimeyer, R. (2000). *Lessons of loss: A guide to coping*. Memphis, TN: Center for the Study of Loss and Transition.

Neimeyer, R. A. (1999). Narrative strategies in grief therapy. *Journal of Constructivist Psychology, 12*(1), 65–85.

Neimeyer, R. A. (2004). Fostering posttraumatic growth: A narrative contribution. *Psychological Inquiry, 15*, 53–59.

Neimeyer, R. A. (2005–2006). Complicated grief and the quest for meaning: A constructivist contribution. *Omega, 52*, 37–52.

Neimeyer, R. A., Burke, L., Mackay, M., & van Dyke Stringer, J. G. (2010). Grief therapy and the reconstruction of meaning: From principles to practice. *Journal of Contemporary Psychotherapy, 40*, 73–83. doi 10.1007/s10879-009-9135-3.

Neimeyer, R. A., Prigerson, H., & Davies, B. (2002). Mourning and meaning. *American Behavioral Scientist, 46*, 235–251.

Neimeyer, R. A., & Raskin, J. D. (Eds.). (2000). *Constructions of disorder: Meaning-making frameworks for psychotherapy*. Washington, DC: American Psychological Association.

Parkes, C. M. (1988). Bereavement as a psychological transition: Processes of adaptation to change. *Journal of Social Issues, 44*, 53–65.

Planchon, L. A., & Templer, D. I. (1996). The correlates of grief after death of pet. *Anthrozoös, 9*, 107–113.

Planchon, L. A., Templer, D. I., Stokes, S., & Keller, J. (2002). Death of a companion cat or dog and human bereavement: Psychosocial variables. *Anthrozoös, 10*, 93–105.

Prigerson, H. G., Maciejewski, P. K., Reynolds, C. F., Bierhals, A. J., Newsom, J. T., Fasiczka, A., et al. (1995). Inventory of complicated grief: A scale to measure maladaptive symptoms and loss. *Psychiatry Research, 59*, 65–79.

Prigerson, H. G., Shear, M. K., Jacobs, S. C., Reynolds, C. F., Maciejewski, P. K., Davidson, J. R. T., et al. (1999). Consensus criteria for traumatic grief: A preliminary empirical test. *British Journal of Psychiatry, 174*, 67–73.

Ryan, R. M., La Guardia, J. G., Solky-Butzel, J., Chirkov, V., & Kim, Y. (2005). On the interpersonal regulation of emotions: Emotional reliance across gender, relationships, and cultures. *Personal Relationships, 12*, 145–163.

Wheeler, I. (2001). Parental bereavement: The crisis of meaning. *Death Studies, 25*, 51–66.

Wrobel, T. A., & Dye, A. L. (2003). Grieving pet death: Normative, gender, and attachment issues. *Omega: Journal of Death & Dying, 47*, 385–393.

Yalom, I. D., & Liberman, M. A. (1991). Bereavement and heightened existential awareness. *Psychiatry, 54*, 334–345.

Subject Index

C. Blazina et al. (eds.), *The Psychology of the Human–Animal Bond,*
DOI 10.1007/978-1-4419-9761-6, © Springer Science+Business Media, LLC 2011

CPSIA information can be obtained at www.ICGtesting.com
Printed in the USA
LVOW11s1413270813

349855LV00002B/33/P